Alzheimer's Disease: A Practical Guide for Clinicians

Alzheimer's Disease: A Practical Guide for Clinicians

Editor: Elena Poole

STATES
ACADEMIC PRESS
www.statesacademicpress.com

www.statesacademicpress.com

STATES
ACADEMIC PRESS

Cataloging-in-Publication Data

Alzheimer's disease : a practical guide for clinicians / edited by Elena Poole.
p. cm.
Includes bibliographical references and index.
ISBN 978-1-63989-788-9
1. Alzheimer's disease. 2. Alzheimer's disease--Treatment.
3. Alzheimer's disease--Diagnosis. I. Poole, Elena.
RC523 .A49 2023
616.831--dc23

States Academic Press,
109 South 5th Street,
Brooklyn, NY 11249, USA

ISBN 978-1-63989-788-9 (Hardback)

Contents

Preface

This book aims to highlight the current researches and provides a platform to further the scope of innovations in this area. This book is a product of the combined efforts of many researchers and scientists, after going through thorough studies and analysis from different parts of the world. The objective of this book is to provide the readers with the latest information of the field.

Alzheimer's disease is a type of brain disorder that affects the memory and thinking abilities. It is a progressive condition that causes brain shrinkage and cell death. The major symptoms of Alzheimer's disease include memory problems, changes in personality and behavior, and mood swings. There is no specific cause for AD. A history of depression, hypertension and head injuries are some of the common risk factors associated with Alzheimer's disease. Its diagnosis involves a physical exam and neurological health assessment. The common diagnostic tests for AD include blood tests, brain imaging and PET scans. Its treatment includes medications to reduce the progression of cognitive decline. This book on Alzheimer's disease is a collective contribution of a renowned group of international experts. It strives to provide a fair idea about this medical condition and to help develop a better understanding of the latest advances within its clinical management.

I would like to express my sincere thanks to the authors for their dedicated efforts in the completion of this book. I acknowledge the efforts of the publisher for providing constant support. Lastly, I would like to thank my family for their support in all academic endeavors.

Editor

1

Pin1 Modulation in Physiological Status and Neurodegeneration: Any Contribution to the Pathogenesis of Type 3 Diabetes?

Marzia Bianchi and Melania Manco *

Research Unit for Multi-factorial Diseases, Obesity and Diabetes, Bambino Gesù Children's Hospital IRCCS (Istituto di Ricovero e Cura a Carattere Scientifico), viale di San Paolo 15, 00146 Rome, Italy; marzia.bianchi@opbg.net

* Correspondence: melania.manco@opbg.net

Abstract: Prolyl isomerases (Peptidylprolyl isomerase, PPIases) are enzymes that catalyze the isomerization between the *cis/trans* Pro conformations. Three subclasses belong to the class: FKBP (FK506 binding protein family), Cyclophilin and Parvulin family (Pin1 and Par14). Among Prolyl isomerases, Pin1 presents as distinctive feature, the ability of binding to the motif pSer/pThr-Pro that is phosphorylated by kinases. Modulation of Pin1 is implicated in cellular processes such as mitosis, differentiation and metabolism: The enzyme is dysregulated in many diverse pathological conditions, i.e., cancer progression, neurodegenerative (i.e., Alzheimer's diseases, AD) and metabolic disorders (i.e., type 2 diabetes, T2D). Indeed, Pin1 KO mice develop a complex phenotype of premature aging, cognitive impairment in elderly mice and neuronal degeneration resembling that of the AD in humans. In addition, since the molecule modulates glucose homeostasis in the brain and peripherally, Pin1 KO mice are resistant to diet-induced obesity, insulin resistance, peripheral glucose intolerance and diabetic vascular dysfunction. In this review, we revise first critically the role of Pin1 in neuronal development and differentiation and then focus on the in vivo studies that demonstrate its pivotal role in neurodegenerative processes and glucose homeostasis. We discuss evidence that enables us to speculate about the role of Pin1 as molecular link in the pathogenesis of type 3 diabetes i.e., the clinical association of dementia/AD and T2D.

Keywords: Alzheimer's disease; brain glucose metabolism; neuronal differentiation; neuronal degeneration; Prolyl isomerases; Pin1; type 2 diabetes; type 3 diabetes

1. Introduction

Prolyl isomerases (Peptidylprolyl isomerase, PPIases) are a class of enzymes that catalyze the *cis/trans* isomerization of the peptide bond between the preceding amino acid and the proline residue (Pro) [1–3]. The presence of Pro's unusual structure lowers the free energy difference and allows these conformational changes [4]. The catalytic activity of PPIases modulates enzyme activity, protein stability and cellular localization by mediating conformational changes of substrates [3,5–9]. Three distinctive groups belong to the class of PPIases: the FKBP (FK506 binding protein), the Cyclophilin and the Parvulin families (Peptidylprolyl *cis/trans* isomerase NIMA-interacting 1 (Pin1) and Par14) [1,3,7,8].

With respect to other PPIases, the distinctive feature of Pin1 is that the Serine (Ser) or the Threonine (Thr) that precedes the Pro residue is phosphorylated accounting for the correct enzyme-substrate recognition [3,9]. The proline-directed kinases phosphorylate Pin1 substrates and induce Pin1-dependent post-phosphorylation conformational changes that impact key proteins. These changes influence cellular functions such as mitosis, differentiation and metabolism. Deregulation of Pin1 substrates has been implied in the onset of various diseases, i.e., cancer, neurodegenerative disorders and metabolic syndromes including type 2 diabetes (T2D) [2–4,10–12].

Expression of Pin1 increases significantly in cell types that undergo active cell division [4,13], depending on cell type, availability of specific substrates, and biological context. Pin1 seems to play a dual role, promoting cell proliferation or even, at the opposite, cell death depending on the biological context. Different capacities result from the adoption of diverse mechanisms of regulation, i.e., gene transcription and protein phosphorylation.

Pin1 serves as molecular "switch" that modulates enzyme activity or an entire signaling pathway [14]. Deeper understanding of function and regulation of Pin1 is essential to appreciate fine mechanisms of signal transduction and integration that are triggered by the propyl isomerase.

In this review, we will discuss the pivotal role of Pin1 in physiological i.e., the neuronal development as well as in neurodegenerative conditions i.e., the Huntinton's, the Parkinson's, the temporal lobe epilepsy (TLE) and the Alzheimer's (AD) diseases.

Then, with regard to AD, important features of the disease phenotype are reduced brain utilization of glucose and impaired glycolytic enzyme activities owing to defective insulin signaling [15]. Therefore AD is deemed as "type 3 diabetes" (T3D) [16] and regarded a metabolic disease. de la Monte defines AD "as a brain form of diabetes in which insulin resistance and deficiency develop either primarily in the brain, or due to systemic insulin resistance disease with secondary involvement of the brain" [17]. Interestingly, in patients with AD, Pin1 seems involved not only in neuronal degeneration but also in brain impaired glucose metabolism. Therefore, Pin1 may be at the crossroad between AD and T2D-associated dementia, contributing to the clinical relationship of these two conditions in the T3D.

2. Pin1 Characterization: Structure, Regulation and Subcellular Localization

Pin1 is a ubiquitous enzyme, with high similarity across species (*Homo sapiens*, *Xenopus laevis*, and *Danio rerio*) that suggests conserved function in vertebrates [4]. X-ray crystallography and solution nuclear magnetic resonance (NMR) studies in extracts of human brain tissues show that Pin1 is a monomeric enzyme of 163 amino acids. Pin1 consists of two functional domains, the WW- at the N-terminus and the PPIase-domains at the C-terminus, covalently fastened by a flexible linker (amino acids 38–53) of 15-residues [9,18]. The linker allows the domains to rotate independently of each other [19,20]. The PPIase domain catalyzes specifically the *cis/trans* isomerization of pSer/pThr-peptidyl-prolyl bonds. The WW domain (type IV) binds, but does not catalyze, similar epitopes [20,21]. Upon Pin1 binding of the specific substrate to the previous phosphorylated S/T-P motifs by proline directed kinases, the two functional domains of Pin1 interact partially with each other in a substrate-dependent manner [20,22,23]. Recognition of the substrate determines a loss of flexibility of residue side-chains in the region between the catalytic loop and the inter-domain surface. The reduced flexibility leads to increased contacts between the two functional domains [23].

Both E2F (E2 factor) [24], a protein involved in the cell cycle regulation, and N1ICD (Notch Intracellular Domain) [25], a protein that regulates Pin1 generating a positive loop in breast cancer cells, are able to activate transcription of Pin1 upon binding. On the contrary, AP4 (Activating Enhancer Binding Protein 4), the brain-selective transcription factor [26], down regulates Pin1 transcription, and the proteasome is responsible of the protein degradation following its ubiquitination [4,27].

Protein kinases regulate the capability of Pin1 to bind substrates. Steps for binding are phosphorylation of S/T-P motifs of substrates by kinases first, and secondly, phosphorylation of specific Ser residues in the Pin1 WW domain. Phosphorylation at the Ser16 residue modulates the ability of Pin1 to bind its substrates in a substrate-dependent manner [3]. In particular, phosphorylation by PKA (Protein kinase A) [28] and Aurora A [29] kinases inhibited the binding of Pin1 to its substrate resulting in mitotic block [28] or progression to G2/M phase [29]. Conversely, both Ser/Thr-kinase RSK2 (ribosomal protein S6 kinase 2) [30] and COT (Cancer Osaka Thyroid) [31] increased the binding of Pin1 to substrates leading to tumor progression.

Other kinases induce post-translational modifications of Pin1 in different Ser residues. The phosphorylation on Ser71 by DAPK1 (Death-associated protein kinase 1), a known tumor suppressor, inhibited Pin1 catalytic activity during the cell cycle progression [32]. MLK3 (Mixed Lineage Kinase 3) is a MAP3K (Mitogen-activated protein kinase kinase kinase) phosphorylated Pin1 on Ser138, thus increasing its activity to drive cell cycle progression [33]. Phosphorylation on Ser65 by PLK1 (Polo-like kinase 1), a regulator of mitotic checkpoints, stabilized Pin1 structure, reducing its ubiquitination and consequently degradation [27].

As to the exact subcellular localization of Pin1, this is not unique. Pin1 subcellular localization seems to vary upon post-translational modification of different Ser residues and different cellular contexts. When the Ser16 residue was phosphorylated and Pin1 modulation was associated with mitotic arrest, Pin1 was found in the nucleus [28,29]. When the same residue was phosphorylated in mouse embryonic fibroblasts and breast cancer cells [30,31], Pin1 was detected out of the nucleus. When Pin1 was phosphorylated on Ser138 enhancing tumorigenesis, Pin1 *trans*-located into the nucleus [33].

Subcellular localization of Pin1 seems to vary in different cell types, tissues and health status. Pin1 localized in the nucleus of cell lines such as SH-SY5Y, but also in the cytoplasm of primary neuron cultures or tissues [4]. Pin1 presented a cytoplasmic localization in axons from cultured DRG (dorsal root ganglia) neurons [34], but it was localized in both compartments at comparable levels in primary cultured mouse cortical neurons [35] and embryonic NPCs (neural stem/progenitor cells) [36]. Ibarra and co-workers found that Pin1 was preferentially localized in the cytoplasm of a number of neuronal cells, but there was nuclear localization in some cases or even nuclear exclusion of Pin1 in some other cases (i.e., in embryos and in adult brain of zebrafish) [4]. In brains from autopsies, PIN1 was found to localize in the nucleus of normal neurons, but both in nuclei and cytoplasm in brains from patients suffering frontotemporal dementias (FTD) [37] or AD [38–40]. In AD patients, Pin1 localized also exclusively in the cytoplasm of neurons of certain brain regions i.e., the hippocampus [38–40].

A sound explanation for the varying cell localization of Pin1 is a dynamic regulation of the enzyme in different cell-types, developmental stages and pathological conditions. Such dynamic regulation might depend on phosphorylation of Pin1 and generation of different isovariants [4]. Indeed, Pin1 showed a number of different phosphorylated isovariants [28–33] that were detectable combining bi-dimensional (2D) denaturant gel electrophoresis followed by western blotting analysis in the zebrafish model at different developmental stages [4].

3. Physiological Role of Pin1 in In Vivo Brain Development

There is a bulk of evidence demonstrating the effects of Pin1 on specific substrates and/or signaling pathways in cell lines. On the contrary, in vivo evidence is limited. We focused on studies performed in in vivo models of mouse and zebrafish to highlight the role of Pin1 in neuronal development.

3.1. Pin1 Expression during Embryogenesis in the Zebrafish

The expression of Pin1 is tightly regulated during embryogenesis. Levels of expression vary during stages of embryogenesis and across different regions of the embryo [4]. Pin1 mRNA was already detected at 1–2 cell-stages, indicating a maternal heredity. Its levels decreased during the next developmental steps. As to regional distribution, analysis of Pin1 mRNA/protein level and distribution provided inconsistent results. In whole mount in situ hybridization (WISH), mRNA levels of Pin1 were higher in head regions (cerebellum, ventricular zone of the diencephalon and thelencephalon) and lower in trunk and tail regions. Levels of Pin1 protein were not different between trunk and head regions [4] in immunofluorescence assays.

3.2. Pin1 Regulates Neuronal Cortical Differentiation: Modulation of the Wnt/β-Catenin Pathway

In 2012, it was demonstrated that Pin1 regulates differentiation of cortical neurons by affecting the Wnt/β-catenin pathway [36]. Pivotal in neurogenesis [36,41], the Wnt/β-catenin pathway works on the two main steps of the neural stem/progenitor cells (NPCs) development: the expansion phase, stimulating proliferation; and the neurogenic phase, regulating the timing and the area of the neuronal differentiation [36,42]. There was no doubt that the β-catenin functionality is regulated by phosphorylation, but the exact mechanism was unclear for long time until β-catenin was identified as specific substrate of Pin1 in NPCs. The researchers used a proteomic approach, glutathione S-transferase (GST)-pull down strategies followed by Electrospray Ionization-Mass Spectrometry (ESI-MS) analysis [36] to demonstrate that Pin1 regulates β-catenin functionality by modulating its conformation after the phosphorylation in the Ser246-Pro motif [36,43]. This occurred in the later phases of neuronal differentiation both in NPCs and mouse brain (Figure 1).

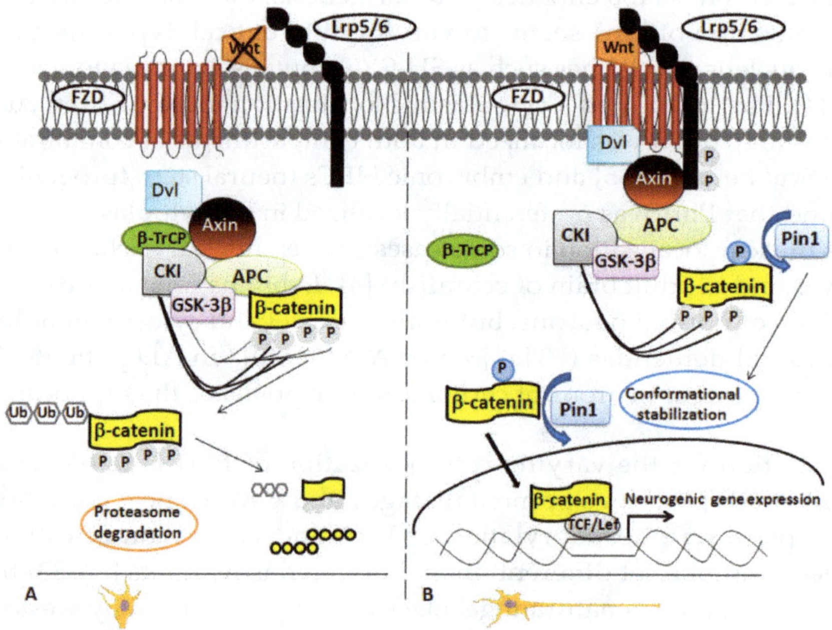

Figure 1. Pin1 modulation of Wnt/β-catenin pathway. **Panel A.** Inactivation of the Wnt/β-catenin pathway. In the absence of Wnt stimulation, levels of β-catenin decrease in the cytoplasm owing to ubiquitination and degradation by the proteasome. Both casein kinase 1α (CK1α) and glycogen synthase kinase-3β (GSK-3β) phosphorylate β-catenin to assemble a complex of proteins (named "destruction complex"). The complex includes scaffold protein axin, adenomatous polyposis coli (APC) and β-transducin repeat-containing E3 ubiquitin protein ligase (β-TrCP). Once phosphorylated, β-catenin is recognized by β-TrCP, ubiquitinated and then degraded. **Panel B.** Activation of the Wnt/β-catenin pathway. A Wnt ligand binds a Frizzled (Fz) receptor and coreceptors LRP5/6 activating the protein Dishevelled (Dvl) mostly by phosphorylation. This modification triggers the recruitment of axin to the phosphorylated tail of LRP and leads to the inhibition of the degradation pathway. Pin1 binds the β-catenin phosphorylated on the Ser246-Pro motif thus downregulating its binding with APC. By doing so, Pin1 catalyzes conformational stabilization of cytoplasmic β-catenin, which gets into the nucleus to regulate the transcription of Wnt target genes.

In NPCs and embryonal mouse cerebral cortex, Pin1 and β-catenin co-localized in both cytosol and nuclei [36].

In Pin1 KO NPCs from embryonal and adult brain, the percentage of differentiated neurons was significantly lower than in WT NPCs [36,44] as evident by using specific markers for neurons and glia cells [36]. Pin1 deficiency did not affect the NPCs proliferation in BrdU assay experiments, but it inhibited specifically cell differentiation into migrating immature neurons at embryonal stage E15.5. These results were consistent with the higher level of Pin1 expression in NPCs at later developmental step. Consistent with this finding, Pin1 KO mice showed an impaired motor activity during the neonatal stage, and this was the result of a specific inhibition of the differentiation of the upper layers neurons in the motor cortex. The authors performed experiments to stimulate/inhibit the signaling in order to confirm the role of Pin1 in the regulation of the Wnt/β-catenin pathway. They observed a rescue of Pin1 KO NPCs phenotype by using constitutively active S33Y β-catenin mutant or NPCs overexpressing Pin1. On the contrary, the truncated TCF4 (DN-TCF4), a dominant-negative mutant of the β-catenin activity, blocked the signaling and resulted in reduced neuronal differentiation [36].

3.3. Pin1 Regulation of Axonal Guidance by Modulation of Microtubule Assembly and Buffering Sema-3A Stimulation

During development of the CNS (central nervous system), axonal growth is tightly regulated by many extracellular mediators that are secreted or bound to cell membranes. The binding of these molecules to their receptors at the active growth cones triggers signaling cascades that modify dynamics of microtubules and result in axonal growth, turn, stop, or retraction [34,45]. Mechanisms of the signaling cascade are not fully understood.

Collapsin response mediator protein 2 (CRMP2), a tubulin heterodimer-binding protein that supports microtubule assembly and axon growth, plays a pivotal role in the cascade [46–48]. The binding affinity of CRMP2 to tubulin regulates the dynamic equilibrium of microtubule assembly-disassembly through phosphorylation by CDK5/GSK-3β (cyclin-dependent kinase 5/glycogen synthase kinase-3β) or Rho kinase [48,49]. In turn, stimulation of growing axons by Sema3A (semaphorin-3A) activates CDK5 [50]. The gene encoding CMRP2 presents two alternative splicing isoforms that differ in their N-terminus: CRMP2B and CRMP2A, a ~100 amino acids longer isoform. The latter was localized in axons rather than dendrites [51,52] and is likely modulated by conformational changes [53]. Balastik and co-authors contributed to the comprehension of this tightly regulated pathway, demonstrating that Pin1 binds and stabilizes CRMP2A. They observed that Pin1 is driven towards the growth cone after stimulation with Sema3A both in vitro and in vivo conditions [34]. Using a proteomic approach, combining GST-pull down followed by SDS-PAGE and tandem mass spectrometry (LC-MS/MS) experiments, they were the first to identify CRMP2A as major target of Pin1 in postnatal neurons. Pin1 stabilized CRMP2A previously phosphorylated by CDK5 selectively in distal axons [34]. Then, they found reduced level of CRMP2A at the growth cone in different experimental models: primary cortical neurons derived from Pin1 KO mice, cell lines knocked down (KD) for Pin1, or after using the specific Pin1 inhibitor (Juglone). In these experiments, Pin1 KO neurons had significantly shorter axons and this phenotype was completely reverted by over expression of CRMP2A. Therefore, they provided robust evidence on the relationship between Pin1 and CRMP2A [34].

Treatment with different concentrations of Sema-3A, and not with lysophosphatidic acid (LPA), a bioactive phospholipid in the Rho-kinase pathway, induced CRMP2 signaling via phosphorylation [54] and collapse of the growth cone both in WT and Pin1 KO primary dorsal root ganglia (DRG) neurons. This observation was associated with a change of Pin1 level and distribution in the growth cone of Pin1 WT. The change was dependent on the stimulation by Sema-3A. These observations confirmed that the catalytic action of Pin1 is specific for the Sema-3A signaling pathway in the vicinity of the growth cone where it co-localizes with CRMP2A [34]. Balastik et al. reported also that Pin1 KO embryos present selective defects of the axon growth that affect several regions of peripheral and CNS, like stunted neurite process and lack of arborization, probably owing to the impaired CRMP2A signaling [55,56]. The authors hypothesized that this uneven neuronal phenotype characterized by axonal defects might be due to compensatory mechanisms put in place for Pin1 deficiency by other members of the CRMP family to rescue reduction of CRMP2A. Indeed, Pin1 expression levels were negatively correlated with susceptibility to neurofibrillary degeneration in different regions of mouse and human brain [34,44].

To confirm in vivo the interplay between Pin1 and Sema-3A signaling, Balastick et al. used a zebrafish model of motor neuron development. Silencing of Sema-3A signaling by using KD of Neuropilin1 (NRP1) induced defects of the motor neuron growth [57,58]. Defects of the motor neuron growth were partially rescued in the simultaneous KD of NRP1 and Pin1. In Pin1 KD silencing of Sema-3A (NRP1 KD) produced a milder phenotype of motor neuron growth defects owing to the reduced stabilization of phosphorylated CRMP2A by Pin1. This would further support the notion that Pin1 regulates the Sema3A-driven axonal guidance. Indeed, Pin1 stabilizes CMRP2A selectively in distal axons and buffers low-level Sema3A stimulation both in vitro and in vivo [34].

4. Role of Pin1 in Neurodegenerative Disorders

The control of mitotic entry and progression is accompanied by the formation of specific phosphoepitopes such as MPM-2 (mitotic protein monoclonal 2), that are formed on Ser or Thr residues next to a Pro residue. Pin1 modulates function and/or dephosphorylation of some of these phosphoproteins, that are mostly recognized by the specific monoclonal antibody MPM-2 [59]. The induction of MPM-2 epitopes is a common feature in a number of neurodegenerative disorders (i.e., AD, FTD with Parkinsonism, progressive supranuclear palsy, corticobasal degeneration, Down's syndrome, and Pick's disease) [44]. Therefore, the presence of MPM-2 epitopes suggests the likely involvement of Pin1's catalytic activity in the pathogenesis of these heterogeneous conditions.

4.1. Huntington's Disease

Pin1 was reported to contribute also to the neurodegeneration seen in a mouse model of Huntington's disease. The expression of mutant Huntingtin (mHtt) determined the phosphorylation of p53 on a Ser46 residue that made it a target site for binding and modulation by Pin1 [60]. The authors hypothesized that this interaction caused the dissociation of p53 from the apoptosis inhibitor iASPP, promoting the p53 activation cascade in striatal neurons. The authors demonstrated that inhibition of Pin1, by using the specific inhibitor PiB, protected in vitro neuronal cells from mHtt-induced apoptosis. Therefore, inhibition of Pin1 might represent a therapeutic target for the treatment of Huntington's disease [60].

4.2. Parkinson's Disease

Lewy bodies (LBs) are aggregates of proteins that represent the histological hallmark of the Parkinson's disease (PD). α-synuclein, a presynaptic neuronal protein of unknown function, is the major constituent of LBs. Post-mortem histochemical analysis of patients' brain revealed the detection of Pin1 in the 50–60% of LBs [61]. Pin1 interacted indirectly and co-localized with α-synuclein in intracellular inclusions. Indeed, Pin1 bound the phosphorylated form of synphilin-1 mediated by casein kinase II (CKII) (player in cell cycle progression) and modulated the interaction between α-synuclein and synphilin-1. In neurons from substantia nigra or locus ceruleus of patients with PD, Pin1 had higher affinity for α-synuclein-synphilin-1 complex than for tau protein (in patients with AD it has the opposite affinity) and did not co-localize with the latter in LBs. Again, we face an example of the diverse modulation of Pin1 depending upon cellular types and biological contexts [61].

4.3. Temporal Lobe Epilepsy

In epileptic mice and patients with TLE, Pin1 was down-regulated as well, suggesting the involvement of the protein also in this disease [62]. Pin1 modulates an important neuronal protein, gephyrin [63], a postsynaptic scaffolding protein that favors the clustering of GABA(A) receptors at inhibitory synapses and that is down expressed in TLE patients [64]. Based on immunofluorescence, Pin1 localized in cytoplasm and cytoplasmic membranes of neurons from hippocampus and neocortex of epileptic patients and pilocarpine-induced epileptic mice [62]. Pin1 expression was down regulated in the hippocampus and cortex of mice with spontaneous recurrent seizures (SRS), compared to controls following the epileptic seizures. The authors performed immunoprecipitation experiments that demonstrated the interaction of Pin1 with NMDAR subunits 2A/2B (NR2A/2B) containing NMDA receptors (NMDARs) and not α-amino-3-hydroxy-5-methyl-4-isoxazole propionic acid receptors (AMPARs). The authors speculated that Pin1 influenced competitively the formation of synapse-associated protein-95/NR2B (PSD95/NR2B) complex thus, negatively affecting NMDAR-mediated synaptic transmission and spine morphology. The reduced expression of Pin1 caused the decreased surface trafficking of NMDARs by promoting NMDARs internalization with the net result of reduced neuronal hyper-excitability. Nevertheless, the fine mechanism by which Pin1 modulates NMDARs internalization remains unclear (Figure 2).

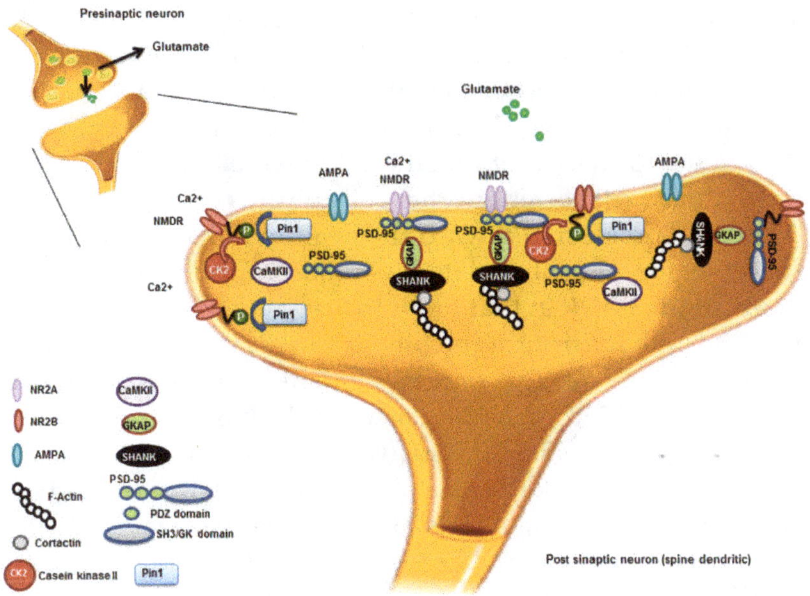

Figure 2. Pin1 regulation of NMDAR complex and synaptic plasticity. Synaptic activation of NMDAR stimulates Ca2$^+$/Calmodulin-dependent protein Kinase II (CaMKII) and casein kinase II (CK2) activity. CK2 phosphorylates the PDZ (postsynaptic density-95(PSD-95)/Discs large/zona occludens-1) ligand of NR2B. Pin1 binds and stabilizes probably the conformational change of NR2B phosphorylated disrupting the interaction between NMDAR on the cell surface and the PDZ domains of PSD-95. This leads to destabilization and internalization of surface NMDAR that influences, in turn, synaptic transmission and spine morphology. NR2A; NR2B; AMPA; F-Actin; Contarctin; CaMKII, Ca2$^+$-Calmodulin dependent protein Kinase II; CK2, casein Kinase 2; PSD-95 presents three PDZ domains, SH3 (Sarc homology 3 domain) and GK (guanylate kinase-like domain) domains; Pin1; GKAP, Guanylate kinase associate protein; Shank, shank protein.

In this disease too, Pin1 with its modulation might represent a target to modulate neuronal hyper-excitability [62].

4.4. Pin1 and Alzheimer's Diseases (AD)

AD is the most frequent form of dementia in the elderly causing progressive cognitive decline and memory loss. AD is characterized by widespread apoptosis of neurons and increased deposition of extracellular plaques and intracellular neurofibrillary tangles (NFTs) within the brain. NFTs are aggregates of microtubules that result from the hyperphosphorylation of tau protein. They are markers of AD: the amount of NFT deposits is correlated with the degree of neurodegeneration [65]. The plaques are primarily comprised of aggregated amyloid-β-peptide (Aβ) derived from the increased processing of the amyloid precursor protein (APP) [66].

Elderly Pin1 KO mice develop a complex phenotype of premature aging characteristics: namely, reduced body size, telomere instability, decreased germ-cell proliferation rate, cognitive impairment and neuronal degeneration that resembles human AD [44,67–70]. Of note, Pin1 KO mice show anomalous behavior and enhanced tau accumulation in the brain. These evidences support the argument that Pin1 dysfunction/deficiency is a pivotal determinant of the AD progression [3].

Level of Pin1 expression increased during neuronal differentiation and remained high during the lifespan [14,44]. In neuronal cells of AD patients, Pin1 was downregulated and the degree of downregulation was inversely correlated with the neuronal loss, since loss the protective ability of the enzyme against degeneration [44]. Pin1 regulated the *cis/trans* conformational changes of tau and APP proteins after their phosphorylation by kinases, such as GSK-3β [71]. Pin1 catalyzed the conformational switch of tau and APP proteins from the dysfunctional *cis*-toward the functional *trans*-structure. As consequence, tau could be dephosphorylated and degraded [39,70,71]. The accumulation of phosphorylated tau in Thr231-Pro motif was an early event in patients affected by mild cognitive impairment (MCI) [71]. In fact, Pin1 co-localized with phosphorylated tau and modulated the assembly of tau and tubulin into microtubules [72]. Pastorino and co-workers demonstrated that Pin1 drove the processing of APP and the formation of nonamyloidogenic βamyloid (Aβ) plaques. Indeed, the over-expression of Pin1 reduced Aβ secretion from cell cultures [70].

Pin1 modulated the APP processing toward the healthy nonamyloidogenic form by catalyzing *cis*-to *trans*-isomerization of the phosphorylated Thr668-Pro motif of APP [70] both directly and inhibiting the phosphorylation of APP in that motif induced by GSK-3β activity [73].

Pin1 inhibited GSK-3β activity trough the binding to a phosphorylated Thr330-Pro motif and catalyzing substrate isomerization [73]. This became evident in H4 neuroglioma cells transfected with WT or mutated construct GSK-3β T330A that did not affect the basal activity of the enzyme. In H4 cells, transfected with the mutated T330A GSK-3β, Pin1 was not able to bind and inhibit GSK-3β activity, thereby increasing the level of toxic amyloidogenic APP processing [73]. It has been speculated that the initial steps of tau phosphorylation have a neuronal protective role against the toxicity exerted by Aβ deposits [74,75], but they become detrimental when the excessive phosphorylation of tau causes the accumulation of NFTs [75]. Thus, the fine regulation of this post-translational modification is central in the pathogenesis of AD.

Alternatively, Pin1 may modulate APP processing to inhibit the phosphorylation of Thr668-Pro motif of APP performed by GSK-3β [73,76] Processing was observed in Pin1 WT or KD cells transfected both with WT or the mutated T330A GSK-3β constructs [73]. When Pin1 KD cells were transfected with both WT and mutated T330A GSK-3β, they showed comparable levels of pThr668, while Pin1 WT cells showed reduced levels of pThr668 only when transfected with WT GSK-3β construct. Therefore, the presence of Pin1 was needed for APP degradation following its binding to the Thr330-Pro motif of GSK-3β, resulting in its inhibition that then reduced phosphorylation of Thr668 [73].

In a molecular model, Pin1 was critical to regulate the active and stable conformation of Akt protein [77], that is an important player in cell survival, growth, migration and proliferation. The Akt signaling cascade is one of the survival pathways activated by neurotrophins through the binding to the tyrosine kinase (Trk) family of receptors. In *post mortem* studies of AD brains, Pin1 and neurotrophins expression levels were reduced in parallel [14]. As Angelucci and Hort hypothesized, another way for Pin1 to determine the fate of neuronal cell survival/death in neurodegenerative disorders might be related to the balance between expression of Pin1 and of neurotrophins (i.e., the brain derived growth factor, BDNF). Pin1 and neurotrophins can modulate the response of p53 [14,78,79], that acts not only as tumor suppressor, but also as a player in neuronal differentiation process [14,80], toward some transcriptional targets. The authors hypothesized that Pin1, modulating Akt and p53 conformation stability, influenced the signal transduction pathways activated by neurotrophins through the Trk receptors binding [14]. In neurodegenerative conditions, the reduced Pin1 expression level determined the reduced activity of neurotrophins-Trk signal transduction pathway causing an increased induction by p53 of neuronal death [14].

Furthermore, Pin1 influenced synaptic plasticity by regulating protein ubiquitination and degradation of postsynaptic density (PSD) proteins. By using a proteomic approach, Xu and collaborators demonstrated the association between Pin1 and Shank proteins at dendritic rafts of neuronal cells and PSD isolated from the synaptosome fractions obtained from the frontal cortical tissues of AD patients and controls [81]. Shank proteins have an "organizing role" in dendritic rafts and PSD. In cultured cortical neurons from Pin1 KO and control mice, Xu and collaborators verified the role of Pin1 in synaptic plasticity, inhibiting both Pin1 (with PiB treatment) and proteasome activity (by using MG132, carbobenzoxy-Leu-Leu-leucinal peptide). Ubiquitinated proteins in the PSD increased after the simultaneous treatment with PiB and MG132. This deregulated pathway determined an enhanced degradation of Shank3 and other PSD proteins, with a consequent alteration in PSD structure from AD brains. Pin1 modulated the NMDA receptor-mediated turnover of Shank proteins. In this regard, Tang and co-workers who studied Pin1 modulation in TLE patients [62], hypothesized that reduced Pin1 activity caused not only misfolded proteins, but also the generation of aberrant synapses contributing to the progression of pre-clinical AD [81].

Despite the role of Pin1 in the pathogenesis of AD, none of the PIN1 polymorphisms have been conclusively associated with delayed AD onset [26,65].

5. Pin1 Links Brain Impaired Glucose Metabolism and Neuronal Degeneration in AD

We speculate that post-translational modulation of Pin1 links AD among neurodegenerative disorders with peripheral and brain impaired glucose metabolism. Pin1 KO mice developed neuronal characteristics of premature aging similar to those observed in human AD i.e., age-related cognitive decline [44,68–70], but also peripheral (in both liver and muscle) and brain impairment of glucose metabolism and altered insulin signaling that resulted in overt glucose intolerance [3].

Autopsy studies in AD brains and intracerebral injected mice with streptozocin (STZ) demonstrated that brain insulin resistance and impaired insulin signaling occur early in the natural history of the disease, even before main clinical and histological characteristics develop. Main features in AD brains and STZ treated mice were cognitive impairment, structural deficits of neuronal cytoskeleton, loss of synaptic connections and increased neuronal apoptosis. Therefore, AD emerged as metabolic brain disease characterized by neuroinflammation and impaired energetic metabolism that lead to neuronal damage [16].

5.1. Type 3 Diabetes

The presence of defective insulin signaling and reduced glucose intake in the brain might be therefore early features that precede the diagnosis of overt cognitive deficits [16].

In *post mortem* brains (i.e., cerebral cortex, hippocampus and hypothalamus), the expression levels of insulin, insulin-like growth factor (IGF) 1, and IGF1 receptors were in AD patients significantly lower than in healthy age-matched individuals [82]. mRNA expression of IGF-2 tended to be different as well. Expression levels were correlated with the degree of cognitive impairment (Braak stages) in AD patients. Differential regional distribution of insulin, IGFs and their receptors was confirmed in primary neuronal cultures from rat fetal brains. Impairment of brain insulin signaling was induced in fetal rat by gestational exposure to ethanol. In this model, there was reduced production of insulin and IGFs as well as reduced expression of their receptors in different areas of the CNS. Reduced synthesis of growth factors in the brain could account for the increased neuronal death. Steen and de la Monte hypothesized that brain insulin resistance manifested as the inability to compensate for reduced secretion of insulin and IGFs with overexpression of their receptors [82]. They speculated a new type of diabetes that they named "type 3 diabetes" [16,17]. T3D would be characteristic of AD patients, affecting glucose metabolism exclusively in the brain or more broadly [75]. The reduced expression of insulin and IGF-1 receptors might explain the insulin resistance registered in the AD brain, thereby affecting negatively the insulin transduction pathway. Insulin/IGF-1 signaling upon binding to receptors activates the auto phosphorylation of receptors at Tyr residues and the activation of docking proteins, named insulin receptor substrates (IRS-1-4) and responsible for signal transduction. The intracellular signal determines the activation of mitogenic functions through MAPK/extracellular signal-regulated kinase

(MAPK/ERK) and metabolic functions through the phosphatidyl-inositol-3-kinase/Akt (PI3K/Akt) pathway that phosphorylates and inactivates GSK-3β. Given the impaired insulin/IGF-1 signal transduction, the expression level of IRS-1 was reduced in tissues from AD brains with respect to controls [82]. As consequence, the decrease of phospho-Akt and the increase of active form of GSK-3β, responsible for tau hyperphosphorylation, increased the apoptotic stimulus and caused mitochondrial dysfunction, thereby increasing mitochondrial-mediated apoptosis and oxidative stress [82].

Insulin and IGFs levels were reduced in brain tissues of AD patients and this was associated with the reduced synthesis of tau [82,83]. Growth factors stimulated tau protein expression in neuroblastoma cells [83]. The condition of brain insulin resistance was characterized by reduced levels of insulin and IGFs, no compensatory hyper-expression of their receptors and therefore a reduced transduction pathway [16,17,82]. de la Monte and collaborators speculated that the brain insulin resistance accounts for most of the molecular, histological and biochemical damages found in AD patients and develops before the onset of the clinical AD phenotype [17].

Therefore, insulin resistance that manifests in patients with T2D as peripheral hyperinsulinemia and increased release of IGF1, defective binding to receptors, impaired insulin signaling in muscle, adipose tissue and liver, could also be characterized in the brain by reduced release of insulin and IGFs and results as well in impaired insulin signaling in the brain. In both cases, impaired signaling causes reduced glucose utilization as determined by clamp and positron emission tomography studies. To further support commonalities in the pathogenesis of T2D and T3D, there is evidence from clinical trials using anti-diabetic dugs (namely analogs of glucagon like peptide 1, GLP1) in patients with T2D and/or AD that demonstrate the amelioration of the cognitive performance in parallel with the improvement of the glucose metabolism [17].

5.2. Pin1 and Insulin Pathways

Pin1 modulated peripheral glucose metabolism influencing independently both insulin secretion and sensitivity. β-cell-specific Pin1 KO (βPin1 KO) mice [84] developed glucose intolerance owing to reduced insulin secretion but preserved peripheral insulin sensitivity. βPin1 KO mice presented reduced β-cell mass as compared to controls suggesting that Pin1 affects β-cells proliferation. Cultured Pin1 KO β-cells had reduced intracellular $Ca2^{+}$ response to glucose- and KCl, despite preserved cellular ATP and insulin content. The mechanism by which Pin 1 influenced $Ca2^{+}$ response implied salt inducible kinase 2 (SIK2) and p35 protein. Pin1 interacted with SIK2, a protein belonging to the AMP-activated protein kinase (AMPK) family that is a key player for insulin secretion. The binding of Pin1 with SIK2 enhanced SIK2 kinase activity that, in turn, promoted p35 protein degradation and down-regulation of the p35-CDK5 (Cyclin-dependent kinase-5) complex activity, a negative regulator of $Ca2^{+}$ influx [84].

Experiments in KO mice, primary human endothelial cells and peripheral blood monocytes (PBMCs) of T2D patients demonstrated that hyperglycemia caused Pin1 upregulation and the latter, in turn, mediated vascular-damage occurring in diabetic patients [85]. Hyperglycemia was associated with reduced methylation of the *Pin1* gene promoter [85], and that is another finding commonly observed also in patients with AD. Indeed, Arosio and collaborators found upregulated *Pin1* gene expression in PBMCs of late onset AD patients and significantly reduced percentage methylation of *Pin1* gene promoter. In PBMCs of these patients, Pin1 quantity and activity tended to be reduced as well [86]. To explain this apparent divergent behavior, Wang [87] suggested that Pin1 reduction contributes first to the accumulation of hyperphosphorylated tau in AD patients, but successively Pin1 is over expressed to compensate for the increased formation of Aβ plaques.

AMPK is the major sensor for cellular energy status. Phosphorylation/dephosphorylation cycles of the α subunit control the activation state of AMPK. In presence of nutrients deficiency, the AMP/ADP molecules bind CBS domain of the γ subunit determining a conformational change of AMPK that protects the α subunit from dephosphorylation by protein-phosphatase 2C (PP2C). Pin1 regulated negatively AMPK, binding its CBS domain in the γ subunit. By doing so, it inhibited the binding of AMP/ADP to the γ subunit of AMPK. Therefore, Pin1 KO mice were resistant to high-fat-diet (HFD) induced obesity [88,89], with the activity level of AMPK in muscle significantly higher than in WT mice [88]. In that interaction with AMPK, Pin1 may represent a therapeutic target also to treat obesity and diabetes.

Indirect evidence in diabetic db/db treated by GLP1-analog demonstrated that PIN1 modulates insulin signaling also at the central level [72,90], being both an insulin receptor substrate-1 (IRS-1) and Akt binding partner [77,89]. About the role of Pin1 on IRS-1 signaling cascades, two hypotheses were formulated. Pin1 isomerase-activity may favor IRS-1 phosphorylation [91], or alternatively the isomerization of IRS-1 may prevent its dephosphorylation by the protein Tyr phosphatase [3]. Although Pin1 interacted with IRS-2, it did not influence its phosphorylation, likely because of a less efficient binding [89,92]. Pin1 isomerization activity induced a reduced response to insulin (insulin resistance), as demonstrated by its association with stress-induced c-Jun N-terminal kinase (JNK) and/or ribosomal protein S6 kinase (S6K), through the modulation of Ser-phosphorylation of IRSs [3,69,93]. In particular, Pin1 increased JNK kinase activity and the phosphorylation level of S6K. In HFD conditions, the Pin1 expression level increased determining the hyper-activation of JNK and S6K. Thus, in this metabolic condition the positive effect of Pin1 on IRS-1 and insulin cascade was abolished causing, instead insulin resistance.

Together with upstream kinases and protein phosphatases, Pin1 influenced the equilibrium between active and stable Akt versus the inactive and unstable form [77]. This modulation represents another way for Pin1 to influence the insulin transduction signaling. In fact, insulin promoted neuronal cytoskeletal dynamics via Akt phosphorylation [94]. Activation of insulin signaling leads usually to the activation of PI3K/Akt pathway. Akt, after being activated through its phosphorylation mainly at Thr308 residue, phosphorylates GSK-3β at Ser9 and inactivates GSK-3β kinase activity [95]. GSK-3β is one of the first enzymes involved in the regulation of glycogen synthase but is also the major protein kinase regulating tau phosphorylation in the brain [96,97] (Figure 3). GSK-3β is inactivated if phosphorylated in Ser9 residue by PI3K/Akt pathway. Its activity was found to be increased in insulin resistance conditions, suggesting that this kinase is pivotal in the regulation of peripheral and brain glucose utilization [75].

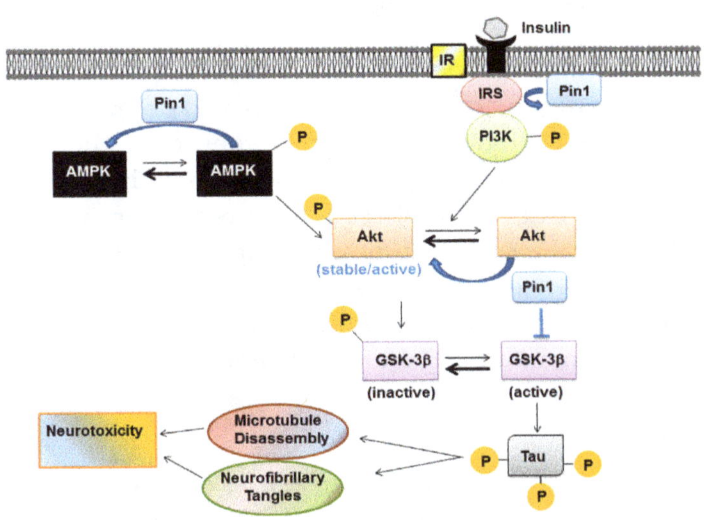

Figure 3. Pin1 in the metabolic pathway acts as a negative regulator of AMPK and modulates the Akt active form. Insulin promotes neuronal cytoskeletal dynamics via Akt phosphorylation. Activation of insulin signaling leads usually to activation of phosphatidyl-inositol-3-kinase/Akt (PI3K/Akt) pathway. After being activated through its phosphorylation mainly at Thr308 residue, Akt phosphorylates glycogen synthase kinase-3β (GSK-3β) at Ser9 and inactivates GSK-3β kinase activity. GSK-3β is also the major protein kinase regulating tau phosphorylation in the brain. Pin1 modulates all these players involved in the signaling cascade.

5.3. Pin1 and GSK-3β(Glycogen Synthase Kinase-3β) Modulation

Hence, Pin1 modulates insulin signaling by acting on Akt [77] and GSK-3β [73] activities. In brain extracts of elderly diabetic db/db mice, Akt activity was down-regulated and GSK-3β activity increased leading to the enhanced phosphorylation of tau protein and formation of NFTs [90]. It may be speculated that, more generally, the oxidative damage occurring in the diabetic brain results in impaired phosphorylation of tau protein and Pin1 modulation is implied. Oxidative modification of Pin1 at Cys113 residue was associated with reduced catalytic activity and expression in hippocampus of patients with MCI and AD too [72,98–100].

The mutual interaction between GSK-3β and Pin1 become evident also in experimental models of hereditary hemochromatosis, whereas homozygous patients carrying the HFE hemocromatosis mutation have enhanced risk of diabetes ("bronze diabetes") if untreated. In SH-SY5Y cells carrying H63D mutation of the HFE gene and in H67D transgenic mice, phosphorylation of Pin1 on Ser16 was increased and resulted in decreased enzyme activity. The treatment with Trolox, an antioxidant, rescued Pin1 activity in both models [101]. In the in vitro model, tau phosphorylation was increased paralleling GSK-3β activity [99], while Pin1 activity was consequently reduced [101]. Conversely, the inhibition of GSK-3β activity by lithium was associated with the increase of Pin1 activity, reinforcing the notion that GSK-3β and Pin1 interact with each other' to influence the ability of Pin1 to modulate its substrates such as tau protein [101,102].

6. Conclusions

The prolyl isomerase Pin1 plays a central role in the switching of proline-directed phosphorylation signaling: it induces the isomerization of the *cis/trans* configuration of protein substrates that are phosphorylated. As molecular "switch" that turns on or off enzyme activities or entire signaling pathways, Pin1 modulates many cellular functions both in physiological processes and pathological conditions (i.e., cancer, neurodegenerative and metabolic diseases). Pin1 exerts different and even opposite effects in vivo that are cell specific, depend upon specific protein substrates and are associated with phosphorylation of distinctive Pin1 binding sites.

Among the various regulatory functions, Pin1 controls neuronal differentiation during brain development by stabilizing β-catenin and synaptic plasticity/degradation of postsynaptic density proteins. Pin1 protects against oxidative damage of neurons, thereby protecting them from neurodegeneration. Indeed, impaired Pin1 function is associated with neurodegeneration and cognitive dysfunction in patients with AD. But Pin1 is also a master regulator of neuronal energy metabolism and interferes particularly with the cell insulin signaling. Because of these dual major roles on neuroprotection and metabolism, we and others speculate that impaired Pin1 function is one of the pivotal molecular links between neurodegeneration and impaired glucose metabolism, both manifesting in patients with dementia. Therefore, we report evidence supporting this hypothesis. There is large overlap between Pin1 and insulin signaling pathways within the brain, with Pin1 influencing insulin signaling.

Therefore, Pin1 may also represent a treatment target to prevent the onset of brain impaired glucose metabolism that is deemed by some researchers as one of the first hints in the pathogenesis of the AD. It may be effective to prevent the onset of or delay the neurodegenerative process, since acting as isomerase, Pin1 catalyzes the conformational switch of tau and APP proteins from the dysfunctional *cis*-toward the functional *trans*-structure and enhances tau dephosphorylation and degradation.

Author Contributions: M.B. and M.M. conceived the review; M.B. write the draft and M.M. revised for intellectual content. Both authors actively contributed in generating figures.

References

1. Gothel, S.F.; Marahiel, M.A. Peptidyl-prolyl *cis-trans* isomerases, a superfamily of ubiquitous folding catalysts. *Cell. Mol. Life Sci.* **1999**, *55*, 423–436. [CrossRef] [PubMed]
2. Reimer, U.; Scherer, G.; Drewello, M.; Kruber, S.; Schutkowski, M.; Fischer, G. Side-chain effects on peptidyl-prolyl *cis/trans* isomerisation. *J. Mol. Biol.* **1998**, *279*, 449–460. [CrossRef] [PubMed]
3. Nakatsu, Y.; Matsunaga, Y.; Yamamotoya, T.; Ueda, K.; Inoue, Y.; Mori, K.; Sakoda, H.; Fujishiro, M.; Ono, H.; Kushiyama, A.; et al. Physiological and Pathogenic Roles of Prolyl Isomerase Pin1 in Metabolic Regulations via Multiple Signal Transduction Pathway Modulations. *Int. J. Mol. Sci.* **2016**, *17*, 1495. [CrossRef] [PubMed]
4. Ibarra, M.S.; Borini Etichetti, C.; di Benedetto, C.; Rosano, G.L.; Margarit, E.; del Sal, G.; Mione, M.; Girardini, J. Dynamic regulation of Pin1 expression and function during zebrafish development. *PLoS ONE* **2017**, *12*, e0175939. [CrossRef] [PubMed]
5. Davies, T.H.; Ning, Y.M.; Sanchez, E.R. A new first step in activation of steroid receptors: Hormone-induced switching of FKBP51 and FKBP52 immunophilins. *J. Biol. Chem.* **2002**, *277*, 4597–4600. [CrossRef] [PubMed]
6. Liu, J.; Farmer, J.D., Jr.; Lane, W.S.; Friedman, J.; Weissman, I.; Schreiber, S.L. Calcineurin is a common target of cyclophilin-cyclosporin A and FKBP-FK506 complexes. *Cell* **1991**, *66*, 807–815. [CrossRef]
7. Lu, K.P.; Finn, G.; Lee, T.H.; Nicholson, L.K. Prolyl *cis-trans* isomerization as a molecular timer. *Nat. Chem. Biol.* **2007**, *3*, 619–629. [CrossRef] [PubMed]
8. Lu, K.P.; Zhou, X.Z. The prolyl isomerase PIN1: A pivotal new twist in phosphorylation signalling and disease. *Nat. Rev. Mol. Cell Biol.* **2007**, *8*, 904–916. [CrossRef] [PubMed]
9. Ranganathan, R.; Lu, K.P.; Hunter, T.; Noel, J.P. Structural and functional analysis of the mitotic rotamase Pin1 suggests substrate recognition is phosphorylation dependent. *Cell* **1997**, *89*, 875–886. [CrossRef]
10. Kim, E.K.; Choi, E.J. Pathological roles of MAPK signaling pathways in human diseases. *Biochim. Biophys. Acta* **2010**, *1802*, 396–405. [CrossRef] [PubMed]
11. MacAulay, K.; Doble, B.W.; Patel, S.; Hansotia, T.; Sinclair, E.M.; Drucker, D.J.; Nagy, A.; Woodgett, J.R. Glycogen synthase kinase 3α-specific regulation of murine hepatic glycogen metabolism. *Cell Metab.* **2007**, *6*, 329–337. [CrossRef] [PubMed]
12. Patrick, G.N.; Zukerberg, L.; Nikolic, M.; de la Monte, S.; Dikkes, P.; Tsai, L.H. Conversion of p35 to p25 deregulates Cdk5 activity and promotes neurodegeneration. *Nature* **1999**, *402*, 615–622. [CrossRef] [PubMed]
13. Bao, L.; Kimzey, A.; Sauter, G.; Sowadski, J.M.; Lu, K.P.; Wang, D.G. Prevalent overexpression of prolyl isomerase Pin1 in human cancers. *Am. J. Pathol.* **2004**, *164*, 1727–1737. [CrossRef]
14. Angelucci, F.; Hort, J. Prolyl isomerase Pin1 and neurotrophins: A loop that may determine the fate of cells in cancer and neurodegeneration. *Ther. Adv. Med. Oncol.* **2017**, *9*, 59–62. [CrossRef] [PubMed]
15. Talbot, K.; Wang, H.Y.; Kazi, H.; Han, L.Y.; Bakshi, K.P.; Stucky, A.; Fuino, R.L.; Kawaguchi, K.R.; Samoyedny, A.J.; Wilson, R.S.; et al. Demonstrated brain insulin resistance in Alzheimer's disease patients is associated with IGF-1 resistance, IRS-1 dysregulation, and cognitive decline. *J. Clin. Investig.* **2012**, *122*, 1316–1338. [CrossRef] [PubMed]
16. De la Monte, S.M.; Wands, J.R. Alzheimer's disease is type 3 diabetes-evidence reviewed. *J. Diabetes Sci. Technol.* **2008**, *2*, 1101–1113. [CrossRef] [PubMed]
17. De la Monte, S.M. Insulin Resistance and Neurodegeneration: Progress Towards the Development of New Therapeutics for Alzheimer's Disease. *Drugs* **2017**, *77*, 47–65. [CrossRef] [PubMed]
18. Verdecia, M.A.; Bowman, M.E.; Lu, K.P.; Hunter, T.; Noel, J.P. Structural basis for phosphoserine-proline recognition by group IV WW domains. *Nat. Struct. Biol.* **2000**, *7*, 639–643. [CrossRef] [PubMed]
19. Bayer, E.; Goettsch, S.; Mueller, J.W.; Griewel, B.; Guiberman, E.; Mayr, L.M.; Bayer, P. Structural analysis of the mitotic regulator hPin1 in solution: Insights into domain architecture and substrate binding. *J. Biol. Chem.* **2003**, *278*, 26183–26193. [CrossRef] [PubMed]
20. Eichner, T.; Kutter, S.; Labeikovsky, W.; Buosi, V.; Kern, D. Molecular Mechanism of Pin1-Tau Recognition and Catalysis. *J. Mol. Biol.* **2016**, *428 Pt A*, 1760–1775. [CrossRef]
21. Labeikovsky, W.; Eisenmesser, E.Z.; Bosco, D.A.; Kern, D. Structure and dynamics of pin1 during catalysis by NMR. *J. Mol. Biol.* **2007**, *367*, 1370–1381. [CrossRef] [PubMed]
22. Jacobs, D.M.; Saxena, K.; Vogtherr, M.; Bernado, P.; Pons, M.; Fiebig, K.M. Peptide binding induces large scale changes in inter-domain mobility in human Pin1. *J. Biol. Chem.* **2003**, *278*, 26174–26182. [CrossRef] [PubMed]

23. Namanja, A.T.; Peng, T.; Zintsmaster, J.S.; Elson, A.C.; Shakour, M.G.; Peng, J.W. Substrate recognition reduces side-chain flexibility for conserved hydrophobic residues in human Pin1. *Structure* **2007**, *15*, 313–327. [CrossRef] [PubMed]
24. Ryo, A.; Liou, Y.C.; Wulf, G.; Nakamura, M.; Lee, S.W.; Lu, K.P. *PIN1* is an E2F target gene essential for Neu/Ras-induced transformation of mammary epithelial cells. *Mol. Cell. Biol.* **2002**, *22*, 5281–5295. [CrossRef] [PubMed]
25. Rustighi, A.; Tiberi, L.; Soldano, A.; Napoli, M.; Nuciforo, P.; Rosato, A.; Kaplan, F.; Capobianco, A.; Pece, S.; Di Fiore, P.P.; et al. The prolyl-isomerase Pin1 is a Notch1 target that enhances Notch1 activation in cancer. *Nat. Cell Biol.* **2009**, *11*, 133–142. [CrossRef] [PubMed]
26. Ma, S.L.; Tang, N.L.; Tam, C.W.; Lui, V.W.; Lam, L.C.; Chiu, H.F.; Driver, J.A.; Pastorino, L.; Lu, K.P. A PIN1 polymorphism that prevents its suppression by AP4 associates with delayed onset of Alzheimer's disease. *Neurobiol. Aging* **2012**, *33*, 804–813. [CrossRef] [PubMed]
27. Eckerdt, F.; Yuan, J.; Saxena, K.; Martin, B.; Kappel, S.; Lindenau, C.; Kramer, A.; Naumann, S.; Daum, S.; Fischer, G.; et al. Polo-like kinase 1-mediated phosphorylation stabilizes Pin1 by inhibiting its ubiquitination in human cells. *J. Biol. Chem.* **2005**, *280*, 36575–36583. [CrossRef] [PubMed]
28. Lu, P.J.; Zhou, X.Z.; Liou, Y.C.; Noel, J.P.; Lu, K.P. Critical role of WW domain phosphorylation in regulating phosphoserine binding activity and Pin1 function. *J. Biol. Chem.* **2002**, *277*, 2381–2384. [CrossRef] [PubMed]
29. Lee, Y.C.; Que, J.; Chen, Y.C.; Lin, J.T.; Liou, Y.C.; Liao, P.C.; Liu, Y.P.; Lee, K.H.; Lin, L.C.; Hsiao, M.; et al. Pin1 acts as a negative regulator of the G2/M transition by interacting with the Aurora-A-Bora complex. *J. Cell Sci.* **2013**, *126 Pt 21*, 4862–4872. [CrossRef]
30. Cho, Y.S.; Park, S.Y.; Kim, D.J.; Lee, S.H.; Woo, K.M.; Lee, K.A.; Lee, Y.J.; Cho, Y.Y.; Shim, J.H. TPA-induced cell transformation provokes a complex formation between Pin1 and 90 kDa ribosomal protein S6 kinase 2. *Mol. Cell. Biochem.* **2012**, *367*, 85–92. [CrossRef] [PubMed]
31. Kim, G.; Khanal, P.; Kim, J.Y.; Yun, H.J.; Lim, S.C.; Shim, J.H.; Choi, H.S. COT phosphorylates prolyl-isomerase Pin1 to promote tumorigenesis in breast cancer. *Mol. Carcinogen.* **2015**, *54*, 440–448. [CrossRef] [PubMed]
32. Lee, T.H.; Chen, C.H.; Suizu, F.; Huang, P.; Schiene-Fischer, C.; Daum, S.; Zhang, Y.J.; Goate, A.; Chen, R.H.; Zhou, X.Z.; et al. Death-associated protein kinase 1 phosphorylates Pin1 and inhibits its prolyl isomerase activity and cellular function. *Mol. Cell* **2011**, *42*, 147–159. [CrossRef] [PubMed]
33. Rangasamy, V.; Mishra, R.; Sondarva, G.; Das, S.; Lee, T.H.; Bakowska, J.C.; Tzivion, G.; Malter, J.S.; Rana, B.; Lu, K.P.; et al. Mixed-lineage kinase 3 phosphorylates prolyl-isomerase Pin1 to regulate its nuclear translocation and cellular function. *Proc. Natl. Acad. Sci. USA* **2012**, *109*, 8149–8154. [CrossRef] [PubMed]
34. Balastik, M.; Zhou, X.Z.; Alberich-Jorda, M.; Weissova, R.; Ziak, J.; Pazyra-Murphy, M.F.; Cosker, K.E.; Machonova, O.; Kozmikova, I.; Chen, C.H.; et al. Prolyl Isomerase Pin1 Regulates Axon Guidance by Stabilizing CRMP2A Selectively in Distal Axons. *Cell Rep.* **2015**, *13*, 812–828. [CrossRef] [PubMed]
35. Baik, S.H.; Fane, M.; Park, J.H.; Cheng, Y.L.; Yang-Wei Fann, D.; Yun, U.J.; Choi, Y.; Park, J.S.; Chai, B.H.; Park, J.S.; et al. Pin1 promotes neuronal death in stroke by stabilizing Notch intracellular domain. *Ann. Neurol.* **2015**, *77*, 504–516. [CrossRef] [PubMed]
36. Nakamura, K.; Kosugi, I.; Lee, D.Y.; Hafner, A.; Sinclair, D.A.; Ryo, A.; Lu, K.P. Prolyl isomerase Pin1 regulates neuronal differentiation via beta-catenin. *Mol. Cell. Biol.* **2012**, *32*, 2966–2978. [CrossRef] [PubMed]
37. Thorpe, J.R.; Mosaheb, S.; Hashemzadeh-Bonehi, L.; Cairns, N.J.; Kay, J.E.; Morley, S.J.; Rulten, S.L. Shortfalls in the peptidyl-prolyl *cis-trans* isomerase protein Pin1 in neurons are associated with frontotemporal dementias. *Neurobiol. Dis.* **2004**, *17*, 237–249. [CrossRef] [PubMed]
38. Holzer, M.; Gartner, U.; Stobe, A.; Hartig, W.; Gruschka, H.; Bruckner, M.K.; Arendt, T. Inverse association of Pin1 and tau accumulation in Alzheimer's disease hippocampus. *Acta Neuropathol.* **2002**, *104*, 471–481. [CrossRef] [PubMed]
39. Lu, P.J.; Wulf, G.; Zhou, X.Z.; Davies, P.; Lu, K.P. The prolyl isomerase Pin1 restores the function of Alzheimer-associated phosphorylated tau protein. *Nature* **1999**, *399*, 784–788. [CrossRef] [PubMed]
40. Ramakrishnan, P.; Dickson, D.W.; Davies, P. Pin1 colocalization with phosphorylated tau in Alzheimer's disease and other tauopathies. *Neurobiol. Dis.* **2003**, *14*, 251–264. [CrossRef]
41. Clevers, H. Wnt/β-catenin signaling in development and disease. *Cell* **2006**, *127*, 469–480. [CrossRef] [PubMed]
42. Hirabayashi, Y.; Itoh, Y.; Tabata, H.; Nakajima, K.; Akiyama, T.; Masuyama, N.; Gotoh, Y. The Wnt/β-catenin pathway directs neuronal differentiation of cortical neural precursor cells. *Development* **2004**, *131*, 2791–2801. [CrossRef] [PubMed]

43. Ryo, A.; Nakamura, M.; Wulf, G.; Liou, Y.C.; Lu, K.P. Pin1 regulates turnover and subcellular localization of β-catenin by inhibiting its interaction with APC. *Nat. Cell Biol.* **2001**, *3*, 793–801. [CrossRef] [PubMed]
44. Liou, Y.C.; Sun, A.; Ryo, A.; Zhou, X.Z.; Yu, Z.X.; Huang, H.K.; Uchida, T.; Bronson, R.; Bing, G.; Li, X.; et al. Role of the prolyl isomerase Pin1 in protecting against age-dependent neurodegeneration. *Nature* **2003**, *424*, 556–561. [CrossRef] [PubMed]
45. Culotti, J.G.; Kolodkin, A.L. Functions of netrins and semaphorins in axon guidance. *Curr. Opin. Neurobiol.* **1996**, *6*, 81–88. [CrossRef]
46. Fukata, Y.; Itoh, T.J.; Kimura, T.; Menager, C.; Nishimura, T.; Shiromizu, T.; Watanabe, H.; Inagaki, N.; Iwamatsu, A.; Hotani, H.; et al. CRMP-2 binds to tubulin heterodimers to promote microtubule assembly. *Nat. Cell Biol.* **2002**, *4*, 583–591. [CrossRef] [PubMed]
47. Inagaki, N.; Chihara, K.; Arimura, N.; Menager, C.; Kawano, Y.; Matsuo, N.; Nishimura, T.; Amano, M.; Kaibuchi, K. CRMP-2 induces axons in cultured hippocampal neurons. *Nat. Neurosci.* **2001**, *4*, 781–782. [CrossRef] [PubMed]
48. Yoshimura, T.; Kawano, Y.; Arimura, N.; Kawabata, S.; Kikuchi, A.; Kaibuchi, K. GSK-3beta regulates phosphorylation of CRMP-2 and neuronal polarity. *Cell* **2005**, *120*, 137–149. [CrossRef] [PubMed]
49. Arimura, N.; Menager, C.; Kawano, Y.; Yoshimura, T.; Kawabata, S.; Hattori, A.; Fukata, Y.; Amano, M.; Goshima, Y.; Inagaki, M.; et al. Phosphorylation by Rho kinase regulates CRMP-2 activity in growth cones. *Mol. Cell. Biol.* **2005**, *25*, 9973–9984. [CrossRef] [PubMed]
50. Sasaki, Y.; Cheng, C.; Uchida, Y.; Nakajima, O.; Ohshima, T.; Yagi, T.; Taniguchi, M.; Nakayama, T.; Kishida, R.; Kudo, Y.; et al. Fyn and Cdk5 mediate semaphorin-3A signaling, which is involved in regulation of dendrite orientation in cerebral cortex. *Neuron* **2002**, *35*, 907–920. [CrossRef]
51. Quinn, C.C.; Chen, E.; Kinjo, T.G.; Kelly, G.; Bell, A.W.; Elliott, R.C.; McPherson, P.S.; Hockfield, S. TUC-4b, a novel TUC family variant, regulates neurite outgrowth and associates with vesicles in the growth cone. *J. Neurosci.* **2003**, *23*, 2815–2823. [CrossRef] [PubMed]
52. Yuasa-Kawada, J.; Suzuki, R.; Kano, F.; Ohkawara, T.; Murata, M.; Noda, M. Axonal morphogenesis controlled by antagonistic roles of two CRMP subtypes in microtubule organization. *Eur. J. Neurosci.* **2003**, *17*, 2329–2343. [CrossRef] [PubMed]
53. Schmidt, E.F.; Strittmatter, S.M. The CRMP family of proteins and their role in Sema3A signaling. *Adv. Exp. Med. Biol.* **2007**, *600*, 1–11. [CrossRef] [PubMed]
54. Goshima, Y.; Nakamura, F.; Strittmatter, P.; Strittmatter, S.M. Collapsin-induced growth cone collapse mediated by an intracellular protein related to UNC-33. *Nature* **1995**, *376*, 509–514. [CrossRef] [PubMed]
55. Arimura, N.; Inagaki, N.; Chihara, K.; Menager, C.; Nakamura, N.; Amano, M.; Iwamatsu, A.; Goshima, Y.; Kaibuchi, K. Phosphorylation of collapsin response mediator protein-2 by Rho-kinase. Evidence for two separate signaling pathways for growth cone collapse. *J. Biol. Chem.* **2000**, *275*, 23973–23980. [CrossRef] [PubMed]
56. Tan, F.; Thiele, C.J.; Li, Z. Collapsin response mediator proteins: Potential diagnostic and prognostic biomarkers in cancers (Review). *Oncol. Lett.* **2014**, *7*, 1333–1340. [CrossRef] [PubMed]
57. Behar, O.; Golden, J.A.; Mashimo, H.; Schoen, F.J.; Fishman, M.C. Semaphorin III is needed for normal patterning and growth of nerves, bones and heart. *Nature* **1996**, *383*, 525–528. [CrossRef] [PubMed]
58. Gu, C.; Rodriguez, E.R.; Reimert, D.V.; Shu, T.; Fritzsch, B.; Richards, L.J.; Kolodkin, A.L.; Ginty, D.D. Neuropilin-1 conveys semaphorin and VEGF signaling during neural and cardiovascular development. *Dev. Cell* **2003**, *5*, 45–57. [CrossRef]
59. Escargueil, A.E.; Larsen, A.K. Mitosis-specific MPM-2 phosphorylation of DNA topoisomerase IIα is regulated directly by protein phosphatase 2A. *Biochem. J.* **2007**, *403*, 235–242. [CrossRef] [PubMed]
60. Grison, A.; Mantovani, F.; Comel, A.; Agostoni, E.; Gustincich, S.; Persichetti, F.; Del Sal, G. Ser46 phosphorylation and prolyl-isomerase Pin1-mediated isomerization of p53 are key events in p53-dependent apoptosis induced by mutant huntingtin. *Proc. Natl. Acad. Sci. USA* **2011**, *108*, 17979–17984. [CrossRef] [PubMed]
61. Ryo, A.; Togo, T.; Nakai, T.; Hirai, A.; Nishi, M.; Yamaguchi, A.; Suzuki, K.; Hirayasu, Y.; Kobayashi, H.; Perrem, K.; et al. Prolyl-isomerase Pin1 accumulates in lewy bodies of parkinson disease and facilitates formation of α-synuclein inclusions. *J. Biol. Chem.* **2006**, *281*, 4117–4125. [CrossRef] [PubMed]
62. Tang, L.; Zhang, Y.; Chen, G.; Xiong, Y.; Wang, X.; Zhu, B. Down-regulation of Pin1 in Temporal Lobe Epilepsy Patients and Mouse Model. *Neurochem. Res.* **2017** *42*, 1211–1218. [CrossRef] [PubMed]

63. Zita, M.M.; Marchionni, I.; Bottos, E.; Righi, M.; del Sal, G.; Cherubini, E.; Zacchi, P. Post-phosphorylation prolyl isomerisation of gephyrin represents a mechanism to modulate glycine receptors function. *EMBO J.* **2007**, *26*, 1761–1771. [CrossRef] [PubMed]
64. Fang, M.; Shen, L.; Yin, H.; Pan, Y.M.; Wang, L.; Chen, D.; Xi, Z.Q.; Xiao, Z.; Wang, X.F.; Zhou, S.N. Downregulation of gephyrin in temporal lobe epilepsy neurons in humans and a rat model. *Synapse (N. Y.)* **2011**, *65*, 1006–1014. [CrossRef] [PubMed]
65. Harris, R.A.; Tindale, L.; Cumming, R.C. Age-dependent metabolic dysregulation in cancer and Alzheimer's disease. *Biogerontology* **2014**, *15*, 559–577. [CrossRef] [PubMed]
66. Zhang, H.; Ma, Q.; Zhang, Y.W.; Xu, H. Proteolytic processing of Alzheimer's beta-amyloid precursor protein. *J. Neurochem.* **2012**, *120*, 9–21. [CrossRef] [PubMed]
67. Atchison, F.W.; Capel, B.; Means, A.R. Pin1 regulates the timing of mammalian primordial germ cell proliferation. *Development* **2003**, *130*, 3579–3586. [CrossRef] [PubMed]
68. Atchison, F.W.; Means, A.R. Spermatogonial depletion in adult Pin1-deficient mice. *Biol. Reprod.* **2003**, *69*, 1989–1997. [CrossRef] [PubMed]
69. Lee, N.Y.; Choi, H.K.; Shim, J.H.; Kang, K.W.; Dong, Z.; Choi, H.S. The prolyl isomerase Pin1 interacts with a ribosomal protein S6 kinase to enhance insulin-induced AP-1 activity and cellular transformation. *Carcinogenesis* **2009**, *30*, 671–681. [CrossRef] [PubMed]
70. Pastorino, L.; Sun, A.; Lu, P.J.; Zhou, X.Z.; Balastik, M.; Finn, G.; Wulf, G.; Lim, J.; Li, S.H.; Li, X.; et al. The prolyl isomerase Pin1 regulates amyloid precursor protein processing and amyloid-beta production. *Nature* **2006**, *440*, 528–534. [CrossRef] [PubMed]
71. Driver, J.A.; Zhou, X.Z.; Lu, K.P. Regulation of protein conformation by Pin1 offers novel disease mechanisms and therapeutic approaches in Alzheimer's disease. *Discov. Med.* **2014**, *17*, 93–99. [PubMed]
72. Butterfield, D.A.; Abdul, H.M.; Opii, W.; Newman, S.F.; Joshi, G.; Ansari, M.A.; Sultana, R. Pin1 in Alzheimer's disease. *J. Neurochem.* **2006**, *98*, 1697–1706. [CrossRef] [PubMed]
73. Ma, S.L.; Pastorino, L.; Zhou, X.Z.; Lu, K.P. Prolyl isomerase Pin1 promotes amyloid precursor protein (APP) turnover by inhibiting glycogen synthase kinase-3β (GSK3β) activity: Novel mechanism for Pin1 to protect against Alzheimer disease. *J. Biol. Chem.* **2012**, *287*, 6969–6973. [CrossRef] [PubMed]
74. Ittner, A.; Chua, S.W.; Bertz, J.; Volkerling, A.; van der Hoven, J.; Gladbach, A.; Przybyla, M.; Bi, M.; van Hummel, A.; Stevens, C.H.; et al. Site-specific phosphorylation of tau inhibits amyloid-β toxicity in Alzheimer's mice. *Science (N. Y.)* **2016**, *354*, 904–908. [CrossRef] [PubMed]
75. Zhang, Y.; Huang, N.Q.; Yan, F.; Jin, H.; Zhou, S.Y.; Shi, J.S.; Jin, F. Diabetes mellitus and Alzheimer's disease: GSK-3β as a potential link. *Behav. Brain Res.* **2018**, *339*, 57–65. [CrossRef] [PubMed]
76. Aplin, A.E.; Gibb, G.M.; Jacobsen, J.S.; Gallo, J.M.; Anderton, B.H. In vitro phosphorylation of the cytoplasmic domain of the amyloid precursor protein by glycogen synthase kinase-3β. *J. Neurochem.* **1996**, *67*, 699–707. [CrossRef] [PubMed]
77. Liao, Y.; Hung, M.C. Physiological regulation of Akt activity and stability. *Am. J. Transl. Res.* **2010**, *2*, 19–42. [PubMed]
78. Brynczka, C.; Labhart, P.; Merrick, B.A. NGF-mediated transcriptional targets of p53 in PC12 neuronal differentiation. *BMC Genom.* **2007**, *8*, 139. [CrossRef] [PubMed]
79. Hu, H.; Wulf, G.M. The amplifier effect: How Pin1 empowers mutant p53. *Breast Cancer Res. BCR* **2011**, *13*, 315. [CrossRef] [PubMed]
80. Tedeschi, A.; Di Giovanni, S. The non-apoptotic role of p53 in neuronal biology: Enlightening the dark side of the moon. *EMBO Rep.* **2009**, *10*, 576–583. [CrossRef] [PubMed]
81. Xu, L.; Ren, Z.; Chow, F.E.; Tsai, R.; Liu, T.; Rizzolio, F.; Boffo, S.; Xu, Y.; Huang, S.; Lippa, C.F.; et al. Pathological Role of Peptidyl-Prolyl Isomerase Pin1 in the Disruption of Synaptic Plasticity in Alzheimer's Disease. *Neural Plast.* **2017**, *2017*, 3270725. [CrossRef] [PubMed]
82. Steen, E.; Terry, B.M.; Rivera, E.J.; Cannon, J.L.; Neely, T.R.; Tavares, R.; Xu, X.J.; Wands, J.R.; de la Monte, S.M. Impaired insulin and insulin-like growth factor expression and signaling mechanisms in Alzheimer's disease—Is this type 3 diabetes? *J. Alzheimer's Dis.* **2005**, *7*, 63–80. [CrossRef]
83. De la Monte, S.M.; Chen, G.J.; Rivera, E.; Wands, J.R. Neuronal thread protein regulation and interaction with microtubule-associated proteins in SH-Sy5y neuronal cells. *Cell. Mol. Life Sci.* **2003**, *60*, 2679–2691. [CrossRef] [PubMed]

84. Nakatsu, Y.; Mori, K.; Matsunaga, Y.; Yamamotoya, T.; Ueda, K.; Inoue, Y.; Mitsuzaki-Miyoshi, K.; Sakoda, H.; Fujishiro, M.; Yamaguchi, S.; et al. The prolyl isomerase Pin1 increases beta-cell proliferation and enhances insulin secretion. *J. Biol. Chem.* **2017**, *292*, 11886–11895. [CrossRef] [PubMed]
85. Paneni, F.; Costantino, S.; Castello, L.; Battista, R.; Capretti, G.; Chiandotto, S.; D'Amario, D.; Scavone, G.; Villano, A.; Rustighi, A.; et al. Targeting prolyl-isomerase Pin1 prevents mitochondrial oxidative stress and vascular dysfunction: Insights in patients with diabetes. *Eur. Heart J.* **2015**, *36*, 817–828. [CrossRef] [PubMed]
86. Arosio, B.; Bulbarelli, A.; Bastias Candia, S.; Lonati, E.; Mastronardi, L.; Romualdi, P.; Candeletti, S.; Gussago, C.; Galimberti, D.; Scarpini, E.; et al. Pin1 contribution to Alzheimer's disease: Transcriptional and epigenetic mechanisms in patients with late-onset Alzheimer's disease. *Neuro-Degener. Dis.* **2012**, *10*, 207–211. [CrossRef] [PubMed]
87. Wang, S.; Simon, B.P.; Bennett, D.A.; Schneider, J.A.; Malter, J.S.; Wang, D.S. The significance of Pin1 in the development of Alzheimer's disease. *J. Alzheimer's Dis.* **2007**, *11*, 13–23. [CrossRef]
88. Nakatsu, Y.; Iwashita, M.; Sakoda, H.; Ono, H.; Nagata, K.; Matsunaga, Y.; Fukushima, T.; Fujishiro, M.; Kushiyama, A.; Kamata, H.; et al. Prolyl isomerase Pin1 negatively regulates AMP-activated protein kinase (AMPK) by associating with the CBS domain in the gamma subunit. *J. Biol. Chem.* **2015**, *290*, 24255–24266. [CrossRef] [PubMed]
89. Nakatsu, Y.; Sakoda, H.; Kushiyama, A.; Zhang, J.; Ono, H.; Fujishiro, M.; Kikuchi, T.; Fukushima, T.; Yoneda, M.; Ohno, H.; et al. Peptidyl-prolyl cis/trans isomerase NIMA-interacting 1 associates with insulin receptor substrate-1 and enhances insulin actions and adipogenesis. *J. Biol. Chem.* **2011**, *286*, 20812–20822. [CrossRef] [PubMed]
90. Ma, D.L.; Chen, F.Q.; Xu, W.J.; Yue, W.Z.; Yuan, G.; Yang, Y. Early intervention with glucagon-like peptide 1 analog liraglutide prevents tau hyperphosphorylation in diabetic db/db mice. *J. Neurochem.* **2015**, *135*, 301–308. [CrossRef] [PubMed]
91. Zhang, J.; Nakatsu, Y.; Shinjo, T.; Guo, Y.; Sakoda, H.; Yamamotoya, T.; Otani, Y.; Okubo, H.; Kushiyama, A.; Fujishiro, M.; et al. Par14 protein associates with insulin receptor substrate 1 (IRS-1), thereby enhancing insulin-induced IRS-1 phosphorylation and metabolic actions. *J. Biol. Chem.* **2013**, *288*, 20692–20701. [CrossRef] [PubMed]
92. Rabiee, A.; Kruger, M.; Ardenkjaer-Larsen, J.; Kahn, C.R.; Emanuelli, B. Distinct signalling properties of insulin receptor substrate (IRS)-1 and IRS-2 in mediating insulin/IGF-1 action. *Cell. Signal.* **2018**, *47*, 1–15. [CrossRef] [PubMed]
93. Park, J.E.; Lee, J.A.; Park, S.G.; Lee, D.H.; Kim, S.J.; Kim, H.J.; Uchida, C.; Uchida, T.; Park, B.C.; Cho, S. A critical step for JNK activation: Isomerization by the prolyl isomerase Pin1. *Cell Death Differ.* **2012**, *19*, 153–161. [CrossRef] [PubMed]
94. Simpson, J.E.; Ince, P.G.; Shaw, P.J.; Heath, P.R.; Raman, R.; Garwood, C.J.; Gelsthorpe, C.; Baxter, L.; Forster, G.; Matthews, F.E.; et al. Microarray analysis of the astrocyte transcriptome in the aging brain: Relationship to Alzheimer's pathology and APOE genotype. *Neurobiol. Aging* **2011**, 32, 1795–1807. [CrossRef] [PubMed]
95. Beale, E.G. Insulin signaling and insulin resistance. *J. Investig. Med.* **2013**, *61*, 11–14. [CrossRef] [PubMed]
96. Hernandez, F.; Lucas, J.J.; Avila, J. GSK3 and tau: Two convergence points in Alzheimer's disease. *J. Alzheimer's Dis.* **2013**, *33* (Suppl. 1), S141–S144. [CrossRef] [PubMed]
97. Takashima, A. GSK-3 is essential in the pathogenesis of Alzheimer's disease. *J. Alzheimer's Dis.* **2006**, *9*, 309–317. [CrossRef]
98. Butterfield, D.A.; Poon, H.F.; St Clair, D.; Keller, J.N.; Pierce, W.M.; Klein, J.B.; Markesbery, W.R. Redox proteomics identification of oxidatively modified hippocampal proteins in mild cognitive impairment: Insights into the development of Alzheimer's disease. *Neurobiol. Dis.* **2006**, *22*, 223–232. [CrossRef] [PubMed]
99. Hall, E.C., 2nd; Lee, S.Y.; Mairuae, N.; Simmons, Z.; Connor, J.R. Expression of the HFE allelic variant H63D in SH-SY5Y cells affects tau phosphorylation at serine residues. *Neurobiol. Aging* **2011**, 32, 1409–1419. [CrossRef] [PubMed]
100. Chen, C.H.; Li, W.; Sultana, R.; You, M.H.; Kondo, A.; Shahpasand, K.; Kim, B.M.; Luo, M.L.; Nechama, M.; Lin, Y.M.; et al. Pin1 cysteine-113 oxidation inhibits its catalytic activity and cellular function in Alzheimer's disease. *Neurobiol. Dis.* **2015**, *76*, 13–23. [CrossRef] [PubMed]

101. Hall, E.C., 2nd; Lee, S.Y.; Simmons, Z.; Neely, E.B.; Nandar, W.; Connor, J.R. Prolyl-peptidyl isomerase, Pin1, phosphorylation is compromised in association with the expression of the HFE polymorphic allele, H63D. *Biochim. Biophys. Acta* **2010**, *1802*, 389–395. [CrossRef] [PubMed]
102. Min, S.H.; Cho, J.S.; Oh, J.H.; Shim, S.B.; Hwang, D.Y.; Lee, S.H.; Jee, S.W.; Lim, H.J.; Kim, M.Y.; Sheen, Y.Y.; et al. Tau and GSK3β dephosphorylations are required for regulating Pin1 phosphorylation. *Neurochem. Res.* **2005**, *30*, 955–961. [CrossRef] [PubMed]

2

Targeted Nutritional Intervention for Patients with Mild Cognitive Impairment: The Cognitive impAiRmEnt Study (CARES) Trial 1

Rebecca Power [1,*], John M. Nolan [1], Alfonso Prado-Cabrero [1], Robert Coen [2], Warren Roche [1], Tommy Power [1], Alan N. Howard [3] and Ríona Mulcahy [4,5,*]

1 Nutrition Research Centre Ireland, School of Health Sciences, Carriganore House, Waterford Institute of Technology West Campus, X91 K0EK Waterford, Ireland; jmnolan@wit.ie (J.M.N.); aprado-cabrero@wit.ie (A.P.-C.); warren.roche@ucdconnect.ie (W.R.); tbpower@wit.ie (T.P.)

2 Mercer's Institute for Research on Ageing, St. James's Hospital, D08 NHY1 Dublin, Ireland; rcoen@stjames.ie

3 Howard Foundation, 7 Marfleet Close, Great Shelford, Cambridge CB22 5LA, UK; alan.howard@howard-foundation.com

4 Age-Related Care Unit, Health Service Executive, University Hospital Waterford, Dunmore Road, X91 ER8E Waterford, Ireland

5 Royal College of Surgeons Ireland, 123 Stephen's Green, Saint Peter's, D02 YN77 Dublin, Ireland

* Correspondence: rpower@wit.ie (R.P.); drriona.mulcahy@hse.ie (R.M.)

Abstract: Omega-3 fatty acids (ω-3FAs), carotenoids, and vitamin E are important constituents of a healthy diet. While they are present in brain tissue, studies have shown that these key nutrients are depleted in individuals with mild cognitive impairment (MCI) in comparison to cognitively healthy individuals. Therefore, it is likely that these individuals will benefit from targeted nutritional intervention, given that poor nutrition is one of the many modifiable risk factors for MCI. Evidence to date suggests that these nutritional compounds can work independently to optimize the neurocognitive environment, primarily due to their antioxidant and anti-inflammatory properties. To date, however, no interventional studies have examined the potential synergistic effects of a combination of ω-3FAs, carotenoids and vitamin E on the cognitive function of patients with MCI. Individuals with clinically confirmed MCI consumed an ω-3FA plus carotenoid plus vitamin E formulation or placebo for 12 months. Cognitive performance was determined from tasks that assessed global cognition and episodic memory. Ω-3FAs, carotenoids, and vitamin E were measured in blood. Carotenoid concentrations were also measured in tissue (skin and retina). Individuals consuming the active intervention (n = 6; median [IQR] age 73.5 [69.5–80.5] years; 50% female) exhibited statistically significant improvements ($p < 0.05$, for all) in tissue carotenoid concentrations, and carotenoid and ω-3FA concentrations in blood. Trends in improvements in episodic memory and global cognition were also observed in this group. In contrast, the placebo group (n = 7; median [IQR] 72 (69.5–75.5) years; 89% female) remained unchanged or worsened for all measurements ($p > 0.05$). Despite a small sample size, this exploratory study is the first of its kind to identify trends in improved cognitive performance in individuals with MCI following supplementation with ω-3FAs, carotenoids, and vitamin E.

Keywords: mild cognitive impairment; nutrition; omega-3 fatty acids; antioxidant; carotenoids; vitamin E; cognition; episodic memory; older adults; ageing

1. Introduction

Given the growing social and economic burden of cognitive decline on society, emphasis is being placed on preventative strategies to delay the onset and reduce the risk of developing dementia, with particular focus on Alzheimer's disease (AD) as it is the most common form of dementia. Mild cognitive impairment (MCI) is often a transitional phase between the cognitive changes that one expects as one ages and very early dementia. It is recognized as a deterioration in cognitive function that exceeds what is anticipated for an individual based on their age and education level. Importantly, these changes in cognition are not significant enough to impact an individual's independence or ability to perform activities of daily living [1]. MCI is difficult to diagnose, and its prognosis is notoriously unpredictable. While the mortality rate is higher in MCI patients in comparison to cognitively healthy individuals [2], it is comparable to dementia mortality rates [3]. Although MCI is a risk factor for AD (with MCI to dementia conversion rates estimated at 3%–15% annually [4]), it is important to note that some individuals with the condition remain stable and do not progress while others may improve (i.e., revert to a cognitively intact state) upon follow-up assessment. This reversion phenomenon is an inherent feature of MCI and may be explained by the heterogeneity of the condition. While reverting from MCI to a cognitively intact state seems like a positive outcome, importantly, a number of studies have shown that these individuals are in fact at a greater risk of cognitive decline in the future [5,6]. Thus, due to the increased risk of mortality and progression to AD, MCI is an important public health concern.

Despite its complex and dynamic nature, MCI offers a window of opportunity to examine the potential of preventative strategies for modifying or delaying disease progression and improving cognitive outcomes. Given that many risk factors (e.g., vascular disease, diabetes, smoking, physical inactivity, social isolation [7–9]) for MCI are modifiable, shifting focus towards preventative strategies seems prudent. Specifically, there is a growing body of evidence to suggest that good nutrition is important for cognitive performance [10–14], and is associated with a reduced risk of MCI and AD [15–18]. Omega-3 fatty acids (ω-3FAs), xanthophyll carotenoids (oxygen-containing, plant-based pigments), and vitamin E are important constituents of a healthy diet. While these specific nutrients are present in brain tissue [19–21], studies have shown that they are depleted in individuals with MCI and AD in comparison to cognitively healthy individuals [22–24]. Therefore, it is likely that specific population groups (e.g., individuals with MCI, very early-stage AD or individuals with a low ω-3FA or carotenoid index) will benefit from targeted nutritional intervention. Indeed, observational [20,25–29] and interventional [30–33] evidence to date suggests that these nutritional compounds can work independently to optimize the neurocognitive environment [34], primarily due to their antioxidant and anti-inflammatory properties. Interestingly, previous exploratory work has shown that a combination of ω-3FAs and xanthophyll carotenoids can work synergistically to improve cognition in older women [35], and maintain function and quality of life in AD patients [36]. To date, however, no interventional studies have examined the potential synergistic effects of a combination of ω-3FAs, xanthophyll carotenoids, and vitamin E on the cognitive health and function of patients with MCI.

The present study, the Cognitive impAiRmEnt Study (CARES), was designed to investigate the impact of targeted nutritional intervention with ω-3FAs, xanthophyll carotenoids, and vitamin E on cognitive function among individuals with MCI. CARES was a parallel group, double-blind, placebo-controlled, randomized clinical trial studying two populations of interest. The first arm of the trial (CARES Trial 1) examined the impact of targeted nutritional supplementation on cognitive function in individuals with MCI, while the second arm of the trial (CARES Trial 2) investigated the impact of targeted nutritional supplementation on cognitive function in cognitively heathy older adults ($\geq$65 years). Herein, exploratory work from CARES Trial 1 is presented and discussed.

2. Materials and Methods

2.1. Study Design

CARES Trial 1 investigated the impact of 12-month supplementation with ω-3FAs, xanthophyll carotenoids, and vitamin E on cognitive function in individuals with MCI. Individuals were initially identified as potentially suitable for enrolment based on a medical assessment performed by consultant geriatricians and psychiatrists of old age in the South-East catchment area of Ireland. Both amnestic and non-amnestic MCI were included. MCI sub-type classification was not performed. A diagnosis of MCI was based on published criteria [37,38]. Specific eligibility criteria included: self or family member reported memory loss; fulfilled criteria for minimal cognitive impairment; functionally independent in activities of daily living; ≥65 years of age; no rapidly progressive or fluctuating symptoms of memory loss; no established diagnosis of early dementia (consumption of cognitive enhancement therapy such as cholinesterase inhibitors or N-methyl-D-aspartate receptor antagonists); no stroke disease (clinical stroke or stroke on CTB); no depression (under active review); no psychiatric illness (under active review of psychotropic medications); no glaucoma (acute angle); no consumption of carotenoid or fish/cod liver oil supplements; and no fish allergy.

2.2. MCI Screening

Prior to enrolment, all individuals who expressed an interest in participating in the trial completed a screening assessment to confirm eligibility. This included assessing cognitive function using the Repeatable Battery for the Assessment of Neurological Status (RBANS) Record Form A and the Montreal Cognitive Assessment (MoCA) version 7.1. Level of functional ability was assessed using the Bristol Activities of Daily Living Scale (BADLS) and the Alzheimer's Questionnaire (AQ). A brief description of each of these assessments is provided below. In the event where an informant was not present during the assessment, a family member or carer was contacted via telephone to complete functional ability assessments. In circumstances where no informant was available, the researcher administered the questionnaires to the patient. Individuals who fulfilled the criteria for each cognitive and functional assessment were invited to participate in the clinical trial. Individuals with borderline scores from the screening assessments were referred to a consensus panel (via email or conference call) consisting of one consultant geriatrician, one psychiatrist of old age and one clinical neuropsychologist for assessment of eligibility [39]. Eligible individuals were then invited to enroll into the study (see Figure 1). Prior to enrolment, written informed consent was obtained from all individuals. Ethical approval was granted by the Research Ethics Committees of the Waterford Institute of Technology and University Hospital Waterford in Waterford, Ireland in December 2015. CARES (trial registration number: ISRCTN10431469) adhered to the tenets of the Declaration of Helsinki and followed the full code of ethics with respect to recruitment, testing and general data protection regulations as set out by the European Parliament and Council of the European Union.

Eligible individuals were randomized to either the active intervention (now commercially known as Memory Health) containing 1 g of fish oil (of which 430 mg docosahexaenoic acid [DHA] and 90 mg eicosapentaenoic acid [EPA]), the xanthophyll carotenoids lutein (L) (10 mg), *meso*-zeaxanthin (MZ) (10 mg) and zeaxanthin (Z) (2 mg), and 15 mg of vitamin E (α-tocopherol), or placebo (sunflower oil) intervention group. These doses were provided via two oval-size capsules. Each capsule contained equal quantities of fish oil, carotenoids and vitamin E (see Table A1 in the Appendix A section). Carotenoid and vitamin E concentrations were manufactured by Industrial Orgánica (Monterrey, Mexico), while fish oil concentrations were manufactured by Epax (Ålesund, Norway; product number: EPAX1050TG/N non-tuna). The complete formula composition and the concentration of fatty acids of total lipids are available in the Appendix A section (Tables A1 and A2, respectively in Appendix A). Individuals were instructed to consume two capsules per day with a meal. Frequent phone calls were made to ensure compliance. Tablet counting was also performed at follow-up. Study visits were conducted at baseline and 12 months at a single site (Nutrition Research

Centre Ireland [NRCI]). Intervention randomization was performed by an electronic trial management system (Trial Controller) designed by our research group (NRCI). This administration system was also used to document patient information (name and contact details), support the organization and management of capsules required for the clinical trial and assist with the scheduling of study visits. The primary outcome measure of CARES Trial 1 was change in cognitive function. Secondary outcome measures included change in the following variables: macular pigment optical volume (MPOV); visual function; serum xanthophyll carotenoid concentrations (L, Z and MZ); serum vitamin E concentrations (α-tocopherol); and plasma ω-3FA concentrations (EPA and DHA). Development of AD was also recorded.

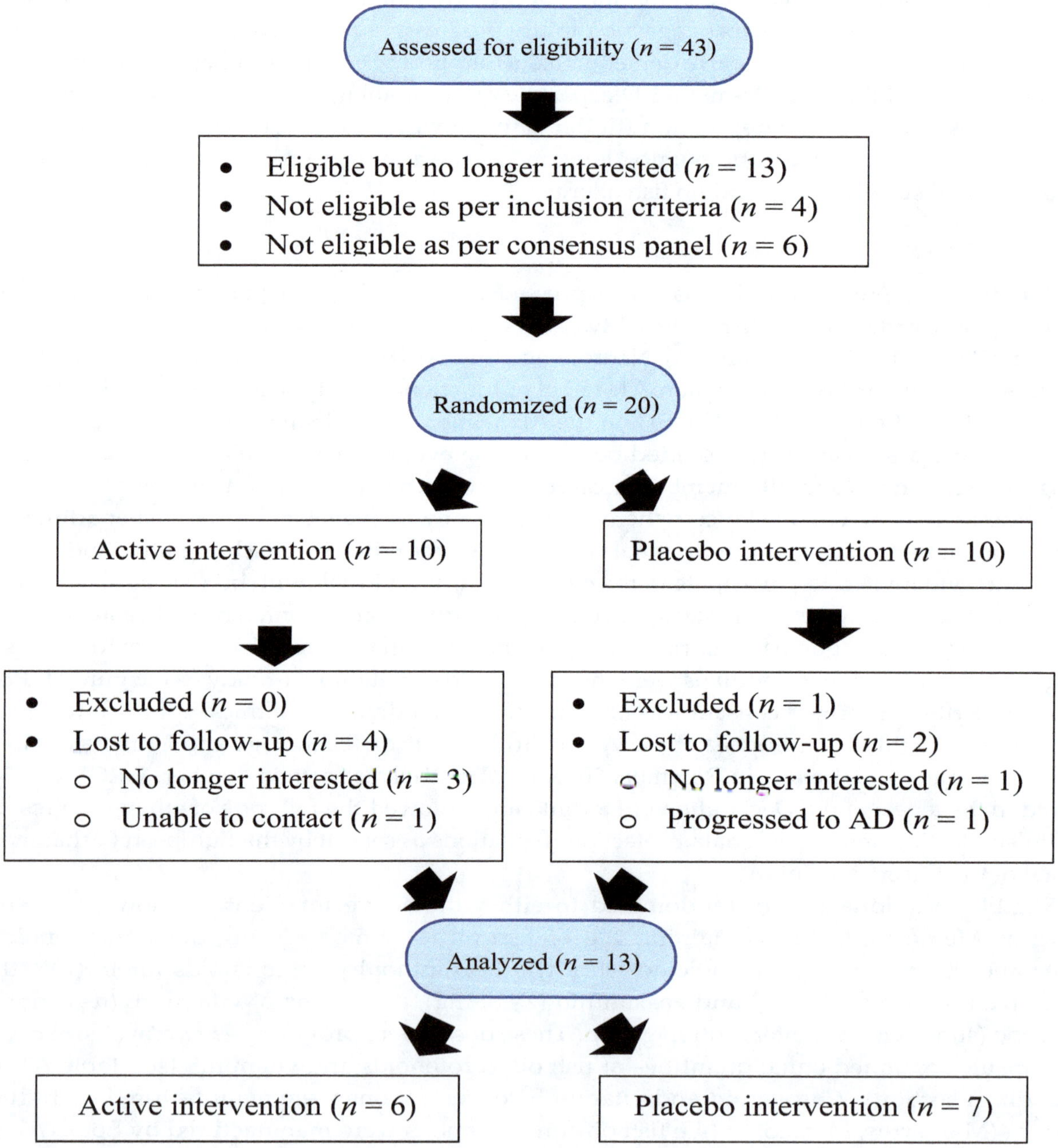

Figure 1. Consolidated Standards of Reporting Trials (CONSORT) flow diagram for the Cognitive impAiRmEnt Study (CARES) Trial 1.

2.3. *Assessing Cognitive Function*

2.3.1. Global Cognition

The MoCA was used at the screening stage to assess global cognition. It is a short (10-min) cognitive screening tool with high sensitivity and specificity for detecting MCI [40]. Thirty items assess multiple cognitive domains including visuospatial abilities, executive function, phonemic fluency, attention, immediate and delayed recall, language and orientation. The RBANS was used to measure global cognition at screening and at 12-month follow-up visits. Five domains of cognition (immediate memory, visuospatial ability, language, attention and delayed memory) were assessed using 12 sub-tests. A composite or "total index/scale score" was also computed. The RBANS takes approximately 30 min to administer and is a core diagnostic tool for detecting and characterizing dementia [41]. The RBANS yields index standard scores that are based on the raw scores of each subtest. RBANS index scores are metrically scaled, with a mean of 100 and a standard deviation (SD) of 15 for each age group. A score of 100 on any of these measures equates to the average performance of individuals of similar age. Scores of 85 and 115 correspond to 1 SD below and above the mean, respectively, while scores of 70 and 130 are 2 SDs below and above the mean. Approximately 68% of all examinees score between 85 and 115, circa 95% score in the 70 to 130 range, and nearly all examinees obtain scores between 55 and 143 [42]. In the present study, scores < 78 and between 19 and 25 for the RBANS and the MoCA, respectively, were desirable for enrolment.

2.3.2. Specific Cognitive Domains

Additional assessments of specific cognitive domains were performed using the Cambridge neuropsychological test automated battery (CANTAB) Connect Research Software (Cambridge Cognition, Cambridge, UK) [43]. This computerized software program was performed on an iPad and required a finger-operated response. This technology has been previously tested and validated in older adult population groups [44]. The CANTAB protocol [45] was followed in the administration of the test battery and was used to assess comprehension, executive function (working memory), attention (reaction time) and episodic memory at baseline and follow-up visits. Table 1 provides an overview of the CANTAB tests performed.

Spatial memory was also assessed at the screening stage only using the 4 mountains test (4MT) [46]. Using a delayed match-to-sample paradigm, memory for the topographical layout of 4 mountains within a computer-generated landscape is tested. Individuals were asked to recall the spatial configuration of a total of 15 sets of computer-generated landscapes from a shifted viewpoint, which is designed to reflect the role of the hippocampus in spatial cognition. This computerized assessment was performed on an iPad and required a finger operated response. The test takes approximately 20 min to complete and has been used previously among individuals with MCI and AD [47]. A study by Moodley and colleagues [48] suggested that a total 4MT score of ≤8 was associated with 100% sensitivity and 90% specificity for detecting early AD when tested in a UK population, and associated with 100% sensitivity and 50% specificity for detection of MCI and AD when tested in an Italian population group.

Table 1. Tasks performed in CARES to assess cognition using the Cambridge neuropsychological test automated battery (CANTAB).

Cognitive Domain	Task	Description	Outcome Measure	Desirable Score	Performance Ranges
Comprehension	MOT	Individuals must touch the flashing cross shown in different locations on the screen.	Latency (speed of response) Total correct Total errors	Lower Higher Lower	- 0–10 0–10
Executive function (working memory)	SWM	The aim of this test is that, by touching the boxes and using a process of elimination, the individual should find one 'token' in each of the boxes and use them to fill up an empty column on the right-hand side of the screen. The key task instruction is that the computer will never hide a token in the same coloured box, so once a token is found in a box the individual should not return to that box to look for another token.	Between errors Total errors Strategy	Lower Lower Lower	0–90 0–90 2–14
Reaction time	RTI	Individuals must press and hold down a touchscreen button at the bottom of the screen. Circles are presented at the top of the screen (one for simple mode, and five for the five-choice mode). In each case, a yellow spot will appear in one of the circles. Individuals must respond to the spot as quickly as they can by letting go of the button and touching inside the circle where the yellow spot appeared.	Simple reaction time Simple movement time Simple error score Five-choice reaction time Five-choice movement time Five-choice error score	Lower Lower Lower Lower Lower Lower	100–5100 100–5100 0–30 100–5100 100–5100 0–30
Episodic memory	PAL	Boxes are displayed on the screen and open one by one in a randomized order to reveal patterns hidden inside. The patterns are then displayed in the middle of the screen, one at a time, and the individual must touch the box where the pattern was originally located. If the individual makes an error, the patterns are re-presented to remind the individual of their locations.	First attempt memory score No. patterns reached Total errors adjusted	Higher Higher Lower	0–20 2–8 0–70

Performance ranges: the minimum and maximum possible score for each measure; Latency: the speed (milliseconds) of response to the stimulus; Total correct: the number of correct responses; Total errors: the distance between the center of the cross and the location touched; Between errors: the number of times the individual revisits a box in which a token has previously been found; Total errors: the number of times a box is selected that is certain not to contain a token and therefore should not have been visited by the individual; Strategy: for problems with six boxes or more. The number of distinct boxes used by the individual to begin a new search for a token, with the same problem; Simple reaction time: the duration between the onset of the stimulus and the time at which the individual released the button. Calculated for correct trials, where the stimulus could appear in one location only; Simple movement time: the time taken to touch the stimulus after the button has been released. Calculated for correct trials, where the stimulus could appear in one location only; Simple error score: the number of trials where the response status is any error (i.e., an inaccurate response, no response, or a premature response) for the assessment trial where stimuli appear on one location only. The error may be an inaccurate response, no response, or a premature response; Five-choice reaction time: the duration between the onset of the stimulus and the release of the button. Calculated for correct, assessed trials where the stimulus could appear in any of the five locations; Five-choice movement time: the time taken to touch the stimulus after the button has been released. Calculated for correct, assessed trials where the stimulus could appear in any of the five locations; Five-choice error score: the number of trials where the response status is any error (i.e., an inaccurate response, no response, or a premature response) for assessment trials where stimuli appear in any of five locations; First attempt memory score: the number of correct box choices that were made on the first attempt during assessment problems; No. patterns reached: the number of patterns on the last problem reached in the task; Total errors adjusted: the number of times the individual chose the incorrect box for a stimulus on assessment problems, plus an adjustment for the estimated no. errors they would have made on any problems, attempts and recalls they did not reach.

2.4. *Assessing Functional Ability*

The BADLS is an informant-based, 20-item questionnaire designed to measure the ability of an individual with dementia to carry out activities of daily living such as washing, dressing, preparing food and using transportation [49,50]. It is sensitive to changes in dementia and is regularly used as an outcome measure in clinical trials, where it is world leading as a dementia-specific measure. This outcome is among those recommended by a consensus recommendation of outcome scales for non-drug interventional studies in dementia [51]. A higher score was desirable for this assessment. The AQ is an informant-based screening tool used to detect cognitive impairment. It is regarded as a time efficient and sensitive measure for detecting MCI using structured interview-based questions. The AQ consists of 21 yes/no questions in a weighted format relevant to five different domains: memory, orientation, functional ability, visuospatial and language. The total score is calculated by summing the number of items with a "yes" response. Clinical symptoms known to be highly predictive of AD are given a greater weight in the total score. A score between 5 and 14 points was desirable for this assessment. The AQ has been previously validated and has shown high sensitivity and specificity for detecting MCI [52,53].

2.5. *Assessing Nutritional Status*

2.5.1. Macular Pigment

The carotenoids L, Z and MZ are preferentially concentrated in the central retina (macula lutea, which is part of the central nervous system) where they are collectively referred to as macular pigment (MP). MP was measured by dual-wavelength autofluorescence (AF) using the Spectralis HRA+OCT MultiColor (Heidelberg Engineering GmbH, Heidelberg, Germany). Pupillary dilation was performed prior to measurement and patient details were entered into the Heidelberg Eye Explorer (HEYEX version 1.7.1.0) software. Dual-wavelength AF in this device uses two excitation wavelengths; one that is well absorbed by MP (486 nm, blue) and one that is not (518 nm, green) [54]. The following acquisition parameters were used: high speed scan resolution, two seconds cyclic buffer size, internal fixation, 30-s movie and manual brightness control. Alignment, focus and illumination were first adjusted in infrared mode. Once the image was evenly illuminated, the laser mode was switched from infrared to blue plus green laser light AF. Using the HEYEX software, the movie images were aligned and averaged, and a MP density map was created. MPOV, calculated as MP average times the area under the curve out to 7° eccentricity [55], is reported here. This system has recently been validated by our research center [56].

2.5.2. Skin Carotenoid Score

Carotenoid concentrations were also measured using the Pharmanex® BioPhotonic Scanner (Salt Lake City, UT, USA). This scanner measures carotenoid levels in human tissue at the skin surface using optical signals (resonant Raman spectroscopy). These signals identify the unique molecular structure of carotenoids, allowing their measurement without interference by other molecular substances. The individual was asked to place a specific point (between the maximal and distal palmar creases, directly below the fifth finger) of their right hand (previously cleaned with hand sanitizer) in front of the scanner's low-energy blue light for 30 s. From this, a skin carotenoid score (SCS) was generated. This provided an indication of the individual's overall antioxidant levels. This was repeated twice more, and an average score was calculated. Based on this result, an individual's score can be classified into three ranges: 0–29,000 = low; 30,000–49,000 = normal; ≥50,000 = high. This technology is safe and has been previously validated [57].

2.6. *Biochemical Analysis of Serum Xanthophyll Carotenoids and Vitamin E*

2.6.1. Serum Extraction

Non-fasting blood samples were collected at each study visit by standard venipuncture techniques. SST II Advance blood collection tubes (8.5 mL) were inverted at least 5 times to ensure thorough mixing of the silica clot activator. The blood samples were left to clot for 30 min at room temperature and then centrifuged at room temperature at 725 g for 10 min in a Gruppe GC12 centrifuge (Desaga Sarstedt, UK) to separate the serum from the whole blood. Following centrifugation, serum was transferred to light-resistant microtubes and stored at circa −80 °C until extraction. Xanthophyll carotenoids and α-tocopherol were extracted from serum samples as previously described [58] and analyzed by high performance liquid chromatography (HPLC).

2.6.2. Lutein, Zeaxanthin and α-Tocopherol Quantification (Assay 1)

The chromatographic analysis of carotenoids and α-tocopherol was performed on an Agilent 1260 Series HPLC (Agilent Technologies Limited, Santa Clara, CA, USA) equipped with a quaternary pump, autosampler, thermostat column compartment and a photodiode array detector monitoring a wavelength of 450 nm for serum carotenoids and 292 nm for α-tocopherol and the internal standard (IS) α-tocopheryl acetate. The dried samples were reconstituted in 0.2 mL of Methanol:MTBE (9:1, *v*/*v*), vortexed at the lowest setting for 1 min and pipetted into HPLC vials containing 0.35 mL glass inserts. 0.1 milliliters of each sample was injected in a C30 carotenoid column (250 × 4.6 mm i.d., 3 μm; YMC Europe, Dinslaken, Germany) with a guard column of the same chemistry. HPLC mobile phase A consisted of methanol:MTBE:water (83:15:2, *v*/*v*), and mobile phase B consisted of methanol:MTBE:water (8:90:2, *v*/*v*), both with 0.1% BHT. At a flow rate of 1 mL min^{-1}, the gradient initiated at 5% solvent B and increased to 20% in the first 12 min, to 55% over the next 8 min and to 95% over the next 7 min. From 27–30 min, solvent B was held at 95%, and then resumed to initial setting within 3 min. Separations were carried out at 16 °C. Total Z from each sample was automatically collected by the fraction collector in amber eppendorfs.

2.6.3. *Meso*-Zeaxanthin Quantification (Assay 2)

Total Z collected in HPLC system 1 was dried in a vacuum centrifuge and re-suspended in 0.2 mL of hexane:isopropanol (90:10, *v*/*v*). 0.1 milliliters of the sample was analyzed on another Agilent 1260 Series HPLC system equipped with a Diode Array Detector, binary pump, degasser, thermostatically controlled column compartment and thermostatically controlled high-performance autosampler. The column used for the separation of the stereoisomers of Z was a Daicel Chiralpak IA-3 column, composed of amylose tris (3,5-dimethylphenylcarbamate) bonded to 3 mm silica gel (250 × 4.6 mm i.d.; Chiral Technologies Europe, Cedex, France). The column was protected with a guard column containing a guard cartridge with the same chemistry of the column. Isocratic elution was performed with hexane:isopropanol (90:10, *v*/*v*) at a flow rate of 0.5 mL min^{-1}. The column temperature was set at 20 °C.

Quantification was performed by constructing a calibration line for each xanthophyll carotenoid analyzed and for α-tocopherol. For each compound of interest, at least five calibration standards were quantified using a UV-Vis spectrophotometer UVmini-1240 (Shimadzu, Kyoto, Japan) with the appropriate molar extinction coefficient (see Appendix A Table A3). These calibrators were analyzed using HPLC system 1 in triplicate, whereas the calibrator of lowest concentration was injected 10 times in order to experimentally calculate the lower limit of quantification (LLOQ) for the compound. The upper limit of quantification (ULOQ) was allocated as the calibrator of highest concentration of each calibration curve analyzed in triplicate (see Appendix A Table A4). Where possible, subject samples that displayed an area in the HPLC chromatogram below the LLOQ or above the ULOQ were re-analyzed in order to obtain an area within the range of the calibration line. If after re-analysis the area of the analyte of interest remained below the LLOQ, this analyte in the subject was marked as 'below LLOQ'.

In order to determine the efficiency and precision of the xanthophyll carotenoid and α-tocopherol quantification methodology, analyte recovery analysis, precision analysis and trueness of sample recovery were performed. Details of this analysis are outlined in the Appendix A section.

2.7. Biochemical Analysis of Plasma Omega-3 Fatty Acids

2.7.1. Plasma Extraction

Lithium heparin blood collection tubes (6 mL) were inverted 8–10 times to ensure thorough mixing and were centrifuged at 4 °C at 3000 rpm for 20 min in a 3–18 K centrifuge (Sigma-Aldrich, St. Louis, MO, USA) to separate red blood cells and plasma. The time of blood collection and time of separation did not exceed 2 h. Following centrifugation, all samples were transferred to light-resistant microtubes and stored at circa −80 °C until the time of analysis. Plasma ω-3FA analysis was performed by gas chromatography (GC). Fatty acid methyl esters (FAME) were prepared as previously described [59]. Briefly, 50 µL of plasma were spiked with 20 µL of 2 mg/mL methyl tricosanoate (Larodan, Solna, Sweden) to assess FAME recovery and saponified with 2 mL of freshly prepared methanolic KOH 0.4 M during 10 min with gentle vortexing at room temperature. The samples were extracted three times with 2 mL of hexane and the combined extracts were dried in a vacuum centrifuge. The pellets were esterified with 2 mL of freshly prepared 5% methanolic sulfuric acid (*v*/*v*) at 80 °C for 30 min in a thermo-block. The FAME produced were extracted three times with 2 mL of hexane and dried in the vacuum centrifuge. The samples were resuspended in 0.4 mL of hexane containing 0.1 mg/mL of methyl heneicosanoate (Larodan) to assess the matrix effect and prepared for GC analysis. Methyl tricosanoate and methyl heneicosanoate 0.1 mg/mL were injected in triplicate to assess recovery and matrix effect, respectively.

2.7.2. DHA and EPA Quantification

FAME were quantified by GC coupled to flame ionization detector (GC-FID) with an Agilent 7890B Gas Chromatographer, using a Thermo 260M142P column (cyanopropylphenyl-based phase, 30 m length, 0.25 mm inner diameter and 0.25 µm film thickness). Nitrogen was used as the carrier gas with a flow rate of 1.5 mL/min and an electronic pressure control at 20.8 psi. Temperature ramp started at 140 °C and was held for 1 min, then followed by an increase of 6 °C min^{-1} until 210 °C, an increase of 2.5 °C min^{-1} until 230 °C and finally an increase of 10 °C min^{-1} until 240 °C, which was maintained for 5 min. Total run time was 26.7 min, with post run temperature at 50 °C and maximum temperature at 250 °C. FAME were identified by comparison with the authentic standard Mixture ME 1220 (Larodan). For FAME quantification, an RF was calculated as follows: a calibration line for methyl docosanoate, methyl undecanoate, methyl heptadecanoate, methyl heneicosanoate, methyl tricosanoate and EPA was prepared with a concentration range of 0.0025–0.5 mg/mL and analyzed in the GC. The resulting calibration lines were forced to pass through the origin of the axes, and the resulting slopes were averaged. The resulting RF was 0.1572 ± 0.0125.

2.8. Additional Biochemical Analysis

Serum and plasma samples were also collected to measure sodium, potassium, chloride, creatinine, total cholesterol, triglycerides, HDL, LDL, folate, vitamin B12, homocysteine, C-reactive protein, thyroid stimulating hormone, and free T4 (see Table A9 in the Appendix A section). One K2EDTA blood collection tube (3 mL) was also used for whole blood analysis. The sample was inverted 8–10 times and refrigerated at 4 °C until sample collection (2–24 h later). This additional analysis was performed by an accredited medical testing service provider (Eurofins Biomnis, Dublin, Ireland).

2.9. Demographic, Health and Lifestyle Data

Demographic, health and lifestyle data, medical history and medication use were recorded via questionnaire. Height and weight measurements were recorded to calculate body mass index (BMI) (kg/m^2). Smoking status was classified into never (smoked < 100 cigarettes in lifetime), past (smoked ≥ 100 cigarettes in lifetime and none in the past year) or current (smoked ≥ 100 cigarettes in lifetime and at least 1 cigarette in the last year) smoker. Alcohol consumption was measured in unit intake per week. One unit of alcohol (10 mL) was the equivalent to one of the following: a single measure of spirits (ABV 37.5%); half a pint of average-strength (4%) lager; two-thirds of a 125 mL glass of average-strength (12%) wine; half a 175 mL glass of average-strength (12%) wine; a third of a 250 mL glass of average-strength (12%) wine. Color fundus photographs were taken to assess the presence of ocular pathology (Zeiss Visucam 200, Carl Zeiss Meditec AG, Jena, Germany).

2.10. Statistical Analysis

The statistical package IBM SPSS version 25 was used and the 5% significance level applied for all analyses. Given that data were not normally distributed, the small sample size and the presence of ranked data, a non-parametric approach was taken. Results were expressed as median (inter quartile range [IQR]) for all variables. Between-group differences (i.e., active versus placebo) were analyzed using Mann–Whitney U, Wilcoxon Signed Rank or Chi-square tests, as appropriate. The Mann–Whitney U test was also used to examine the significance of change in nutrition variables over time between active and placebo intervention groups. Significance values were not computed to examine change in cognition or vision variables over time between both groups due to a lack of statistical power and the small magnitude of change over time observed for these variables. As an alternative, the average percentage change per subject was reported. Of note, percentage change could not be calculated for some variables (e.g., episodic memory) as baseline values were recorded as 0. Thus, the average change per subject was reported.

3. Results

3.1. Baseline Results

Table 2 presents the baseline demographic, health and lifestyle data for active and placebo intervention groups. Table 3 presents the baseline cognitive function and functional ability for active and placebo intervention groups. Baseline variables were statistically comparable between both groups, with the exception of the number of between errors (p = 0.006) and total errors (p = 0.012) made at stage 8 of the SWM tasks, which were significantly higher in the active group. Additionally, creatinine levels were significantly higher in the active group at baseline (p = 0.008), but were within normal ranges (see Table A9 in the Appendix A section). No comprehension or sensorimotor difficulties were observed during the CANTAB assessment (see Materials and Methods section), as the motor screening task (MOT) latency assessment was completed by all individuals at baseline and follow-up. No adverse events were reported by individuals in the active or placebo intervention groups during the trial.

3.2. Observed Change in Nutritional Status

Table 4 summarizes the observed change in nutrition variables for both groups following the 12-month intervention period. Figure 2A–C illustrate the observed changes in MPOV, serum L concentrations and plasma DHA concentrations, respectively. Individuals in the active intervention group exhibited statistically significant improvements in MPOV (62% improvement versus 2% decline for active and placebo groups, respectively; p = 0.001) and SCS (79% improvement versus 2% improvement for active and placebo groups, respectively; p = 0.014) in comparison to individuals in the placebo group. In terms of biochemical response, individuals in the active intervention group exhibited statistically significant improvements in serum carotenoid concentrations of L and MZ, as well as statistically significant improvements in plasma concentrations of DHA (p < 0.05, for all) in comparison to individuals receiving placebo. Serum Z and plasma EPA levels increased in both groups; however, results were not statistically significant (p > 0.05, for all). A mixed response to vitamin E supplementation was observed in blood, where levels decreased (−4%) over 12 months in the active intervention group and increased slightly (+1%) in the placebo group.

3.3. Observed Change in Global Cognition

Table 5 shows trends in improvements (ranging from 6% to 18%) in global cognition (as per the RBANS assessment tool) in the active intervention group after 12 months. Specifically, trends in improvements were observed in the immediate memory, attention and delayed memory domains, as well as the total scale score. minor declines were denoted in the visuospatial and language domains (both by 1%). Global cognition results were mixed in the placebo group. Immediate memory, visuospatial and attention domains of the RBANS remained unchanged while language, delayed memory and total scale scores improved after 12 months. Further analysis of the RBANS delayed memory domain in the placebo group suggested that the observed improvement (i.e., a 14% improvement) was driven by one subject. When this subject was removed, an improvement of 4% was denoted. As an example, Figure 3 shows the change in individual scores recorded for the immediate memory domain of the RBANS in both groups.

Table 2. Baseline demographic, health and lifestyle data of active and placebo intervention groups.

Variable	Active (n = 10) Median (IQR)	Placebo (n = 9) Median (IQR)	Sig.
Demographic data			
Age (years)	73.5 (69.5–80.5)	72.0 (69.5–75.5)	0.549
Sex ([n]; [% female])	5 (50.0%)	8 (88.9%)	0.069
Education (years)	17.5 (15.5–21.0)	15.0 (15.0–16.5)	0.095
Health and lifestyle data			
Medications	6.0 (3.0–8.3)	5.0 (2.0–5.5)	0.133
Exercise (min/week)	217.0 (0–326.3)	210.0 (45.0–375.0)	0.720
Smoking ([n]; [%])			0.463
Never	5 (50%)	6 (66.7%)	
Past	5 (50%)	3 (33.3%)	
Current	0	0	
Alcohol consumption ([n]; [%])			0.473
0 units	5 (50.0%)	4 (44.4%)	
1 unit	3 (30.0%)	2 (22.2%)	
2–5 units	0	2 (22.2%)	
6–10 units	2 (20.0%)	1 (11.2%)	
>10 units	0	0	
BMI (kg/m^2)	26.3 (25.8–30.7)	26.7 (25.1–27.8)	0.720
Nutritional status			
MPOV	6987 (2969–9080)	4682 (3740–7311)	0.497
SCS	4.20 (3.75–5.60)	4.65 (4.23–5.40)	0.541
Serum L	1.72 (1.03–2.21)	1.32 (1.04–1.86)	0.815
Serum Z	1.34 (1.06–1.55)	2.03 (1.14–2.12)	0.236
Serum MZ	2.50 (1.85–3.50)	2.15 (1.48–3.78)	0.743
Serum vitamin E	11.0 (8.10–15.55)	8.65 (7.33–11.80)	0.236
Plasma DHA	0.80 (0.55–5.10)	0.45 (0.30–1.10)	0.236
Plasma EPA	1.52 (0.97–2.15)	1.08 (0.95–1.84)	0.541
Folate	12.10 (10.85–14.20)	11.90 (10.88–13.78)	0.888
Vitamin B_{12}	14.10 (12.55–15.15)	12.90 (12.48–13.38)	0.236

Data displayed are median (inter quartile range) for numeric data and actual number and percentages for categorical data; Education: age (years) completed formal education; Medications: the number of prescribed medications consumed; Alcohol consumption: units/week: MPOV: a volume of macular pigment calculated as macular pigment average times the area under the curve out to 7° eccentricity (measured using the Heidelberg Spectralis®). SCS: skin carotenoid score (measured using the Pharmanex BioPhotonic Scanner). Serum lutein, zeaxanthin, *meso*-zeaxanthin and vitamin E concentrations are expressed in µmol/L; Plasma docosahexaenoic acid and eicosapentaenoic acid concentrations expressed in µmol/L; Serum folate concentrations expressed in ng/mL; Serum vitamin B_{12} concentrations expressed in pg/mL. Serum carotenoid and vitamin E data were not available for two individuals in the active intervention and one individual in the placebo group. Plasma DHA and EPA were not available for one individual in the active intervention and one individual in the placebo group.

Table 3. Baseline cognitive function and functional ability data of active and placebo intervention groups.

Variable	Active (*n* = 10) Median (IQR)	Placebo (*n* = 9) Median (IQR)	Sig.
Global cognition			
MoCA	21.0 (18.8–24.0)	21.0 (19.0–24.0)	0.842
RBANS immediate memory	78.0 (64.0–82.5)	85.0 (72.5–98.5)	0.156
RBANS visuospatial	101.0 (92.0–109.0)	100.0 (91.5–110.5)	0.842
RBANS language	89.0 (84.5–93.0)	88.0 (82.0–92.0)	0.661
RBANS attention	81.0 (71.0–98.5)	79.0 (77.0–89.5)	0.905
RBANS delayed memory	75.0 (47.0–87.5)	71.0 (58.0–87.0)	<0.999
RBANS total scale	78.0 (75.0–84.0)	82.0 (73.5–85.0)	0.497
4 mountains test	6.5 (6.0–7.8)	7.0 (5.5–7.5)	0.905
Comprehension			
Latency	1165.9 (812.9–1322.2)	1152.8 (991.75–1301.5)	0.842
Total errors	0	0	0.720
Working memory			
Between errors			
Stage 4	1.0 (0.8–2.0)	(1.0–2.5)	0.497
Stage 6	6.0 (4.3–7.5)	6.0 (6.0–7.0)	0.497
Stage 8	16.0 (15.0–17.0)	12.5 (11.0–14.0)	0.006
All stages	21.5 (21.0–26.5)	20.0 (18.0–22.5)	0.182
Total errors			
Stage 4	(0.8–2.0)	2.0 (1.0–2.5)	0.447
Stage 6	6.0 (4.3–7.5)	6.0 (6.0–7.0)	0.497
Stage 8	16.5 (15.0–17.3)	13.0 (11.0–14.8)	0.012
All stages	21.5 (21.0–28.3)	22.0 (18.0–22.5)	0.447
Strategy	10.0 (9.0–11.3)	9.0 (8.5–10.0)	0.315
Reaction time			
Simple reaction time	382.4 (370.7–463.6)	372.9 (354.9–411.5)	0.356
Simple movement time	296.5 (249.6–336.6)	318.9 (277.3–352.3)	0.497
Simple error score	2.0 (0.8–3.5)	1.0 (0–3.0)	0.400
Five-choice reaction time	458.1 (415.7–510.3)	435.1 (406.5–485.5)	0.549
Five-choice movement time	310.3 (286.5–367.0)	313.0 (294.2–335.4)	<0.999
Five-choice error score	0.5 (0–1.3)	1.0 (0–2.0)	0.549
Episodic memory			
First attempt memory score	4.0 (3.5–5.5)	4.0 (2.5–6.5)	0.905
No. patterns reached	6.0 (4.0–6.5)	6.0 (4.0–6.0)	0.549
Total errors adjusted stage 2	0 (0–0.3)	0 (0–0.5)	0.905
Total errors adjusted stage 4	6.0 (2.3–8.8)	6.0 (0.5–9.5)	0.780
Total errors adjusted stage 6	18.5 (12.3–20.0)	20.0 (14.5–20.0)	<0.999
Total errors adjusted stage 8	28.0 (25.3–28.0)	28.0 (28.0–28.0)	0.720
Total errors adjusted all stages	52.5 (42.8–59.0)	48.0 (45.0–58.0)	0.780
Functional ability			
BADLS	20.0 (15.5–20.0)	20.0 (20.0–20.0)	0.243
AQ	8.0 (4.8–13.8)	5.0 (2.5–8.0)	0.113

Data displayed are median (inter quartile range); MoCA: Montreal Cognitive Assessment; RBANS: Repeatable Battery for the Assessment of Neuropsychological Status; BADLS: Bristol Activities of Daily Living Scale; AQ: Alzheimer's Questionnaire.

Table 4. Change in nutritional status over 12 months between active and placebo intervention groups.

Variable	Active Intervention					Placebo Intervention					
	n	Baseline Median (IQR)	12 Months Median (IQR)	%Δ	Outcome	*n*	Baseline Median (IQR)	12 Months (Median (IQR)	%Δ	Outcome	Sig.
Nutrition											
MPOV	6	6987 (2947–9080)	10,363 (5488–12,906)	+62	Improved	7	4682 (3838–7264)	4300 (3827–7277)	−2	Declined	**0.001**
SCS	6	27,250 (18,250–36,705)	37,000 (30,000–60,250)	+79	Improved	7	17,000 (15,000–35,000)	21,000 (14,000–38,000)	+2	Improved	**0.014**
Serum L	5	0.152 (0.107–0.217)	0.562 (0.339–1.388)	+421	Improved	7	0.104 (0.067–0.188)	0.133 (0.067–0.168)	+5	Improved	**0.003**
Serum Z	5	0.059 (0.036–0.078)	0.075 (0.056–0.125)	+58	Improved	7	0.037 (0.035–0.051)	0.042 (0.037–0.049)	+1	Improved	0.247
Serum MZ	5	0	0.068 (0.031–0.234)	-	Improved	7	0	0	0	Unchanged	**0.003**
Serum vit. E	5	23.988 (20.346–30.264)	23.015 (21.010–31.802)	−4	Declined	7	24.426 (22.007–26.274)	24.704 (23.074–26.093)	+1	Improved	>0.999
Plasma DHA	5	235.730 (153.115–258.315)	291.910 (262.170–406.650)	+59	Improved	7	200.480 (165.230–212.230)	234.630 (204.150–267.680)	+17	Improved	**0.048**
Plasma EPA	5	164.500 (90.000–199.070)	178.410 (178.410–205.425)	+6	Improved	7	129.530 (127.550–146.620)	147.020 (108.080–201.850)	+13	Improved	0.639

Data displayed are median (inter quartile range); %Δ: average percentage change per subject; Sig.: Level of significance of the observed change over time between active and placebo intervention groups; MPOV, a volume of macular pigment calculated as macular pigment average times the area under the curve out to 7° eccentricity (measured using the Heidelberg Spectralis®); SCS: skin carotenoid score (obtained using the Pharmanex BioPhotonic Scanner); Serum lutein, zeaxanthin, *meso*-zeaxanthin and vitamin E concentrations are expressed in μmol/L; Plasma docosahexaenoic acid and eicosapentaenoic acid concentrations expressed in μmol/L.

Table 5. Average percentage change in global cognition over 12 months between active and placebo intervention groups.

Variable	Active Intervention					Placebo Intervention				
	n	Baseline Median (IQR)	12 Months Median (IQR)	%Δ	Outcome	*n*	Baseline Median (IQR)	12 Months (Median (IQR)	%Δ	Outcome
Global cognition (RBANS)										
Immediate memory	6	78.0 (73.3–82.5)	91.0 (81.3–100.8)	+18	Improved	7	94.0 (85.0–100.0)	90.0 (81.0–103.0)	0	Unchanged
Visuospatial	6	107.0 (101.5–110.8)	105.0 (101.5–112.0)	−1	Declined	7	96.0 (87.0–109.0)	96.0 (84.0–109.0)	0	Unchanged
Language	6	91.0 (88.0–96.0)	89.0 (88.0–93.0)	−1	Declined	7	88.0 (82.0–92.0)	92.0 (72.0–105.0)	+2	Improved
Attention	6	84.5 (68.0–103.8)	91.0 (79.0–100.0)	+7	Improved	7	79.0 (75.0–85.0)	79.0 (79.0–94.0)	0	Unchanged
Delayed memory	6	85.0 (63.3–96.5)	86.0 (63.0–106.3)	+12	Improved	7	71.0 (60.0–93.0)	90.0 (78.0–98.0)	+14	Improved
Total scale	6	82.0 (78.0–91.5)	87.0 (82.3–99.3)	+6	Improved	7	82.5 (76.3–87.3)	88.5 (78.5–91.3)	+3	Improved

Data displayed are median (inter quartile range); %Δ: average percentage change per subject; RBANS: Repeatable Battery for the Assessment of Neuropsychological Status.

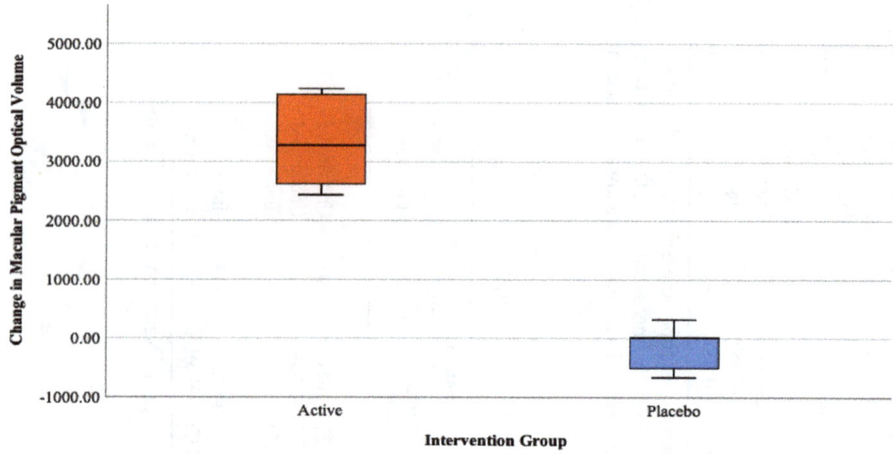

(**A**)

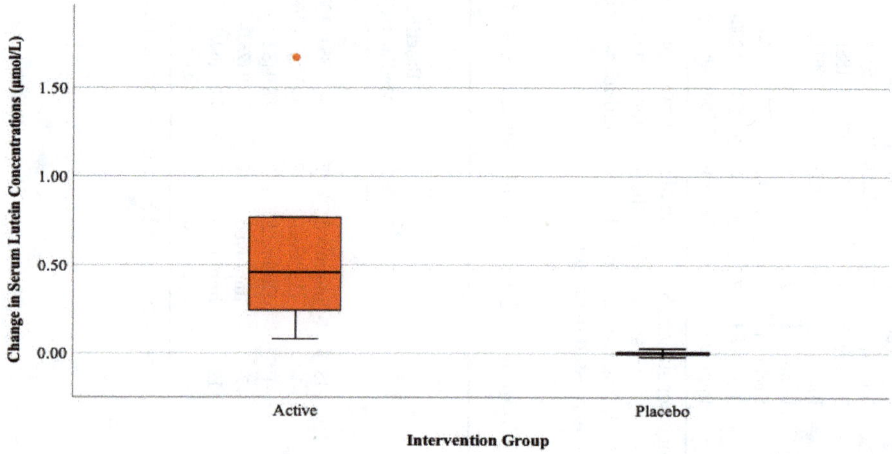

(**B**)

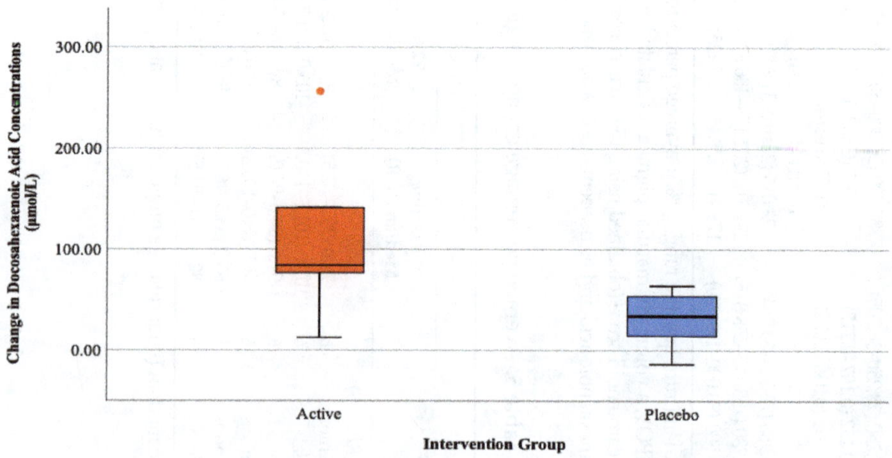

(**C**)

Figure 2. (**A**) Box plots illustrating change in MPOV over 12 months for active and placebo intervention groups. (**B**) Box plot illustrating change in serum lutein over 12 months for active and placebo intervention groups. (**C**) Box plot illustrating change in plasma DHA over 12 months for active and placebo intervention groups.

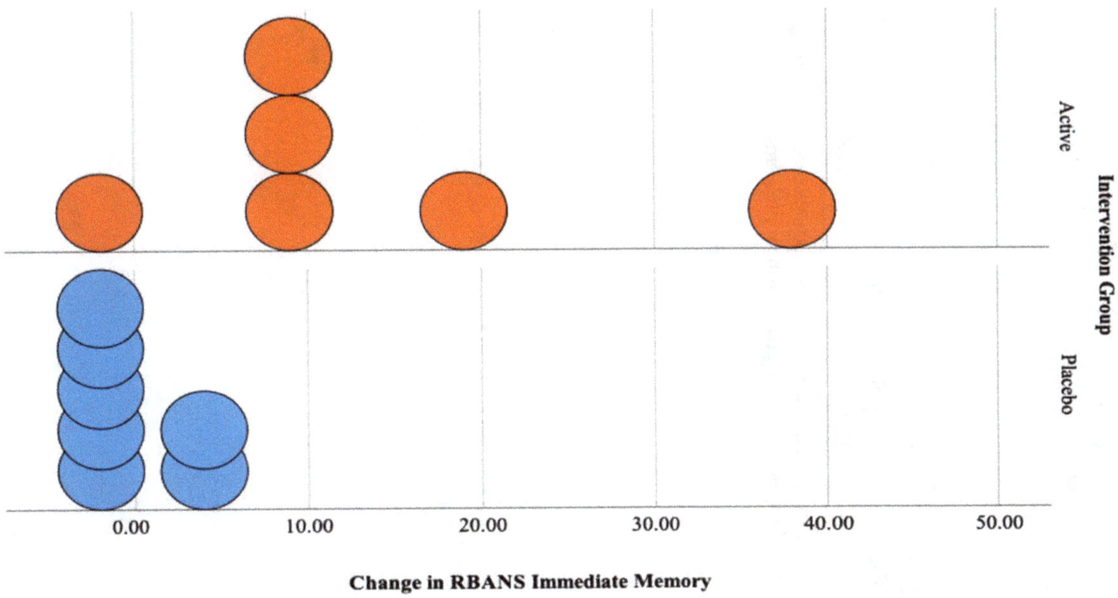

Figure 3. Dot plots illustrating change in individual scores recorded for the immediate memory domain of the RBANS for active and placebo intervention groups.

3.4. *Observed Change in Episodic Memory*

Table 6 shows trends in improvements in episodic memory in the active intervention group where individuals consuming the nutritional supplement recorded fewer errors at the latter (and more challenging) stages of the paired associated learning (PAL) task in comparison to individuals in the placebo group where scores either remained unchanged or worsened. A minimal improvement (+1%) in the first attempt memory score was also observed among individuals in the active group while individuals in the placebo group declined slightly (by 1%).

3.5. *Observed Change in Working Memory*

Table 7 summaries the observed changes in working memory following the 12-month intervention period. For both groups, all tasks that assessed working memory either remained unchanged or worsened over the 12-month study period, with the exception of the number of between and total errors made at stage 8 which improved slightly (by two points each) among individuals in the active intervention group and the number of total errors made at stage 4 of the SWM task, which improved slightly (by one point) among individuals in the placebo group. Of note, individuals in the placebo group recorded significantly fewer between and total errors at stage 8 of the SWM tasks at baseline.

3.6. *Observed Change in Reaction Time*

Table 7 also shows the observed changes in reaction time following the 12-month intervention period. Results for reaction times were also mixed for both groups. Trends in improvements in simple reaction time were observed in both groups (by an average of 2 milliseconds [ms]). In addition, trends in improvements in five-choice reaction time (by an average of 20 ms) were observed among individuals in the active intervention group while declines (by an average of 12 ms) were recorded among individuals receiving placebo. Both simple and five-choice movement times declined in both groups (by an average of 13 ms and 29 ms for active and placebo groups, respectively) with overall trends suggesting a lesser decline among individuals in the active intervention group. Finally, error scores for all reaction time assessments remained unchanged with the exception of the number of errors made during the five-choice reaction time assessment, which declined (by one point) in the placebo group (see Table 7).

Table 6. Average change per subject in episodic memory, working memory and reaction time over 12 months between active and placebo intervention groups.

Variable	Active Intervention					Placebo Intervention			
	n	Baseline Median (IQR)	12 Months Median (IQR)	Δ	Outcome	Baseline Median (IQR)	12 Months (Median (IQR)	Δ	Outcome
Episodic memory (PAL)									
First attempt memory score	6	4.5 (3.3–7.5)	6.5 (2.0–9.8)	+1	Improved	4.0 (3.0–6.0)	3.0 (2.0–6.0)	−1	Declined
Total errors adjusted stage 2	6	0 (0–1.3)	0 (0)	−1	Improved	0 (0)	0 (0–2.0)	−1	Improved
Total errors adjusted stage 4	6	6.0 (2.3–3.0)	7.5 (2.0–11.8)	+2	Declined	6.0 (0–10.0)	8.0 (4.0–10.0)	+2	Declined
Total errors adjusted stage 6	6	15.0 (7.0–18.5)	14.0 (5.8–20.0)	−1	Improved	20.0 (15.0–20.0)	20.0 (15.0–20.0)	0	Unchanged
Total errors adjusted stage 8	6	28.0 (15.3–28.0)	20.5 (8.8–28.0)	−4	Improved	28.0 (28.0–28.0)	28.0 (28.0–28.0)	0	Unchanged
Total errors adjusted all stages	6	54.5 (24.8–54.5)	39.5 (17.8–59.8)	−4	Improved	48.0 (47.0–58.0)	51.0 (48.0–58.0)	+2	Declined

Data displayed are median (inter quartile range); Δ: average change per subject; PAL: paired associated learning; First attempt memory score: the number of correct box choices that were made on the first attempt during assessment problems; Total errors adjusted: the number of times the individual chose the incorrect box for a stimulus on assessment problems, plus an adjustment for the estimated no. errors they would have made on any problems, attempts and recalls they did not reach.

Table 7. Average change per subject in working memory and reaction time over 12 months between active and placebo intervention groups.

Variable	Active Intervention					Placebo Intervention				
	n	Baseline Median (IQR)	12 Months Median (IQR)	Δ	Outcome	*n*	Baseline Median (IQR)	12 Months (Median (IQR)	Δ	Outcome
Working memory (SWM)										
Between errors stage 4	6	1.0 (0.8–2.0)	1.5 (0.8–2.5)	+1	Declined	7	2.0 (1.0–3.0)	2.0 (0–3.0)	0	Unchanged
Between errors stage 6	6	5.5 (2.0–7.5)	6.0 (5.5–8.8)	+2	Declined	7	6.0 (6.0–7.0)	9.0 (6.0–10.0)	+1	Declined
Between errors stage 8	5	17.0 (15.0–17.0)	16.0 (10.0–18.0)	−2	Improved	5	12.0 (10.5–15.5)	13.0 (12.5–18.0)	+2	Declined
Between errors all stages	5	21.0 (20.0–24.0)	26.0 (15.5–27.0)	−2	Improved	5	20.0 (19.0–23.5)	21.0 (20.0–24.0)	+2	Declined
Total errors stage 4	6	1.0 (0.8–2.0)	1.5 (0.8–2.5)	+1	Declined	7	2.0 (1.0–3.0)	2.0 (0–3.0)	−1	Improved
Total errors stage 6	6	5.5 (2.0–7.5)	6.0 (5.5–9.0)	+2	Declined	7	6.0 (6.0–7.0)	10.0 (6.0–11.0)	+2	Declined
Total errors stage 8	5	17.0 (15.0–18.5)	16.0 (10.5–19.0)	−2	Improved	5	12.0 (10.5–16.5)	15.0 (12.5–18.0)	+2	Declined
Total errors all stages	5	21.0 (20.0–25.5)	26.0 (16.0–28.0)	0	Unchanged	5	22.0 (13.5–22.8)	22.5 (20.5–24.3)	+4	Declined
Strategy	5	10.0 (8.5–12.0)	10.0 (8.5–11.5)	0	Unchanged	5	9.0 (6.8–10.5)	9.0 (9.0–10.5)	+1	Declined
Attention (RTI)										
Simple reaction time	6	381.1 (364.4–463.6)	397.3 (342.8–453.9)	−2	Improved	7	389.7 (340.4–430.6)	369.2 (355.3–448.7)	−2	Improved
Simple movement time	6	302.9 (181.9–432.5)	316.0 (244.7–433.5)	+13	Declined	7	318.9 (274.6–337.7)	344.2 (246.3–449.8)	+29	Declined
Simple error score	6	1.5 (0–2.8)	1.0 (0–2.5)	0	Unchanged	7	1.0 (0–3.0)	1.0 (1.0–3.0)	0	Unchanged
Five-choice reaction time	6	483.7 (420.5–519.5)	445.7 (429.1–477.4)	−20	Improved	7	435.1 (391.2–479.0)	450.7 (393.4–488.3)	+12	Declined
Five-choice movement time	6	316.6 (279.2–443.8)	333.2 (261.8–417.4)	+13	Declined	7	310.5 (289.1–320.0)	332.8 (323.3–416.4)	+29	Declined
Five-choice error score	6	1.0 (0–2.3)	0 (0–3.3)	0	Unchanged	7	1.0 (0–2.0)	1.0 (0–3.0)	+1	Declined

Data displayed are median (inter quartile range); Δ: average change per subject. SWM: spatial working memory; Between errors: the number of times the individual revisits a box in which a token has previously been found; Total errors: the number of times a box is selected that is certain not to contain a token and therefore should not have been visited by the individual; Strategy: for problems with six boxes or more. The number of distinct boxes used by the individual to begin a new search for a token, with the same problem; RTI: reaction time; Simple reaction time: the duration between the onset of the stimulus and the time at which the individual released the button. Calculated for correct trials, where the stimulus could appear in one location only; Simple movement time: the time taken to touch the stimulus after the button has been released. Calculated for correct trials, where the stimulus could appear in one location only; Simple error score: the number of trials where the response status is any error (i.e., an inaccurate response, no response, or a premature response) for the assessment trial where stimuli appear on one location only. The error may be an inaccurate response, no response, or a premature response; Five-choice reaction time: the duration between the onset of the stimulus and the release of the button. Calculated for correct, assessed trials where the stimulus could appear in any of the five locations; Five-choice movement time: the time taken to touch the stimulus after the button has been released. Calculated for correct, assessed trials where the stimulus could appear in any of the five locations; Five-choice error score: the number of trials where the response status is any error (i.e., an inaccurate response, no response, or a premature response) for assessment trials where stimuli appear in any of five locations.

4. Discussion

Given that ω-3FAs, xanthophyll carotenoids, and vitamin E are present in brain tissue, and given their ability to attenuate mechanisms involved in the pathogenesis of AD (namely oxidative stress and neuro-inflammation), it is likely that they play an important neuroprotective role by maintaining and optimizing cognition and reducing the risk of cognitive decline. Importantly, previous studies have shown that cognitively impaired individuals are deficient in these key nutritional compounds in comparison to cognitively healthy individuals. Therefore, it is likely that specific population groups, such as individuals with MCI, will benefit from nutritional intervention. CARES Trial 1 was a parallel group, double-blind, placebo-controlled, randomized clinical trial designed to examine the effect of targeted nutritional intervention on cognitive performance among individuals with MCI. Following 12-month supplementation with a combination of ω-3FAs (DHA and EPA), xanthophyll carotenoids (L, Z and MZ), and vitamin E (α-tocopherol), this exploratory study identified trends in improved performance in episodic memory, immediate memory, attention and delayed memory among individuals with clinically confirmed MCI.

4.1. *Significance and Interpretation of Findings*

This exploratory study is the first of its kind to examine the impact of a combination of ω-3FAs, xanthophyll carotenoids, and vitamin E on cognition in individuals with MCI. Previous studies have examined the effects of varying combinations of nutritional compounds on the cognitive health of individuals with MCI (see [60] for a review). While many of the studies included in the review performed by Solfrizzi and colleagues [60] observed reductions in brain atrophy in individuals with MCI, no positive effects on cognition were found, with the exception of [61] where improvements in the dementia rating scale were reported following 6-month consumption of a combination of vitamin B_{12}, α-tocopherol, s-adenosylmethionine, N-acetylcysteine and acetyl-L-carnitine. Interestingly, supplementation with ω-3FAs alone have yielded positive results among individuals with MCI. A meta-analysis of 15 interventional trials suggested a benefit of DHA supplementation in terms of improving episodic memory among mildly impaired individuals [62]. Other studies have also reported benefits in memory (episodic, short-term, working, and immediate verbal), processing speed, and attention [63–65] following ω-3FA supplementation. In contrast, supplementation with vitamin E is less promising as, currently, no improvements in cognitive performance have been observed in MCI samples [66] and none have examined the impact of xanthophyll carotenoid supplementation alone on cognition in individuals with MCI. Importantly, to date, none have examined the potential synergistic effect of the ω-3FAs DHA and EPA, the xanthophylls L, Z and MZ, and vitamin E in the α-tocopherol form on cognitive function among individuals with MCI.

In the present exploratory study, individuals with MCI in the active intervention group responded positively to 12-month nutritional supplementation in terms of statistically significant improvements in tissue carotenoid concentrations, as well as statistically significant increases in blood concentrations of serum L, serum MZ and plasma DHA. Of note, individuals in the active intervention group responded poorly to vitamin E (α-tocopherol) supplementation. Reasons underlying the poor vitamin E response following supplementation remain unclear. While in accordance with international recommended dietary allowances (RDAs) [67,68], it is possible that the daily dosage of vitamin E (i.e., 15 mg) used in the present study was too low (in comparison to other interventional studies (e.g., [69,70]) to have any meaningful effect.

Most of the positive outcomes identified in the present exploratory study relate to performance in tasks assessing memory. Memory deficits, which involve difficulties with the encoding, storage and retrieval of information, are commonplace among individuals with MCI. Specifically, impairment in episodic memory has been frequently documented in MCI and is an inherent feature of amnestic MCI [71,72]. Episodic memory refers to the ability to learn, store and retrieve information about experiences that occurred at a particular time and place (e.g., remembering where you parked your car in a multi-story carpark, remembering the details of a family event attended in the past few weeks [73]).

Encoding, retention and retrieval difficulties are likely due to changes in the relevant neurocircuitry including frontal, temporal and medial temporal lobe regions, the hippocampus and adjacent cortical areas [74,75].

4.2. Neurobiological Mechanisms

The brain is a lipid-dense organ containing large amounts of ω-3FAs (and DHA in particular) [76]. Additionally, xanthophyll carotenoids selectively accumulate in brain tissue including frontal and temporal cortices. Ω-3FAs are considered to play an important role in neurological health. It has been suggested that DHA plays an important role in the control and resolution of neuro-inflammation. This role is performed by a number of pathways, including being converted into bioactive lipid metabolites such as endocannabinoid epoxides (molecules that are responsible for antiangiogenic effects, vasodilatory actions, and regulation of platelet aggregation) [77]. It has also been suggested that DHA downregulates the expression of genes involved in the synthesis of pro-inflammatory eicosanoids produced from the ω-6FA arachidonic acid [78]. Despite EPA being stored in the brain in low amounts, it has been demonstrated that this fatty acid is important for neural efficiency. This suggests that EPA may positively influence pathways that regulate high-order cognitive functions [79]. It has also been suggested that EPA can facilitate enzymatic processes required to inhibit neuronal damage from inflammation and oxidative stress [80].

Additionally, xanthophyll carotenoids are premised to be neuroprotective primarily owing to their antioxidant properties. Due to their conjugated double-bond structure, carotenoids are efficient scavengers of reactive oxygen species [81]. The lipid solubility of carotenoids also enables them to reduce the susceptibility of cellular membranes and lipoproteins to oxidative damage through free-radical scavenging [82]. L and Z have been shown to positively impact neural efficiency [83,84] and cellular communication via gap junctions [85]. Carotenoids can also combat inflammation. For example, it has been shown that carotenoids are involved in the modulation of inflammatory cells and pro-inflammatory enzymes, the downregulation of pro-inflammatory molecule production, and the attenuation of inflammatory gene expression [86].

While it cannot be asserted that improvements in specific cognitive domains (as a result of supplementation for example) necessarily negates any pre-existing risk for going on to develop AD, nevertheless it is reasonable to hypothesize that the observed improvements in the encoding and memory retrieval process among individuals consuming the nutritional intervention may reflect favorable changes in the physiological functionality, structural integrity and synaptic activity of brain regions involved in memory, and that these favorable changes may be attributable to the enrichment of the aforementioned nutritional compounds. Moreover, the observed trends in improvements in cognitive outcomes may help to favorably alter the risk profile of these individuals for further cognitive decline in the future by enriching the neurocognitive environment.

4.3. Strengths and Limitations

Strengths of CARES Trial 1 include a comprehensive assessment of MCI using sensitive and validated diagnostic measurement tools at screening, enrolment and follow-up assessments. Furthermore, the use of a consensus panel provided in-depth characterization of all individuals and the implementation of robust inclusion and exclusion criteria ensured a clean dataset. The interpretation, analysis and generalizability of results from CARES Trial 1 were limited due to the lack of statistical power in the trial. In order to ensure sufficient statistical power to test the proposed research hypothesis, CARES Trial 1 aimed to recruit 60 individuals with MCI. In order to achieve this target (and allowing for a 10% attrition rate), it was anticipated that a large number of individuals would have to be screened. Despite increased attempts, the identification and recruitment of individuals with MCI proved extremely challenging. The high rate (30%) of individuals who chose not to participate (despite their eligibility) and high attrition rate (as illustrated in Figure 1) were unforeseen and highlights the challenges of conducting research in the MCI population. A number of attempts were made to address the challenges of identifying and enrolling individuals with MCI. These included widening the recruitment catchment area from one city (i.e., Waterford, Ireland) to the entire South-East region of Ireland and hosting briefing meetings with the relevant consultant geriatricians and psychiatrists of old age in the region. Repeated written communication was also carried out to remind the relevant consultant geriatricians and psychiatrists of old age in the region about the clinical trial (including the project aims and inclusion criteria). Despite increased attempts, MCI baseline numbers remained low and drop-out rates remained high.

The small sample size of CARES Trial 1 also precluded the study from comparing MCI subtypes (i.e., amnestic versus non-amnestic) and examining potential relationships between nutritional status and cognitive outcomes. CARES Trial 1 may also be subject to selection bias, given that individuals were primarily recruited from the clinic setting. Finally, depressive symptoms were not assessed at screening. However, depression under active review was part of the exclusion criteria and may counteract this perceived limitation. Despite these limitations, this exploratory study provides encouraging preliminary data. We have shown that individuals with MCI respond (in tissue and in blood) to targeted nutritional supplementation. Additionally, we have observed trends in improved performance in tasks assessing episodic memory and global cognition (namely immediate memory, delayed memory and attention).

5. Conclusions

In conclusion, the present exploratory study has identified trends in improved performance in episodic memory and global cognition among individuals with clinically confirmed MCI following 12-month targeted nutritional supplementation with a combination of ω-3FAs, xanthophyll carotenoids, and vitamin E. Despite the heterogeneity of MCI, studying individuals with this condition provides a unique opportunity to examine the efficacy of nutrition as a preventative approach in slowing the progression of cognitive impairment and improving cognitive-related outcomes. Given that there has been little clinical success with pharmacological strategies for cognitive decline and AD and given that current thinking surrounding the amyloid hypothesis is being challenged by many in the scientific community [87], shifting focus towards preventative approaches is timely and warranted. The results of the present study are highly promising and highlight the potential of nutrition as a preventative strategy for modifying or delaying MCI progression and improving cognitive outcomes. MCI presents a unique opportunity to examine the potential of nutrition for improving cognitive outcomes in individuals at an early stage of impairment. Despite the small sample size, this exploratory interventional work has not only addressed a gap in the literature but has also shown that individuals with clinically confirmed MCI respond positively to targeted nutritional supplementation. Larger-scaled and appropriately powered interventional trials are clearly warranted to confirm this finding and to explore interactions between nutritional compounds and cognitive status.

Author Contributions: Data curation and formal analysis: R.P., J.M.N., W.R.; investigation, project administration, visualization: R.P., J.M.N.; methodology: R.P., J.M.N., A.P.-C., R.C., T.P., R.M.; resources: R.P., J.M.N., R.M.; writing—original draft: R.P., J.M.N., A.P.-C., R.M.; writing—review & editing: R.P., J.M.N., A.P.-C., R.C., A.N.H., R.M.; supervision: A.P.-C., R.M.; validation: A.P.-C., W.R.; software: W.R.; formula analysis: T.P.; conceptualization: A.N.H., R.M.; funding acquisition: A.N.H. All authors have read and agreed to the published version of the manuscript.

Acknowledgments: The authors thank Michael Kirby (University Hospital Waterford, Waterford, Ireland) for his contribution to the consensus panel. The authors also thank Catherine Kelly and Lisa O'Brien (Whitfield Pharmacy, Waterford, Ireland) for the management of the trial supplements and Eurofins Biomnis (Dublin, Ireland) for performing the additional biochemical assessments for the trial.

APC has also been involved in a Commercialization Fund Programme from Enterprise Ireland to develop a biotechnological process to produce carotenoids and the fatty acids EPA and DHA. APC is currently supported by VistaMilk SFI Research Centre to develop commercial dairy products enriched in carotenoids. Robert Coen: RC declares no conflict of interest. Warren Roche: WR declares no conflict of interest. Tommy Power: TB declares no conflict of interest. Alan N. Howard: ANH is trustee of Howard Foundation. ANH is also a director of Nutriproducts Ltd. which trades in nutraceuticals on behalf of the Howard Foundation. ANH was involved in design of the study, and the reviewing of the manuscript. Ríona Mulcahy: RM does consultancy work on behalf of the Howard Foundation.

Appendix A

Table A1. Composition of formulation used in CARES Trial 1 (mg/capsule).

Compound Family	Compound	Formulated	Actual
Fatty Acids	Palmitic acid (16:0)		55.44 ± 1.39
	Palmitoleic acid (16:1)		0.84 ± 0.02
	Stearic acid (18:0)		31.60 ± 1.02
	Oleic acid (18:1n9c)		40.24 ± 0.74
	Vaccenic acid (18:1n9t)		6.26 ± 0.06
	Linoleic acid (18:2n6)		28.57 ± 0.78
	α-Linolenic acid (18:3n3)		1.55 ± 0.03
	Eicosenoic acid (20:1n7, n9, n11)		41.16 ± 0.94
	Homo-γ-linolenic acid (20:3)		1.45 ± 0.04
	Arachidonic acid (20:4n6)		14.20 ± 0.20
	Eicosapentaenoic acid (20:5n3)	45	47.89 ± 0.69
	Docosapentaenoic acid (22:5n3)		11.37 ± 0.18
	Docosahexaenoic acid (22:6n3)	215	258.03 ± 2.75
Carotenoids	Lutein	5	5.18 ± 0.06
	Zeaxanthin	1	1.75 ± 0.03
	meso-zeaxanthin	5	6.48 ± 0.24
Vitamin E	α-tocopherol	7.5	6.12 ± 0.04
	Total mg		558.15

Data presented as mean ± SD. Formulations analyzed in triplicate (three capsules analyzed). Average capsule content calculated gravimetric analysis, 0.666 ± 0.001 g (n = 3).

Table A2. Concentration of fatty acids (mean ± SD, μmol/L) of plasma total lipids.

	Placebo		Active	
	V1	V2	V1	V2
Miristic acid	158.39 ± 117.06	200.19 ± 98.13	166.02 ± 89.64	147.14 ± 76.60
Palmitic acid	4040.87 ± 689.23	3976.31 ± 504.27	4088.68 ± 855.16	3794.24 ± 832.03
Palmitoleic acid	208.07 ± 80.91	223.47 ± 59.86	231.43 ± 159.19	231.81 ± 153.37
Stearic acid	1144.93 ± 154.75	1150.95 ± 105.75	1017.71 ± 186.56	938.33 ± 132.44
Oleic acid	2368.04 ± 686.01	2693.92 ± 645.78	2383.20 ± 752.13	2405.17 ± 638.84
Vaccenic acid	138.70 ± 21.46	155.97 ± 25.73	148.20 ± 46.87	137.51 ± 45.76
Linoleic acid	2398.38 ± 409.88	2584.15 ± 206.55	2452.42 ± 186.15	2428.33 ± 276.07
γ-linolenic acid	54.37 ± 19.81	51.36 ± 21.40	41.45 ± 20.50	39.65 ± 20.23
α-linolenic acid	88.09 ± 32.29	96.32 ± 46.64	112.40 ± 29.93	101.14 ± 14.93
Eicosenoic acid	493.59 ± 85.53	373.54 ± 46.86	479.94 ± 85.43	369.29 ± 33.35
Homo-γ-linolenic acid	162.94 ± 39.32	166.81 ± 43.94	134.27 ± 36.82	127.83 ± 19.35
Arachidonic acid	789.65 ± 197.72	842.89 ± 271.43	628.37 ± 208.69	588.96 ± 241.35
Eicosapentaenoic acid (EPA)	141.06 ± 43.75	167.51 ± 90.72	148.53 ± 58.71	155.60 ± 60.72
Docosapentaenoic acid (DPA)	55.21 ± 6.88	59.49 ± 16.69	50.74 ± 5.78	49.03 ± 13.64
Docosahexaenoic acid (DHA)	199.96 ± 43.11	231.64 ± 47.20	211.72 ± 56.47	325.91 ± 97.80

Data presented as mean ± SD.

Table A3. Calibration standards used to quantify xanthophyll carotenoids and vitamin E.

	Molecular Weight	Maximum Wavelength	Extinction Coefficient	Solvent	Reference
Lutein	568.88	444	144.8×10^3	Ethanol	[88]
Zeaxanthin	568.88	450	144.2×10^3	Ethanol	[89]
β-cryptoxanthin	552.85	450	135.7×10^3	Hexane	[90]
α-tocopherol	430.71	292	326.5	Ethanol	[91]

Molecular weight (g mol^{-1}); Maximum wavelength (nm); Extinction coefficient (L mol^{-1} cm^{-1}).

Table A4. Regression line, lower and upper limits of quantification for xanthophyll carotenoids and vitamin E.

Compound	Equation	R^2	LLOQ (n = 10)	ULOQ (n = 3)
Lutein	$y = 0.0827x + 0.3409$	0.9997	0.069 ± 0.0007	2.514 ± 0.003
Zeaxanthin	$y = 0.0793x + 1.4721$	0.9998	0.048 ± 0.0003	2.487 ± 0.007
β-cryptoxanthin	$y = 0.0909x + 1.9363$	0.9997	0.071 ± 0.0005	2.460 ± 0.007
α-tocopherol	$y = 0.00254x + 0.04380$	0.9992	4.053 ± 0.0913	69.469 ± 1.011

LLOQ: lower limit of quantification expressed in μmol/L; ULOQ; upper limit of quantification expressed in μmol/L.

Appendix A.1 Analyte Recovery Analysis

L was used as a representative of carotenoid recovery efficiency; recovery efficiency of α-tocopherol was also assessed. To do this, the respective authentic standard was added to a pooled serum sample in a concentration of 85% to 110% ULOQ. The concentration of the analyte was determined by HPLC in this spiked sample, as well as in the pooled serum and in the prepared authentic standard separately. The percentage of recovery of the analyte of interest was determined by adding the area of the analyte in the prepared authentic standard and in the pooled serum, and dividing it by the area of the analyte in the spiked sample. This determination was performed in triplicate for each analyte and on three different days. The efficiency of the recovery of L (Table A5) was 99.4 ± 2.9 % without adjusting with the IS, and 121.6 ± 0.7 adjusting with the IS, at a concentration 92.3 ± 10.4 % of ULOQ (n = 3). The efficiency of recovery of α-tocopherol (Table A6) was 88.2 ± 2.1 % without adjusting with the IS, and 104.1 ± 5.8 % adjusting with the IS, at a concentration of 100.5 ± 11.1 % of ULOQ (n = 3). These results suggested that the method performed to quantify L was exhaustive in terms of L extraction and re-suspension prior to HPLC analysis, but incomplete in this sense for α-tocopherol. Therefore, we did not to use the IS to correct carotenoid concentrations, but used it to correct α-tocopherol concentrations in the samples analysed.

Table A5. Lutein recovery assay.

Assay	% ULOQ	% Recovery No IS	% Recovery with IS
1	81.6	99.4	122.4
2	93.0	102.2	120.9
3	102.4	96.5	121.6
Average	92.3 ± 10.4	99.3 ± 2.9	121.6 ± 0.7

ULOQ; upper limit of quantification; IS: internal standard.

Table A6. α-tocopherol recovery assay.

Assay	%ULOQ	% Recovery No IS	% Recovery with IS
1	88.4	86.1	97.5
2	108.8	90.2	108.6
3	103.5	88.3	106.1
Average	100.2 ± 10.6	88.2 ± 2.1	104.1 ± 5.8

ULOQ; upper limit of quantification; IS: internal standard.

Appendix A.2 HPLC Precision Analysis

The HPLC analysis of the samples were completed in four independent batches, each one performed on a different day. Intra-day and inter-day precision of carotenoid and α-tocopherol analysis were evaluated and quantified in an independently pooled serum sample that was analysed at the beginning, middle and end of each daily analysis. L and α-tocopherol were analysed over runs as witnesses of precision of HPLC analysis. L concentration in the pooled serum averaged 0.151 ± 0.004 µmol/L (Table A7), which is roughly twice the concentration of the LLOQ. Intra-day precision in each day of analysis, expressed as the co-efficient of variation (CV) of the concentration of each analyte was below 5% in L and α-tocopherol, which is below the 15% limit recommended by EMA [92]. Inter-day precision was calculated averaging compound concentration of the pooled samples in each day of analysis. The highest inter-day variability was for α-tocopherol (8.33%, Table A7), which is also below the 15% limit recommended by EMA.

Table A7. Intra-day and inter-day precision of lutein and α-tocopherol in human serum.

µmol/L (n; CV)	Intra-Day 1 (n = 3)	Intra-Day 2 (n = 4)	Intra-Day 3 (n = 3)	Intra-Day 4 (n = 2)	Inter-Day
Lutein	0.148 ± 0.007 (CV = 4.98%)	0.156 ± 0.003 (CV = 1.89%)	0.153 ± 0.003 (CV = 1.65%)	0.147 ± 0.002 (CV = 1.05%)	0.151 ± 0.004 (CV = 2.71%)
α-tocopherol	26.123 ± 1.095 (CV = 4.19%)	29.031 ± 0.881 (CV = 3.03%)	27.210 ± 0.697 (CV = 2.56%)	23.745 ± 1.057 (CV = 4.45%)	26.527 ± 2.209 (CV = 8.33%)

CV: co-efficient of variation.

Appendix A.3 Trueness of Xanthophyll Carotenoid Quantification

Trueness was assessed with the Certified Standard Material NIST SRM 968f, fat-soluble vitamins in frozen human serum in two different concentrations (level 1 and level 2) using our calibration lines. Only α-tocopherol was below the consensus value for level 1 by 17%; the rest of the compounds were within the limits set by NIST [93] (see Table A8). The IS was not used to calculate carotenoid concentrations, but it was used to calculate α-tocopherol concentration.

Table A8. Trueness of xanthophyll carotenoid quantification.

Compound	NIST Concentration (µmol/L)	
	Level 1 (NIST Consensus Values)	Level 2 (NIST Consensus Values)
Total lutein	0.035 (0.036 ± 0.010)	0.075 (0.087 ± 0.037)
Total lutein + zeaxanthin	0.053 (0.052 ± 0.006)	0.106 (0.115 ± 0.019)
β-cryptoxanthin	0.030 (0.030 ± 0.008)	0.038 (0.044 ± 0.017)
α-tocopherol	4.114 (5.15 ± 0.21)	11.508 (11.85 ± 0.73)

NIST: National Institute of Standards and Technology. Experimental vs. Consensus values (in brackets) equated to the mean of the value of the compound ± expanded uncertainty ($U_{95\%}$).

Table A9. Additional biochemical assessments measured in active and placebo intervention groups.

Variable	Active (n = 10) Median (IQR)	Placebo (n = 9) Median (IQR)	Sig.
Cholesterol (mmol/L)	4.20 (3.75–5.60)	4.65 (4.23–5.40)	0.541
Triglycerides (mmol/L)	1.72 (1.03–2.21)	1.32 (1.04–1.86)	0.815
HDL (mmol/L)	1.34 (1.06–1.55)	2.03 (1.14–2.12)	0.236
LDL (mmol/L)	2.50 (1.85–3.50)	2.15 (1.48–3.78)	0.743
Homocysteine (μmol/L)	11.0 (8.10–15.55)	8.65 (7.33–11.80)	0.236
C-reactive protein (mg/L)	0.80 (0.55–5.10)	0.45 (0.30–1.10)	0.236
TSH (ulUml)	1.52 (0.97–2.15)	1.08 (0.95–1.84)	0.541
Free T4 (pmol/L)	12.10 (10.85–14.20)	11.90 (10.88–13.78)	0.888
Haemoglobin (g/dL)	14.10 (12.55–15.15)	12.90 (12.48–13.38)	0.236
Sodium (mmol/L)	138.0 (137.50–140.0)	139.0 (138.0–140.0)	0.743
Potassium (mmol/L)	4.15 (3.88–4.83)	4.20 (4.05–4.50)	0.999
Chloride (mmol/L)	101.0 (98.0–104.0)	102.0 (97.0–103.75)	0.999
Creatinine (μmol/L)	74.0 (70.0–86.50)	63.5 (57.5–68.75)	**0.008**

Data displayed are median (inter quartile range): HDL: high-density lipoprotein; LDL: low-density lipoprotein; Free T4: Free thyroxine; TSH: thyroid stimulating hormone. Additional biochemical assessments were not obtained for one individual in the active intervention group and one individual in the placebo group.

References

1. Petersen, R.C.; Roberts, R.O.; Knopman, D.S.; Boeve, B.F.; Geda, Y.E.; Ivnik, R.J.; Smith, G.E.; Jack, C.R., Jr. Mild cognitive impairment: Ten years later. *Arch. Neurol.* **2009**, *66*, 1447–1455. [CrossRef]
2. Bae, J.B.; Han, J.W.; Kwak, K.P.; Kim, B.J.; Kim, S.G.; Kim, J.L.; Kim, T.H.; Ryu, S.H.; Moon, S.W.; Park, J.H.; et al. Impact of Mild Cognitive Impairment on Mortality and Cause of Death in the Elderly. *J. Alzheimers Dis.* **2018**, *64*, 607–616. [CrossRef]
3. Ganguli, M.; Dodge, H.H.; Shen, C.; Pandav, R.S.; DeKosky, S.T. Alzheimer disease and mortality: A 15-year epidemiological study. *Arch. Neurol.* **2005**, *62*, 779–784. [CrossRef]
4. Farias, S.T.; Mungas, D.; Reed, B.R.; Harvey, D.; DeCarli, C. Progression of mild cognitive impairment to dementia in clinic- vs community-based cohorts. *Arch. Neurol.* **2009**, *66*, 1151–1157. [CrossRef]
5. Roberts, R.O.; Knopman, D.S.; Mielke, M.M.; Cha, R.H.; Pankratz, V.S.; Christianson, T.J.; Geda, Y.E.; Boeve, B.F.; Ivnik, R.J.; Tangalos, E.G.; et al. Higher risk of progression to dementia in mild cognitive impairment cases who revert to normal. *Neurology* **2014**, *82*, 317–325. [CrossRef]
6. Lopez, O.L.; Becker, J.T., Chang, Y.F; Sweet, R.A.; DeKosky, S.T.; Gach, M.H.; Carmichael, O.T.; McDade, E.; Kuller, L.H. Incidence of mild cognitive impairment in the Pittsburgh Cardiovascular Health Study-Cognition Study. *Neurology* **2012**, *79*, 1599–1606. [CrossRef]
7. Cheng, G.; Huang, C.; Deng, H.; Wang, H. Diabetes as a risk factor for dementia and mild cognitive impairment: A meta-analysis of longitudinal studies. *Intern. Med. J.* **2012**, *42*, 484–491. [CrossRef]
8. Livingston, G.; Sommerlad, A.; Orgeta, V.; Costafreda, S.G.; Huntley, J.; Ames, D.; Ballard, C.; Banerjee, S.; Burns, A.; Cohen-Mansfield, J.; et al. Dementia prevention, intervention, and care. *Lancet* **2017**, *390*, 2673–2734. [CrossRef]
9. DeCarlo, C.A.; MacDonald, S.W.; Vergote, D.; Jhamandas, J.; Westaway, D.; Dixon, R.A. Vascular Health and Genetic Risk Affect Mild Cognitive Impairment Status and 4-Year Stability: Evidence From the Victoria Longitudinal Study. *J. Gerontol. B. Psychol. Sci. Soc. Sci.* **2016**, *71*, 1004–1014. [CrossRef]
10. Valls-Pedret, C.; Sala-Vila, A.; Serra-Mir, M.; Corella, D.; de la Torre, R.; Martinez-Gonzalez, M.A.; Martinez-Lapiscina, E.H.; Fito, M.; Perez-Heras, A.; Salas-Salvado, J.; et al. Mediterranean Diet and Age-Related Cognitive Decline: A Randomized Clinical Trial. *Jama. Intern. Med.* **2015**, *175*, 1094–1103. [CrossRef]
11. Pelletier, A.; Barul, C.; Feart, C.; Helmer, C.; Bernard, C.; Periot, O.; Dilharreguy, B.; Dartigues, J.F.; Allard, M.; Barberger-Gateau, P.; et al. Mediterranean diet and preserved brain structural connectivity in older subjects. *Alzheimers Dement.* **2015**, *11*, 1023–1031. [CrossRef] [PubMed]

12. Zamroziewicz, M.K.; Barbey, A.K. The Mediterranean diet and healthy brain aging: Innovations from nutritional cognitive neuroscience. In *Role of the Mediterranean Diet in the Brain and Neurodegenerative Diseases*; Farooqui, T., Farooqui, A.A., Eds.; Elsevier Publishing Company: New York, NY, USA, 2017.
13. Zwilling, C.E.; Talukdar, T.; Zamroziewicz, M.K.; Barbey, A.K. Nutrient biomarker patterns, cognitive function, and fMRI measures of network efficiency in the aging brain. *Neuroimage* **2019**, *188*, 239–251. [CrossRef] [PubMed]
14. Hardman, R.J.; Kennedy, G.; Macpherson, H.; Scholey, A.B.; Pipingas, A. Adherence to a Mediterranean-Style Diet and Effects on Cognition in Adults: A Qualitative Evaluation and Systematic Review of Longitudinal and Prospective Trials. *Front. Nutr.* **2016**, *3*, 22. [CrossRef] [PubMed]
15. Otaegui-Arrazola, A.; Amiano, P.; Elbusto, A.; Urdaneta, E.; Martinez-Lage, P. Diet, cognition, and Alzheimer's disease: Food for thought. *Eur. J. Nutr.* **2014**, *53*, 1–23. [CrossRef]
16. Lourida, I.; Soni, M.; Thompson-Coon, J.; Purandare, N.; Lang, I.A.; Ukoumunne, O.C.; Llewellyn, D.J. Mediterranean diet, cognitive function, and dementia: A systematic review. *Epidemiology* **2013**, *24*, 479–489. [CrossRef]
17. Roberts, R.O.; Geda, Y.E.; Cerhan, J.R.; Knopman, D.S.; Cha, R.H.; Christianson, T.J.; Pankratz, V.S.; Ivnik, R.J.; Boeve, B.F.; O'Connor, H.M.; et al. Vegetables, unsaturated fats, moderate alcohol intake, and mild cognitive impairment. *Dement. Geriatr. Cogn. Disord.* **2010**, *29*, 413–423. [CrossRef]
18. Singh, B.; Parsaik, A.K.; Mielke, M.M.; Erwin, P.J.; Knopman, D.S.; Petersen, R.C.; Roberts, R.O. Association of mediterranean diet with mild cognitive impairment and Alzheimer's disease: A systematic review and meta-analysis. *J. Alzheimer Dis.* **2014**, *39*, 271–282. [CrossRef]
19. Craft, N.E.; Haitema, T.B.; Garnett, K.M.; Fitch, K.A.; Dorey, C.K. Carotenoid, tocopherol, and retinol concentrations in elderly human brain. *J. Nutr. Health. Aging* **2004**, *8*, 156–162.
20. Johnson, E.J.; Vishwanathan, R.; Johnson, M.A.; Hausman, D.B.; Davey, A.; Scott, T.M.; Green, R.C.; Miller, L.S.; Gearing, M.; Woodard, J. Relationship between serum and brain carotenoids,-tocopherol, and retinol concentrations and cognitive performance in the oldest old from the Georgia Centenarian Study. *J. Aging Res.* **2013**, *2013*, 951786. [CrossRef]
21. Singh, M. Essential fatty acids, DHA and human brain. *Indian. J. Pediatr.* **2005**, *72*, 239–242. [CrossRef]
22. Rinaldi, P.; Polidori, M.C.; Metastasio, A.; Mariani, E.; Mattioli, P.; Cherubini, A.; Catani, M.; Cecchetti, R.; Senin, U.; Mecocci, P. Plasma antioxidants are similarly depleted in mild cognitive impairment and in Alzheimer's disease. *Neurobiol. Aging* **2003**, *24*, 915–919. [CrossRef]
23. Cunnane, S.C.; Schneider, J.A.; Tangney, C.; Tremblay-Mercier, J.; Fortier, M.; Bennett, D.A.; Morris, M.C. Plasma and brain fatty acid profiles in mild cognitive impairment and Alzheimer's disease. *J. Alzheimers Dis.* **2012**, *29*, 691–697. [CrossRef]
24. Nolan, J.; Loskutova, E.; Howard, N.A.; Moran, R.; Mulcahy, R.; Stack, J.; Bolger, M.; Dennison, J.; Akuffo, K.; Owens, N.; et al. Macular Pigment, Visual Function, and Macular Disease among Subjects with Alzheimer's Disease: An Exploratory Study. *J. Alzheimers Dis.* **2014**, *42*, 1191–1202. [CrossRef]
25. Feeney, J.; O'Leary, N.; Moran, R.; O'Halloran, A.M.; Nolan, J.M.; Beatty, S.; Young, I.S.; Kenny, R.A. Plasma Lutein and Zeaxanthin Are Associated With Better Cognitive Function Across Multiple Domains in a Large Population-Based Sample of Older Adults: Findings from The Irish Longitudinal Study on Aging. *J. Gerontol. A. Biol. Sci. Med. Sci.* **2017**, *72*, 1431–1436. [CrossRef]
26. Zamroziewicz, M.K.; Paul, E.J.; Zwilling, C.E.; Johnson, E.J.; Kuchan, M.J.; Cohen, N.J.; Barbey, A.K. Parahippocampal Cortex Mediates the Relationship between Lutein and Crystallized Intelligence in Healthy, Older Adults. *Front. Aging Neurosci.* **2016**, *8*, 297. [CrossRef]
27. Wu, S.; Ding, Y.; Wu, F.; Li, R.; Hou, J.; Mao, P. Omega-3 fatty acids intake and risks of dementia and Alzheimer's disease: A meta-analysis. *Neurosci. Biobehav. Rev.* **2015**, *48*, 1–9. [CrossRef]
28. Talukdar, T.; Zamroziewicz, M.K.; Zwilling, C.E.; Barbey, A.K. Nutrient biomarkers shape individual differences in functional brain connectivity: Evidence from omega-3 PUFAs. *Hum. Brain. Mapp.* **2019**, *40*, 1887–1897. [CrossRef]
29. Bowman, G.L.; Dodge, H.H.; Mattek, N.; Barbey, A.K.; Silbert, L.C.; Shinto, L.; Howieson, D.B.; Kaye, J.A.; Quinn, J.F. Plasma omega-3 PUFA and white matter mediated executive decline in older adults. *Front. Aging Neurosci.* **2013**, *5*, 92. [CrossRef]
30. Power, R.; Coen, R.F.; Beatty, S.; Mulcahy, R.; Moran, R.; Stack, J.; Howard, A.N.; Nolan, J.M. Supplemental Retinal Carotenoids Enhance Memory in Healthy Individuals with Low Levels of Macular Pigment in A Randomized, Double-Blind, Placebo-Controlled Clinical Trial. *J. Alzheimers Dis.* **2018**, *61*, 947–961. [CrossRef]

31. Hammond, B.R., Jr.; Miller, L.S.; Bello, M.O.; Lindbergh, C.A.; Mewborn, C.; Renzi-Hammond, L.M. Effects of Lutein/Zeaxanthin Supplementation on the Cognitive Function of Community Dwelling Older Adults: A Randomized, Double-Masked, Placebo-Controlled Trial. *Front. Aging Neurosci.* **2017**, *9*, 254. [CrossRef]
32. Kulzow, N.; Witte, A.V.; Kerti, L.; Grittner, U.; Schuchardt, J.P.; Hahn, A.; Floel, A. Impact of Omega-3 Fatty Acid Supplementation on Memory Functions in Healthy Older Adults. *J. Alzheimers Dis.* **2016**, *51*, 713–725. [CrossRef]
33. Yurko-Mauro, K.; McCarthy, D.; Rom, D.; Nelson, E.B.; Ryan, A.S.; Blackwell, A.; Salem, N., Jr.; Stedman, M. Beneficial effects of docosahexaenoic acid on cognition in age-related cognitive decline. *Alzheimers Dement.* **2010**, *6*, 456–464. [CrossRef]
34. Power, R.; Prado-Cabrero, A.; Mulcahy, R.; Howard, A.; Nolan, J.M. The Role of Nutrition for the Aging Population: Implications for Cognition and Alzheimer's Disease. *Annu. Rev. Food. Sci. Technol.* **2019**, *10*, 619–639. [CrossRef]
35. Johnson, E.J.; McDonald, K.; Caldarella, S.M.; Chung, H.Y.; Troen, A.M.; Snodderly, D.M. Cognitive findings of an exploratory trial of docosahexaenoic acid and lutein supplementation in older women. *Nutr. Neurosci.* **2008**, *11*, 75–83. [CrossRef]
36. Nolan, J.M.; Mulcahy, R.; Power, R.; Moran, R.; Howard, A.N. Nutritional Intervention to Prevent Alzheimer's Disease: Potential Benefits of Xanthophyll Carotenoids and Omega-3 Fatty Acids Combined. *J. Alzheimers Dis.* **2018**, *64*, 367–378. [CrossRef]
37. Petersen, R.C.; Smith, G.E.; Waring, S.C.; Ivnik, R.J.; Tangalos, E.G.; Kokmen, E. Mild cognitive impairment: Clinical characterization and outcome. *Arch. Neurol.* **1999**, *56*, 303–308. [CrossRef]
38. Winblad, B.; Palmer, K.; Kivipelto, M.; Jelic, V.; Fratiglioni, L.; Wahlund, L.O.; Nordberg, A.; Bäckman, L.; Albert, M.; Almkvist, O.; et al. Mild cognitive impairment—Beyond controversies, towards a consensus: Report of the International Working Group on Mild Cognitive Impairment. *J. Intern. Med.* **2004**, *256*, 240–246. [CrossRef]
39. Dubois, B.; Albert, M.L. Amnestic MCI or prodromal Alzheimer's disease? *Lancet Neurol.* **2004**, *3*, 246–248. [CrossRef]
40. Nasreddine, Z.S.; Phillips, N.A.; Bedirian, V.; Charbonneau, S.; Whitehead, V.; Collin, I.; Cummings, J.L.; Chertkow, H. The Montreal Cognitive Assessment, MoCA: A brief screening tool for mild cognitive impairment. *J. Am. Geriatr. Soc.* **2005**, *53*, 695–699. [CrossRef]
41. Randolph, C.; Tierney, M.C.; Mohr, E.; Chase, T.N. The Repeatable Battery for the Assessment of Neuropsychological Status (RBANS): Preliminary clinical validity. *J. Clin. Exp. Neuropsychol.* **1998**, *20*, 310–319. [CrossRef]
42. Randolph, C. *RBANS. Update: Repeatable Battery for the Assessment of Neuropsychological Status Manual*; NCS Pearson; PsychCorp: Bloomington, MN, USA, 2012.
43. Cambridge Cognition. *CANTAB Connect Research: Admin Application User Guide v1.6*; Cambridge Cognition Limited: Cambridge, UK, 2019.
44. Zygouris, S.; Tsolaki, M. Computerized cognitive testing for older adults: A review. *Am. J. Alzheimers Dis. Other. Demen.* **2015**, *30*, 13–28. [CrossRef] [PubMed]
45. Cambridge Cognition. *Product Overview: CANTAB Connect Research v11.10*; Cambridge Cognition Limited: Cambridge, UK, 2019.
46. Chan, D.; Gallaher, L.M.; Moodley, K.; minati, L.; Burgess, N.; Hartley, T. The 4 Mountains Test: A Short Test of Spatial Memory with High Sensitivity for the Diagnosis of Pre-dementia Alzheimer's Disease. *J. Vis. Exp.* **2016**. [CrossRef]
47. Bird, C.M.; Chan, D.; Hartley, T.; Pijnenburg, Y.A.; Rossor, M.N.; Burgess, N. Topographical short-term memory differentiates Alzheimer's disease from frontotemporal lobar degeneration. *Hippocampus* **2010**, *20*, 1154–1169. [CrossRef] [PubMed]
48. Moodley, K.; minati, L.; Contarino, V.; Prioni, S.; Wood, R.; Cooper, R.; D'Incerti, L.; Tagliavini, F.; Chan, D. Diagnostic differentiation of mild cognitive impairment due to Alzheimer's disease using a hippocampus-dependent test of spatial memory. *Hippocampus* **2015**, *25*, 939–951. [CrossRef]
49. Bucks, R.S.; Ashworth, D.L.; Wilcock, G.K.; Siegfried, K. Assessment of activities of daily living in dementia: Development of the Bristol Activities of Daily Living Scale. *Age. Ageing* **1996**, *25*, 113–120. [CrossRef] [PubMed]

50. Bucks, R.S.; Haworth, J. Bristol Activities of Daily Living Scale: A critical evaluation. *Expert. Rev. Neurother.* **2002**, *2*, 669–676. [CrossRef]
51. Moniz-Cook, E.; Vernooij-Dassen, M.; Woods, R.; Verhey, F.; Chattat, R.; De Vugt, M.; Mountain, G.; O'Connell, M.; Harrison, J.; Vasse, E.; et al. A European consensus on outcome measures for pyschosocial intervention research in dementia care. *Aging Ment. Health.* **2008**, *12*, 14–29. [CrossRef]
52. Sabbagh, M.N.; Malek-Ahmadi, M.; Kataria, R.; Belden, C.M.; Connor, D.J.; Pearson, C.; Jacobson, S.; Davis, K.; Yaari, R.; Singh, U. The Alzheimer's questionnaire: A proof of concept study for a new informant-based dementia assessment. *J. Alzheimers Dis.* **2010**, *22*, 1015–1021. [CrossRef]
53. Malek-Ahmadi, M.; Davis, K.; Belden, C.; Laizure, B.; Jacobson, S.; Yaari, R.; Singh, U.; Sabbagh, M.N. Validation and diagnostic accuracy of the Alzheimer's questionnaire. *Age. Ageing.* **2012**, *41*, 396–399. [CrossRef]
54. Trieschmann, M.; Heimes, B.; Hense, H.W.; Pauleikhoff, D. Macular pigment optical density measurement in autofluorescence imaging: Comparison of one- and two-wavelength methods. *Graefes. Arch. Clin. Exp. Ophthalmol.* **2006**, *244*, 1565–1574. [CrossRef]
55. Roche, W.; Green-Gomez, M.; Moran, R.; Nolan, J. The physics of using the Heidelberg Spectralis dual-wavelength autofluorescence method for the measurement of macular pigment volume. *J. Alzheimers Dis.* **2018**, *64*, 1019–1048.
56. Green-Gomez, M.; Bernstein, P.S.; Curcio, C.A.; Moran, R.; Roche, W.; Nolan, J. Standardizing the Assessment of Macular Pigment Using a Dual-Wavelength Autofluorescence Technique. *Transl. Vis. Sci. Technol.* **2019**, *8*, 41. [CrossRef] [PubMed]
57. Zidichouski, J.A.; Mastaloudis, A.; Poole, S.J.; Reading, J.C.; Smidt, C.R. Clinical validation of a noninvasive, Raman spectroscopic method to assess carotenoid nutritional status in humans. *J. Am. Coll. Nutr.* **2009**, *28*, 687–693. [CrossRef] [PubMed]
58. Meagher, K.A.; Thurnham, D.I.; Beatty, S.; Howard, A.N.; Connolly, E.; Cummins, W.; Nolan, J.M. Serum response to supplemental macular carotenoids in subjects with and without age-related macular degeneration. *Br. J. Nutr.* **2013**, *110*, 289–300. [CrossRef] [PubMed]
59. Benner, B.A.; Schantz, M.M.; Powers, C.D.; Schleicher, R.L.; Camara, J.E.; Sharpless, K.E.; Yen, J.H.; Sniegoski, L.T. Standard Reference Material (SRM) 2378 fatty acids in frozen human serum. Certification of a clinical SRM based on endogenous supplementation of polyunsaturated fatty acids. *Anal. Bioanal. Chem.* **2018**, *410*, 2321–2329. [CrossRef]
60. Solfrizzi, V.; Agosti, P.; Lozupone, M.; Custodero, C.; Schilardi, A.; Valiani, V.; Santamato, A.; Sardone, R.; Dibello, V.; Di Lena, L.; et al. Nutritional interventions and cognitive-related outcomes in patients with late-life cognitive disorders: A systematic review. *Neurosci. Biobehav. Rev.* **2018**, *95*, 480–498. [CrossRef]
61. Remington, R.; Lortie, J.J.; Hoffmann, H.; Page, R.; Morrell, C.; Shea, T.B. A Nutritional Formulation for Cognitive Performance in Mild Cognitive Impairment: A Placebo-Controlled Trial with an Open-Label Extension. *J. Alzheimers Dis.* **2015**, *48*, 591–595. [CrossRef]
62. Yurko-Mauro, K.; Alexander, D.D.; Van Elswyk, M.E. Docosahexaenoic acid and adult memory: A systematic review and meta-analysis. *PLoS ONE* **2015**, *10*, e0120391. [CrossRef]
63. Lee, L.K.; Shahar, S.; Chin, A.V.; Yusoff, N.A. Docosahexaenoic acid-concentrated fish oil supplementation in subjects with mild cognitive impairment (MCI): A 12-month randomised, double-blind, placebo-controlled trial. *Psychopharmacology* **2013**, *225*, 605–612. [CrossRef]
64. Mazereeuw, G.; Lanctot, K.L.; Chau, S.A.; Swardfager, W.; Herrmann, N. Effects of omega-3 fatty acids on cognitive performance: A meta-analysis. *Neurobiol. Aging* **2012**, *33*, 1482.e1417–1429. [CrossRef]
65. Bo, Y.; Zhang, X.; Wang, Y.; You, J.; Cui, H.; Zhu, Y.; Pang, W.; Liu, W.; Jiang, Y.; Lu, Q. The n-3 Polyunsaturated Fatty Acids Supplementation Improved the Cognitive Function in the Chinese Elderly with Mild Cognitive Impairment: A Double-Blind Randomized Controlled Trial. *Nutrients* **2017**, *9*. [CrossRef] [PubMed]
66. Farina, N.; Llewellyn, D.; Isaac, M.G.E.K.; Tabet, N. Vitamin E for Alzheimer's dementia and mild cognitive impairment. *Cochrane. Database Syst. Rev.* **2017**, *4*, CD002854. [CrossRef] [PubMed]
67. European Food Safety Authority. Scientific Opinion on Dietary Reference Values for vitamin E as α-tocopherol. *Efsa. J.* **2015**, *13*. [CrossRef]
68. Institute of Medicine. *Dietary Reference Intakes for Vitamin C, Vitamin E, Selenium, and Carotenoids*; The National Academies Press: Washington, DC, USA, 2000.
69. Dysken, M.W.; Sano, M.; Asthana, S.; Vertrees, J.E.; Pallaki, M.; Llorente, M.; Love, S.; Schellenberg, G.D.;

McCarten, J.R.; Malphurs, J.; et al. Effect of vitamin E and memantine on functional decline in Alzheimer disease: The TEAM-AD VA cooperative randomized trial. *JAMA* **2014**, *311*, 33–44. [CrossRef]

70. Kryscio, R.J.; Abner, E.L.; Caban-Holt, A.; Lovell, M.; Goodman, P.; Darke, A.K.; Yee, M.; Crowley, J.; Schmitt, F.A. Association of Antioxidant Supplement Use and Dementia in the Prevention of Alzheimer's Disease by Vitamin E and Selenium Trial (PREADViSE). *JAMA Neurol.* **2017**, *74*, 567–573. [CrossRef]
71. Andrés, P.; Vico, H.; Yáñez, A.; Siquier, A.; Ferrer, G.A. Quantifying memory deficits in amnestic mild cognitive impairment. *Alzheimers Dement.* **2019**, *11*, 108–114. [CrossRef]
72. Irish, M.; Lawlor, B.A.; Coen, R.F.; O'Mara, S.M. Everyday episodic memory in amnestic mild cognitive impairment: A preliminary investigation. *BMC Neurosci.* **2011**, *12*, 80. [CrossRef]
73. Hasselmo, M.E. *How We Remember: Brain Mechanisms of Episodic Memory*; MIT Press: Cambridge, MA, USA, 2011.
74. Nyberg, L. Functional brain imaging of episodic memory decline in ageing. *J. Intern. Med.* **2017**, *281*, 65–74. [CrossRef]
75. Nyberg, L.; McIntosh, A.R.; Cabeza, R.; Habib, R.; Houle, S.; Tulving, E. General and specific brain regions involved in encoding and retrieval of events: What, where, and when. *Proc. Natl. Acad. Sci. USA* **1996**, *93*, 11280–11285. [CrossRef]
76. Weiser, M.J.; Butt, C.M.; Mohajeri, M.H. Docosahexaenoic Acid and Cognition throughout the Lifespan. *Nutrients* **2016**, *8*, 99. [CrossRef]
77. McDougle, D.R.; Watson, J.E.; Abdeen, A.A.; Adili, R.; Caputo, M.P.; Krapf, J.E.; Johnson, R.W.; Kilian, K.A.; Holinstat, M.; Das, A. Anti-inflammatory ω-3 endocannabinoid epoxides. *Proc. Natl. Acad. Sci. USA* **2017**, *114*, E6034–E6043. [CrossRef] [PubMed]
78. Smedt-Peyrusse, V.D.; Sargueil, F.; Moranis, A.; Harizi, H.; Mongrand, S.; Layé, S. Docosahexaenoic acid prevents lipopolysaccharide-induced cytokine production in microglial cells by inhibiting lipopolysaccharide receptor presentation but not its membrane subdomain localization. *J. Neurochem.* **2008**, *105*, 296–307. [CrossRef] [PubMed]
79. Bauer, I.; Crewther, S.; Pipingas, A.; Sellick, L.; Crewther, D. Does omega-3 fatty acid supplementation enhance neural efficiency? A review of the literature. *Hum. Psychopharmacol.* **2014**, *29*, 8–18. [CrossRef] [PubMed]
80. Okabe, N.; Nakamura, T.; Toyoshima, T.; Miyamoto, O.; Lu, F.; Itano, T. Eicosapentaenoic acid prevents memory impairment after ischemia by inhibiting inflammatory response and oxidative damage. *J. Stroke. Cereb. Dis.* **2011**, *20*, 188–195. [CrossRef] [PubMed]
81. Sakai, C.; Ishida, M.; Ohba, H.; Yamashita, H.; Uchida, H.; Yoshizumi, M.; Ishida, T. Fish oil omega-3 polyunsaturated fatty acids attenuate oxidative stress-induced DNA damage in vascular endothelial cells. *PLoS ONE* **2017**, *12*, e0187934. [CrossRef] [PubMed]
82. Bouayed, J.; Bohn, T. Dietary Derived Antioxidants: Implications on Health, Nutrition, Well-Being and Health. Available online: https://www.intechopen.com/books/nutrition-well-being-and-health/dietary-derived-antioxidants-implication-on-health (accessed on 31 March 2020).
83. Bovier, E.R.; Hammond, B.R. A randomized placebo-controlled study on the effects of lutein and zeaxanthin on visual processing speed in young healthy subjects. *Arch. Biochem. Biophys.* **2015**, *572*, 54–57. [CrossRef] [PubMed]
84. Lindbergh, C.A.; Mewborn, C.M.; Hammond, B.R.; Renzi-Hammond, L.M.; Curran-Celentano, J.M.; Miller, L.S. Relationship of Lutein and Zeaxanthin Levels to Neurocognitive Functioning: An fMRI Study of Older Adults. *J. Int. Neuropsychol. Soc.* **2016**, 1–12. [CrossRef]
85. Sohl, G.; Maxeiner, S.; Willecke, K. Expression and functions of neuronal gap junctions. *Nat. Rev. Neurosci.* **2005**, *6*, 191–200. [CrossRef]
86. Guest, J.; Grant, R. Carotenoids and Neurobiological Health. *Adv. Neurobiol.* **2016**, *12*, 199–228. [CrossRef]
87. Kametani, F.; Hasegawa, M. Reconsideration of Amyloid Hypothesis and Tau Hypothesis in Alzheimer's Disease. *Front. Neurosci.* **2018**, *12*, 25. [CrossRef] [PubMed]
88. Strain, H.H. *Leaf Xanthophylls*; Carnegie Institution of Washington: Washington, DC, USA, 1938.
89. Zhang, J.; Burgess, J.G. Enhanced eicosapentaenoic acid production by a new deep-sea marine bacterium Shewanella electrodiphila MAR441T. *PLoS ONE* **2017**, *12*, e0188081. [CrossRef] [PubMed]
90. Britton, G. *Carotenoids Volume 1B: Spectroscopy*; Britton, G., Ed.; Birkhauser Verlag: Basel, Switzerland, 1995.
91. Gueguen, S.; Herbeth, B.; Siest, G.; Leroy, P. An Isocratic Liquid Chromatographic Method with Diode-Array Detection for the Simultaneous Determination of alpha-Tocopherol, Retinol, and Five Carotenoids in

Human Serum. *J. Chromatogr. Sci.* **2002**, *40*, 69–76. [CrossRef] [PubMed]

92. European Medicines Agency. *Guideline on Bioanalytical Method Validation*; European Medicines Agency: Amsterdam, The Netherlands, 2011.
93. Brown, J.M.; Duewer, D.L.; Burdette, C.Q.; Sniegoski, L.T.; Yen, J.H. *Certification of Standard Reference Material® 968f Fat-Soluble Vitamins in Frozen Human Serum*; Special Publication, Report Number 260-188; National Institute of Standards and Technology: Gaithersburg, MD, USA, 2017.

3

Advantages and Pitfalls in Fluid Biomarkers for Diagnosis of Alzheimer's Disease

Syed Haris Omar [1,2,*] **and John Preddy** [1,2]

1 Rural Clinical School, Faculty of Medicine, University of New South Wales, Wagga Wagga, NSW 2650, Australia; j.preddy@unsw.edu.au

2 Murrumbidgee Local Health District, NSW Health, Wagga Wagga, NSW 2650, Australia

* Correspondence: haris.omar@unsw.edu.au or syedharisomar@gmail.com

Abstract: Alzheimer's disease (AD) is a commonly occurring neurodegenerative disease in the advanced-age population, with a doubling of prevalence for each 5 years of age above 60 years. In the past two decades, there has been a sustained effort to find suitable biomarkers that may not only aide with the diagnosis of AD early in the disease process but also predict the onset of the disease in asymptomatic individuals. Current diagnostic evidence is supportive of some biomarker candidates isolated from cerebrospinal fluid (CSF), including amyloid beta peptide (Aβ), total tau (*t*-tau), and phosphorylated tau (p-tau) as being involved in the pathophysiology of AD. However, there are a few biomarkers that have been shown to be helpful, such as proteomic, inflammatory, oral, ocular and olfactory in the early detection of AD, especially in the individuals with mild cognitive impairment (MCI). To date, biomarkers are collected through invasive techniques, especially CSF from lumbar puncture; however, non-invasive (radio imaging) methods are used in practice to diagnose AD. In order to reduce invasive testing on the patients, present literature has highlighted the potential importance of biomarkers in blood to assist with diagnosing AD.

Keywords: Alzheimer's disease; cerebrospinal fluid; amyloid beta peptide; total tau; phosphorylated tau; diagnosis

1. Introduction

Alzheimer's disease (AD) is one of the most common neurodegenerative disease in an ageing population. AD is the most common cause of dementia and is characterized by cognitive impairment and the impedance of daily activities, including communication, decision making and behavioral changes [1]. It has been shown that the frequency of AD doubles for each 5 years of life above the age of sixty years. It is predicted that by 2050, 130 million globally will be symptomatic from AD [2]. In terms of risk factors, advanced age is the most important risk for the sporadic or late onset of AD as well as the presence of APOE e4 alleles. Inherited mutations in chromosome 11 amyloid precursor protein (APP), Presenilin-1 ($PSEN_1$), and Presenilin-2 ($PSEN_2$) are prevalent in the less common familial form of AD. In addition, women are more prone to AD compared with men, early menopause is also risk factor for AD. Cardiovascular disease and diabetes mellitus type-2 are associated with an increased risk of AD. The exact pathophysiology of AD is still under investigation; however, the deposition of senile plaques, neurofibrillary tangles (NFTs), and astrogliosis are cardinal features [3]. Moreover, studies have shown that pathological involvement of oxidative stress, neuron degeneration induced synaptic alteration, inflammation and microgliosis are important in the pathogenesis of AD [4]. Despite almost 3 decades of research into the exact molecular mechanism causing AD, unfortunately, none of the hypothesis completely answers the question. The still amyloid cascade hypothesis suggests a core pathological role of amyloid beta in AD [5]. The presence of Aβ peptides in cerebral and peripheral tissues mainly consists of amino acids and their sequences ranging from 1 to 43. $A\beta_{42}$ is very prone to aggregate and proceed to form the senile plaques found in hippocampus, neocortex and in the cerebrovasculature region [6]. Another highly aggregated peptide called tau (which undergoes extensive hyperphosphorylation) is responsible for the formation of neurofibrillary tangles inside neurons and ultimately results in extensive brain and nerve damage [7]. Currently, approved drugs only provided symptomatic relief for patients with AD without modifying the disease or slowing disease progression. However, for the treatment of mild cognitive impairment (MCI), there is no FDA-approved drugs available and suggested to consider off-label treatment, such as an acetylcholinesterase (AChE) inhibitor, which has provided a modest impact but is also associated with the risk of side effects. In order to reduce the side effects, research has been undertaken to modify the chemical moiety of drugs with compatible substitutes and also focused on natural products with the potential to act as disease modifying agents [8,9]. Several natural products including curcumin, ginkgolides, resveratrol, oleuropein etc. have been shown to be effective against AD pathology in vitro or in vivo models but have not shown success in randomized trails [10–13]. Lifestyle modification, including exercise and dietary modification, especially the Mediterranean diet (MedDi) and Mediterranean-Dietary Approaches to Stop Hypertension (DASH) diet Intervention for Neurological Delay (MIND) diet, have been associated with improved cognition among elderly subjects [14].

It has been shown that pathological changes of AD occur long before the appearance of clinical symptoms. Therefore, it is important to establish a diagnosis as early as possible especially for people above the age 60 years. Biomarkers offer essential tools for AD diagnosis, monitoring, early detection, therapeutic intervention, as well as prevention of inaccurate diagnoses. Body fluid biomarkers in cerebrospinal fluid (CSF) and blood have shown potential for AD diagnosis, individual prognosis and patient stratification. Despite the availability of numerous theoretical and clinical diagnostic tools, AD is still poor diagnosed, especially in the early stage of the disease. AD has a prolonged pre-symptomatic prodromal phase; however, the lack of specific biomarker, procedural and methodological inconsistencies, inconsistent cut-off values as well as a lack of assay standardization, have thwarted attempts to establish a diagnosis and treat AD during this early phase.

2. Search Methods

Potential studies were identified in electronic database PubMed, Embase, ScienceDirect, Cochrane Library, SpringerLink, Scopus and Google Scholar using combination of following keywords "Alzheimer's Disease", "biomarkers" and "Alzheimer's disease", "cerebrospinal fluid", "CSF", "invasive biomarkers", "non-invasive biomarkers", "plasma biomarkers", "blood biomarkers", "plasma amyloid", "plasma tau", "inflammatory biomarkers", "imaging biomarkers", "proteomic biomarkers", "salivary biomarkers", "olfactory biomarkers" and "ocular biomarkers". Selected studies published between 1990 and May 2020 were included to ensure that all randomized trial, pilot studies, and critical reviews or systematic reviews published evidence on potential Alzheimer's disease biomarkers for three decades were encompassed. The preclinical studies, in vitro studies, published media, as well as duplicate articles were excluded due to being outside the scope of the clinical study aim.

3. Biomarkers in Alzheimer's Disease

A biomarker is usually characterized by substances (synthetic molecules, specified cells, proteins, enzymes, hormones or genetic material) or imaging finding, which is used as a metric characteristic to indicate the presence of a specific physiological state and may assist with establishing a diagnosis well before a clinical diagnosis can be made. Furthermore, the use of biomarkers is increasingly for assisting with the prognosis and diagnosis of AD, reflected by a tremendous increase in research from 1980 to current time (Figure 1).

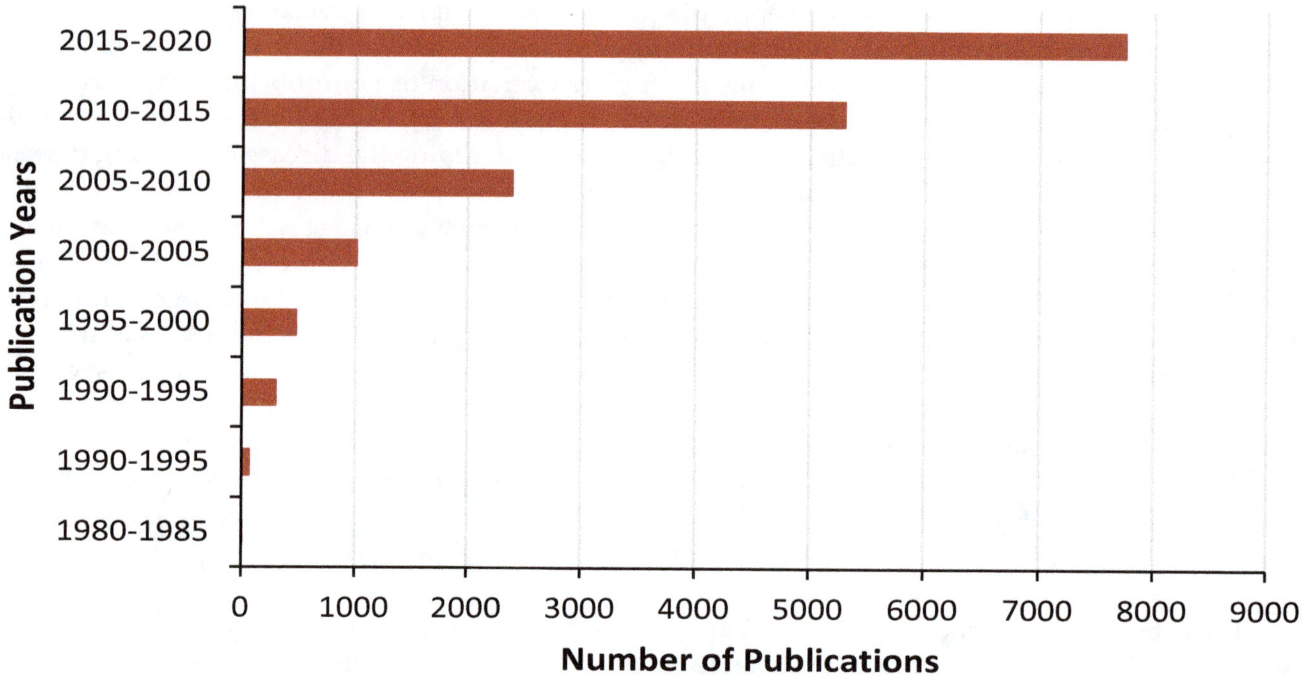

Figure 1. Publications statistics for "Biomarkers in Alzheimer's disease", source PubMed.

On the basis of AD pathogenesis and clinical condition, a set of diagnostic criteria were established in 1984, which was updated by the National Institute on Aging and Alzheimer's Association (NIA-AA) [15]. The updated NIA-AA guideline was mainly based upon the pathophysiological advancement in clinical, imaging, and research technologies in AD. Similarly, based upon clinical *probable*, *possible*, or *definite* symptoms, National Institute on Neurological and Communicative Disorder and Stroke and the Alzheimer's Disease and Related Disorders Association (NINCDS-ADRDA) have also published a diagnostic criteria for AD [16]. The clinical conditions of AD are considered to fall into three stages; however, some studies have expanded this to 1–5 or 1–7 stages. Of all the stages of AD, the prodromal period has the longest duration. This has resulted in a revision of NIA-AA diagnostic criteria, which are mainly based upon the identification of biomarkers, including CSF and imaging as valid diagnostic tools [17]. Based on modern diagnosis criteria, three sets of biomarkers are used as diagnostic tools, including Aβ peptide (A), tau peptide (T) and neurodegeneration (N), which are classified as A/T/N framework (Table 1) of AD diagnosis [17].

Table 1. Biomarkers based upon National Institute on Aging and Alzheimer's Association (NIA-AA) classification [17].

NIA-AA Classification	Alzheimer's Disease Biomarkers	Biomarkers Significance in AD
Amyloid (A) aggregates	CSF $A\beta_{42}$, $A\beta_{42}/A\beta_{40}$ ratio & Amyloid PET	↓ CSF $A\beta_{42}$ & $A\beta_{42}/A\beta_{40}$
Tau (T) aggregates	CSF phosphorylated tau & Tau PET	↑ CSF p-tau
Neurodegeneration (N)	CSF total tau & Anatomic MRI FDG PET	↑ t-tau

NIA-AA: National Institute on Aging and Alzheimer's Association; ↑: increase; ↓: decrease; CSF: cerebrospinal fluid; Aβ: β-amyloid; PET: positron emission tomography; FDG: fluorodeoxyglucose; MRI: magnetic resonance imaging.

4. Biomarkers Based upon Alzheimer's Disease Stages

Stage 1: assigned to the individuals who do not have functional impairment but might have cognitive impairment, which can only be detected through neuropsychological sensitive instruments. There is increasing evidence that certain biomarkers can predict the pathological changes at an early preclinical phase, namely the presence of amyloid imaging and a reduced CSF $A\beta_{42}$ concentration.

Early diagnosis based on biomarkers may assist with the approval of AD treatment, which could provide clinical benefits and improve outcomes [18]. Further trials are required to evaluate the reliability of clinical measurement and access the potential improvement with the drug-placebo conclusion.

Stage 2: Presence of biomarkers that predict pathophysiological changes of AD, a subtle cognitive effect, but no functional deficits in the patients, which can be detected with the use of sensitive instruments; however, they do not fulfil the criteria for dementia. According to the FDA guidance, sensitive neuropsychological testing should be considered alongside biomarker changes to diagnose AD stage 2 [18].

Stage 3: Pathophysiological biomarkers are present, and patients have started to have difficulty in doing some daily tasks which are measurable. This stage of the disease corresponds with mild cognitive impairment, whereas the first two stages are preclinical.

Stage 4, Stage 5 and Stage 6: Pathophysiological biomarkers are present with the consecutive stages of mild, moderate, and severe AD dementia with worsening cognitive impairment.

Assessment of Stages in AD

From the FDA classification of stages in Alzheimer's disease, stage 1 and 2 should be considered critical and monitored seriously. However, from stage 3 onwards, AD patients have similar pathophysiological biomarkers and ongoing cognitive decline. There are two basic questions that stem from the stages of AD. Which biomarkers may predict the presence of stage 1 and stage 2 AD in individuals? Secondly, from the treatment perspective, how can we establish the clinical effect of current FDA-approved drugs for patients with stage-1 AD, which is preclinical (based on the presence of amyloid and reduced CSF $A\beta_{42}$ concentration) without evidence of cognitive decline? There is a need to evaluate predictive biomarkers and establish whether changes in biomarkers is a predictor of treatment success.

5. Biomarkers through Invasive Diagnostic Methods

5.1. Cerebrospinal Fluid Biomarkers

Cerebrospinal fluid (CSF) is a clear liquid that is present in the subarachnoid space and ventricular system of the brain and spinal cord. The volume of CSF in the body varies between 125 and 150 mL. The composition of CSF can demonstrate minor biochemical change in the brain. Currently, CSF is considered an excellent biologic fluid that may contain potential biomarkers for AD, which may be able to identify without going through autopsy or biopsy. Furthermore, the presence and concentration of biomarkers may change in parallel to AD progression. The three most suggestive biomarkers in AD are $A\beta$, total tau (t-tau), and phosphorylated tau (p-tau) (Table 2). It has been suggested that CSF biomarkers did not vary with severity with stable levels noted in the follow-up patients with clinical AD [19].

Table 2. Established diagnostic biomarkers in the cerebrospinal fluid CSF of Alzheimer's disease (AD) [a] [20] and showed 85% sensitivity cutoff values for AD dementia diagnosis [21].

Biomarkers	Controls (pg/mL)	AD (pg/mL)	% Sensitivity (AD-Control)	% Sensitivity (MCI-Control)
$A\beta_{42}$	794 ± 20	<500 *	73 (≥75 years)	60 (≥75 years)
tau peptide	136 ± 89 (21–50 years)	[b]	74 (≤64 years)	65 (≤64 years)
	243 ± 127 (51–70 years)	>450	53 (65–74 years)	49 (65–74 years)
	341 ± 171 (>71 years)	>600 *	61 (≥75 years)	46 (≥75 years)
p-tau-181	23 ± 2	>60	37 (≥75 years)	30 (≥75 years)

[a] Data obtained using innogenetics single 96-well ELISA kits. [b] This is not relevant for sporadic AD, because it is only for patients >60 years of age. * $p < 0.001$.

5.1.1. CSF Aβ Biomarker

The amyloid isoforms $A\beta_{40}$ and $A\beta_{42}$ concentration in CSF are considered to be the most dependable biomarkers for the diagnosis of the AD disease. The production of both amyloid isoforms $A\beta_{40}$ and $A\beta_{42}$ was 24% higher for mutation carriers than noncarriers in the autosomal dominant AD patients. However, it was suggested that the fractional turnover rate of $A\beta_{42}$ was noted 65% higher in mutation carriers [22]. Interestingly, it was also reported that there is no change in CSF $A\beta_{40}$, while it is present in a 10-fold higher concentration than $A\beta_{42}$ in the CSF of AD patients. It was suggested that $A\beta_{42}$ be used as a proxy of total Aβ concentration. The amyloidogenic protein is found throughout the human body, and studies showed that $A\beta_{42}$ concentrations in CSF often correlate with Aβ levels in the patient's brain [23]. It was found that the $A\beta_{42}$ concentration was significantly reduced in CSF, which is a consequence of its presence in fibrils and plaques in the brains of patients with AD [24–26]. There are variations in quantification; however, it was found that $A\beta_{42}$ concentration declined by 50% in CSF of patients with AD as a result of its deposition in the brain parenchyma [27].

The underlying mechanisms of the reduction CSF $A\beta_{42}$ is not clear; however, few studies have suggested that it is due to the excessive hydrophobic aggregation of $A\beta_{42}$ sequestration in plaques, a reduction in its diffusion from interstitial fluid to CSF and/or decreased Aβ clearance as a consequence of an impaired blood–brain barrier [28,29]. It was reported that the other isoform of amyloid peptides, $A\beta_{38}$, was also found to have an increased concentration in CSF. Furthermore, the ratio of $A\beta_{42}/A\beta_{38}$ closely corresponds with imaging findings in patients with AD and thus results in a robust biomarkers for AD pathogenesis, which is more useful than the concentration of $A\beta_{42}$ alone in CSF [30,31]. In contrast, several studies have reported that the $A\beta_{40}$ concentration was unchanged in CSF from patients with AD and does not correlate with amyloid deposits in the brain [32]. In spite of the discrepancy in the diagnosis of CSF $A\beta_{40}$ levels, several studies supported a decrease CSF $A\beta_{42/40}$ ratio in the diagnosis of MCI patients compared to controls [33]. Because of the observed Aβ isoforms ratio and their positive relationship with AD pathogenesis, the NIA-AA has accepted $A\beta_{42}$ concentration as well as a comparative ratio of $A\beta_{42}/A\beta_{40}$ as important biomarkers in the diagnostic guideline for AD [17].

5.1.2. Assessment of CSF $A\beta_{42}$ Biomarker

CSF $A\beta_{42}$ biomarkers support a diagnosis of AD in its preclinical stage and are predictors of disease progression in cognitively unimpaired individuals and in those with MCI. One of the main limitations of CSF sampling is its invasive collection technique i.e., through lumbar puncture compared with blood sampling. Post lumbar puncturing, headache as most common adverse effect.

Most of the studies showed a significant decline in $A\beta_{42}$ levels as diagnostic biomarker and agreed that upto 40% reduction was observed in AD patients when compared with those of healthy individuals [34]. In contrast to the reduction of $A\beta_{42}$ concentration in CSF, some of the past studies have shown an unchanged $A\beta_{42}$ concentration [35] and an elevated level [36] in CSF $A\beta_{42}$ concentration compared to AD patients and healthy controls. CSF $A\beta_{42}$ was found to reach the plateau state early in the disease progression and produce a conflicting outcome, which demonstrates a process of preceding aggregation of Aβ mainly detected with amyloid PET analysis. There is a lack of standard protocol and universal agreement because of the varying biomarker concentrations and contradictory outcomes, which required further investigation in the age- and stage-matched individuals considering prodromal stage individuals with different ethnic groups. It has been demonstrated that CSF $A\beta_{42/40}$ ratio may predict abnormal cortical amyloid deposition (visualized with PET) compared with CSF $A\beta_{42}$. However, this diagnosis could result as false positive (low CSF $A\beta_{42}$) or false negative (high CSF $A\beta_{42}$) in fewer patients [25]. Further studies have been reported the presence of oligomers formation prior to the formation of Aβ fibrils in the pathogenesis of AD and suggested oligomers as potential early target in the prodromal stages, which required further confirmation in randomized trial as early diagnostic biomarker.

5.1.3. CSF Tau Biomarker

The Aβ and tau peptides have been suggested to interact mutually and prompt both aggregation and toxicity followed by proposed mechanisms including Aβ encourage tau pathology or tau induces Aβ toxicity, or synergistic toxicity exists between Aβ and tau [37,38]. Basically, tau is a microtubule associated protein have a pivotal action in intracellular transportation. Tau proteins classified as p-tau representing hyperphosphorylation, and t-tau representing several isomers of the tau protein. It was suggested that the hyperphosphorylation occur at threonine-231 (p-tau_{231}), threonine-181 (p-tau_{181}), and at serine-199 (p-tau_{199}). The involvement of p-tau in the assembly of neurofibrillary tangles represented as 'T' marker, and their presence in the CSF proving a sign of neuronal death as 'N' marker [39,40]. It was reported that CSF p-tau_{231} was involved in the neurofibrillary neocortical pathology [40], and showed a significant increase in concentration correlated with a decline in cognitive performance and conversion to AD [41]. The concentration of t-tau in CSF was found to be highly age dependent and observed <300 pg/mL in 21–50 years, <450 pg/mL in 51–70 years, and <500 ng/L in 71–93 years age group of normal cognitive healthy individuals [42]. Several lines of studies have supported the results of significant rise in CSF tau peptide concentration in AD patients [39,43]. In particular, p-tau and t-tau were found to be increased by 200% 300% concentration in AD compared with nondemented elderly subjects [27,44]. Tau pathology cause an elevated level of CSF t-tau and p-tau and strongly associated with cognitive decline compared to the amyloid pathology.

Furthermore, the degree of neurodegeneration and neuronal/axonal damage in AD patients' brains marked by the presence of considerable CSF t-tau concentrations and constituted in the A,T,N Framework as a marker of 'N' [17,45,46]. A systematic review included 15 studies showed the presence and accuracy of CSF t-tau in seven studies, while six studies have showed the presence and accuracy of the CSF p-tau in mild cognitive impaired patients [47].

The intermediate filaments known as neurofilament light (NfL) were found to be present in the axons cytoplasm and may interfere with cytoplasmic function of axonal homeostasis as well as synaptic transmission. Studies have shown the presence of elevated NfL in AD patients and suggested end results of neuronal and axon damages [48]. More pronouncedly, the increase level of NfL could serve as a risk factor for MCI. However, elevated NfL levels were also recognized as a biomarker in other neurodegenerative diseases having marked axonal degeneration, white matter injury, or both, such as frontotemporal dementia, amyotrophic lateral sclerosis, Creutzfeldt–Jakob disease, multiple sclerosis and traumatic brain injury. A few post-mortem studies have reported significant elevated NfL levels in patients with amyotrophic lateral sclerosis and frontotemporal dementia more than the AD patients and suggested that NfL could be used for differentiation of two types of dementia [49]. Due to non-specificity in disease diagnosis, NfL is less popular as confirmatory biomarkers compared to Aβ and tau in AD.

5.1.4. Assessment of CSF Tau Biomarker

The increase in both CSF t-tau and p-tau concentrations are well settled in AD compared with controls, specifically the intensity of neuronal injury and neurodegeneration are indicated by CSF t-tau in AD. The concentration of CSF t-tau was reported two to three folds higher in patients with AD compared to the normal controls [34]. Still, it is not confirmed about the agreement in distinct tau phosphorylation sites for AD. Most studies have showed the significant rise in tau concentration with aging as well as in patients with AD; however, few studies have reported contradictory information and showed no significant change in the CSF tau level in normal healthy aged individuals [50]. It was postulated that the incidence of tau phosphorylation and the building of neurofibrillary tangles inside neuron is a results of cellular protective mechanism against oxidative stress and suggesting normal physiological pathway rather than a toxic pathway [51]. It is still unknown about the inconsistent results for tau analysis and required to develop a new technique for consistent outcome. It has been suggested that, due to the presence of heterogeneity in trial subjects, the consistency of the result varies and not being reproducible. Thus, there is a requirement to agree on one productive model for the diagnosis of CSF tau biomarkers and run the trial in a large cohort that can be reproducible or verify in a repetitive/confirmatory trial.

5.2. Blood Biomarkers in AD

Blood is a most commonly accessible biological sample than other body fluids such as CSF and offer inexpensive clinical diagnosis or screening methods and even convenient for getting reproducible results in clinical trials. In cardiovascular disease and cancer diagnosis and research, biofluid blood has been established as biomarkers; therefore, it may perform as a critical measure in the early diagnosis of AD [52]. Due to the presence of Aβ in the prodromal stage of AD and their ability to pass through the blood–brain barrier, for diagnostic purposes, Aβ received a considerable amount of attention as a potential blood biomarker.

5.2.1. Plasma Aβ Biomarker

In order to evaluate and understand amyloid clearance, studies reported a significant decline in amyloid clearance using the stable isotope labelling kinetic method in late-onset AD patient [53]. Both $A\beta_{40}$ and $A\beta_{42}$ production were found to be increased by 24% in individuals with mutation carriers than noncarriers autosomal dominant form of AD (ADAD), and, furthermore, the $A\beta_{42}$ fractional turnover rate was 65% faster deposition in mutation carriers individuals [22]. Several studies have reported the existence of Aβ in blood plasma and showed the rise of both $A\beta_{40}$ [54] and $A\beta_{42}$ [55] levels. In contrast, studies have also reported a fall in both $A\beta_{40}$ [56,57] and $A\beta_{42}$ [58] concentrations in individuals susceptible to AD. More recently, a comprehensive meta-analysis study showed the inconsistency in plasma for both $A\beta_{42}$ and $A\beta_{40}$ in AD [59]. In order to achieve consistency and accuracy in the biomarker analysis, trials based on immunoprecipitation-mass-spectrometry-based assays for evaluation showed a significant decline in both $A\beta_{40}$ and $A\beta_{42}$ concentration in plasma $A\beta_{42}/A\beta_{40}$ ratio (in the line with CSF test) with approximately 90% of diagnostic accuracy [60,61].

5.2.2. Assessment of Plasma Aβ Biomarkers in AD

Blood considered as highly complex fluid connective tissue containing cellular components and several compounds, such as proteinases nature compounds, genetic materials, and metabolites, appear in plasma. The primary barrier for inconsistency in the biomarkers analysis results was suggested due to the presence of low blood Aβ concentration as well as victims of matrix effects. In addition, a lack in assay sensitivity, specificity and methods selectivity are responsible for inconsistency in Aβ finding as biomarkers in blood. In general, biomarkers localized in the brain are not easily available in blood because of the restriction of movement through the blood–brain barrier, poor expression of AD pathology biomarkers in blood and the interference of blood containing endogenous antibodies with the assay reagents that finally resulted in a false rise and fall of measurement. There is a need to develop the analytical sensitive plasma-based assay, which can minimize the event of reaction of biomarkers such as Aβ with the reagent, and careful validation work. A few attempts have been made to analyze Aβ in blood through a new diagnostic technique; however, such attempts were unable to resolve the cerebral expression of Aβ including plasma protein and blood platelets [62] but still represent an important step forward.

5.2.3. Plasma Tau Biomarker

Studies have been reported that the elevated plasma tau levels but with overlapping ranges of results across diagnostic groups of AD patients compared with the normal control [63]. It has been suggested that the plasma tau is a late-stage marker of AD and did not show any change in the plasma of the MCI-stage individual followed by missing the interrelationship between tau levels in plasma and CSF due to the differential regulation of tau in both fluids [63]. Further study showed a positive associations between increased plasma tau level and AD hallmarks [64]. The elevated level of plasma total tau and $pTau_{181}$ were investigated in patients with dementia compared to the cognitively unimpaired individuals [65]. In general, total tau protein concentration was found to be approximately seven times higher than p-tau$_{181}$ in human plasma. Based on immunomagnetic reduction technique, a study evaluated the concentration ratios of p-tau$_{181}$ to t-tau in plasma are 14.4% for healthy controls, 13.6% for patients with MCI due to AD, and 19.5% for very mild AD, respectively, and suggested that p-tau$_{181}$ in plasma can be used to differentiate memory disorder/cognitive decline in early-stage AD patients [66]. Further study based on the evaluation of plasma p-tau$_{181}$ as a biomarker using ultrasensitive immunoassay methods showed a significantly higher plasma p-tau$_{181}$ level in the AD group compared with the control group [67]. A recent study measured plasma-phosphorylated tau concentration and found a significantly higher concentration in the AD group compared with age-matched cognitively normal controls [68]. Tau hyperphosphorylation-induced neuronal damage was also investigated and suggested the presence of neurofilament as biomarker for neurodegeneration in AD [69]. Neurofilament was measured by using an ultrasensitive immunoassay method and showed increased serum neurofilament light (NfL) concentration in familial AD prior to symptomatic disease [70]. In the line of the previous report, a recent study outcome showed an early rise of serum neurofilament light in the presymptomatic phase of familial AD and continue to increase in neurofilament light level, respectively [71]. Increased plasma neurofilament light was found in MCI and AD dementia patients compared with controls and correlated with poor cognition [72].

NfL in plasma well determined, reported their elevated levels in the serum of familial AD patients usually appear a decade ahead to the onset of symptom and well correlated with whole-brain atrophy intensity through MRI and an assessment of cognition [73]. In addition, a high level of NfL was determined in plasma of MCI compared to AD patients and healthy controls, which can be used as a determinant assay to easily distinguish individual between MCI and AD [72].

5.2.4. Assessment of Plasma Tau Biomarkers in AD

In the past two decades, it is still in debate that tau pathology starts early in normal cognitive individuals upon ageing (>60 years) than Aβ pathology. However, research based on tau pathophysiology have showed high consistency in the increase level of tau protein (neurofilament light, p-tau$_{181}$, and total tau as biomarkers) and easily detected in serum. In contrast, Aβ (Aβ_{40}, Aβ_{42} and Aβ_{42}/Aβ_{40} as biomarkers) protein appearance in blood do not show those consistent results in early stage of AD progression regardless with the determination techniques. It was suggested that ultrasensitive immunoassays granted the accurate quantification of tau in blood. Further research is required to justify and validate tau protein as an early diagnostic biomarker in AD.

6. Biomarkers through Non-Invasive Diagnostic Methods

6.1. Cognitive Biomarkers

Currently, non-invasive diagnostic criteria for AD based on a group of assessments, including individual clinical history, cognitive and neuropsychological state and clinical rating score resulted from Mini-Mental State Examination (MMSE), Clinical Dementia Rating (CDR) and the Wechsler Memory Scale (WMS) Logical Memory (LM) test [74]. According to the MMSE score (0–30), if an individual has received a score between 20 and 24, then suggested mild dementia, followed by a score between 13 and 20 suggest moderate dementia and have a score less than 12 designated severe dementia [75]. A study evaluated the accuracy of the MMSE for diagnosing dementia subtypes in people aged 65 years who do not examine earlier for dementia and supported the diagnostic use of MMSE as part of the process for deciding whether or not someone has dementia [76]. The LM test consist of LM-I (immediate recall), LM-II (delayed recall), and LM Recognition (delayed recognition), used to investigate and measure verbal episodic memory in individuals [77]. The LM-I directed individual to immediately recall details of two short passages, while LM-II phase based on recall the passages after a 20 to 30-min delay. The LM recognition phase test provided questionnaire-based evaluation on an earlier provided passage in the form of yes or no.

6.2. Assessment of Cognitive Biomarkers

Several studies have indicated the psychometric limitations of MMSE analysis, including large ceiling and floor effects, and sensitivity to practice effects, limiting the clinical efficacy of MMSE in MCI and AD dementia investigation. Moreover, the scoring system in MMSE was found to lack accuracy in the investigation of individuals with MCI or mild AD dementia. The LM subtest is not only useful for distinguishing certain types of dementia such as AD dementia but is also known as a tool that can detect subtle memory changes in the individuals with MCI [78].

6.3. Imaging Biomarkers

The imaging of the brain in the diagnosis of AD has been used as a second line of diagnostic criteria, including magnetic resonance imaging (MRI), functional MRI (fMRI) and positron emission tomography (PET). In a clinical setting, current guidelines follow the structural imaging, i.e., magnetic resonance imaging (MRI) or computerized tomography (CT), mainly required for the evaluation of patients presenting with a cognitive/dementia syndrome [79]. In order to investigate the visualization of AD-linked cortical atrophy and changes in brain connectivity, MRI is used to provide a structural and functional imaging technique [80]. In addition, fMRI investigation provided the functional connectivity of the brain such as abnormality in the hippocampus [81]. Positron emission tomography (PET) is an advanced imaging technique using compounds labelled with short-lived positron-emitting radionuclides to detect Aβ associated metabolic activity and plaques deposition in AD [82]. Commonly used PET tracers, including Pittsburgh Compound-B (PiB) and Fluoro-2-deoxy-D-glucose (FDG), have a high sensitivity and specificity of diagnosis, particularly in the early stages, and are utilized in imaging biomarkers of amyloid plaque progression in individuals [83].

6.4. Assessment of Imaging Biomarkers

In a clinical setting for AD diagnosis, imaging techniques are often used as a second or third line of investigation due to the unavailability of imaging facility at every center, especially in rural areas. Imaging require rigorous measurement, expertise to interpret the findings and burden of high cost, preventing their frequent use in the routine clinical assessment of individual during their first visit. ^{18}F-FDG-PET analysis may differentiate dementia from normal aging and is used as an indicator biomarker for neurodegeneration; however, it is unable to track down pathology at an early stage of AD. In addition, the current practicing guidelines and expert opinions suggested that amyloid PET analysis was unable to anticipate the trajectory of AD disease progression for an individual patient [84,85]. Moreover, it is also uncertain how effective the PET analysis is at characterizing differences across the pathophysiological phase of AD.

7. Promising Biomarkers in AD

7.1. Proteomic or Enzymatic Biomarkers in AD

In order to investigate novel protein and their capacity to predict AD, an early study analyzed 120 plasma proteins and discovered 18 signaling proteins, which showed 90% of accuracy in diagnosis for AD patients and 91% for MCI patients [86]. Further studies have been reported a total of 1590 AD-related proteins, including 296 proteins encoded with 115 up-regulated and 181 down-regulated genes, and supposed to be blood-secretory proteins involved in the pathogenesis of AD [87]. It was suggested that around 35 AD-related proteins are consistent, including four key proteins (APP, apolipoprotein E, PSEN-1, and PSEN-2) involved in AD pathology [87]. Synaptic proteins such as synaptosomal-associated protein 25 (SNAP-25) and synaptotagmin-1 (SYT1) were found to be significantly increased in the CSF of AD dementia and prodromal AD patients; however, SNAP-25 and SYT1 were specified to decline in cortical areas [88,89]. To facilitate early diagnosis in AD, a protein profiling of blood samples in mild AD patients showed a downregulation of apolipoprotein A_1, α-2-HS-glycoprotein, and afamin, while, apolipoprotein A_4 and the fibrinogen gamma chain were identified upregulated [90].

The CSF BACE1 enzymatic activity and protein concentration has been elevated in AD patients [91], and represented as an indicator biomarker of MCI [92]. In support of elevated BACE1 activity, a study reported a significant rise in plasma BACE1 activity by 53.2% in subjects with MCI and by 68.9% in patients with AD and suggesting plasma BACE1 activity as a diagnostic biomarker [93]. The study focused on plasma-based biomarkers showed a significantly elevated level of BACE1, and soluble forms of APP were observed in AD patient [94]. Further study showed the presence of increased BACE1 enzymatic activity along with the increase in phospholipase-A_2 activity in platelets and brains of patient with AD [95]. One of the main interests for determining BACE1 biomarker is the development of specific BACE1 inhibitors, which may help in the reduction of amyloid production. It is unfortunate that the present plasma BACE1 investigation as biomarkers have not demonstrated a consistent result in terms of significant rise in BACE1 in AD patients compared to normal individuals. In search of other proteomic or enzymatic biomarker, the protein kinases such as glycogen synthase kinase 3β (GSK-3β) has been observed in tau protein hyperphosphorylation, and reported significantly elevated in plasma of MCI and AD patients compared with aged-matched controls [96] as well as their elevated level was also observed in white blood cells of AD and MCI patients compared with healthy individuals [97].

7.2. Assessment of Proteomic or Enzymatic Biomarkers

Several studies have shown the presence of proteins in plasma or serum, including albumin, lipoproteins, Aβ autoantibodies, fibrinogen, immunoglobulin, apolipoprotein-J, apolipoprotein-E, transthyretin, α-2-macroglobulin, serum amyloid p-component, plasminogen and amylin were found to be strongly interferes with the estimation of specific protein biomarkers. It was found that studies that have been conducted on proteomic or enzymatic biomarkers were only in cohorts with unmatched age patients and a target single protein or enzymatic marker; therefore, such studies were required to be focused on proteomics and enzymatic research in individuals with MCI and AD compared to aged-matched controls. Proteomic or enzymatic biomarkers could be an excellent and potential candidate for blood biomarkers as diagnostic tools, but due to the presence of low concentration and the incidence of protein-protein interactions in plasma result the inconsistency in outcomes.

Therefore, it is difficult to replicate due to the lack of specificity and accuracy involved in the current methods of investigation. Thus, the development of highly sensitive and reproducible novel methods that might have the capability to detect the plasma biomarkers in low concentration with accuracy is required.

7.3. Inflammatory Biomarkers in AD

Inflammation is one of the major cellular events considered at the initial pathogenic factor causing neurodegeneration in AD mainly through the activation of microglia. Out of the several investigated inflammatory biomarkers, the diminished C-reactive protein (CRP) level and increased level of triggering receptor expressed on myeloid cells-2 (TREM-2) were observed in the CSF of the patient with AD compared to the normal elderly controls [98]. Moreover, the reduced levels of plasma CRP was also observed in AD patients compared to MCI or normal cognition individuals [99]. The estimation of TREM-2 in CSF and blood is a marker of microglia response. Several studies have investigated the concentration of TREM-2 and reported their increased levels in CSF of AD patient, which was mainly associated with tau pathology compared to the controls [100,101].

Further studies have shown polymorphism in about 23 cytokines, and their 13 types were found to be observed in AD pathogenesis, including interleukins, TNF-α, TGF-β and IFN-γ [102]. Pro-inflammatory cytokines such as TNF-α level were significantly increased followed by decrease in the anti-inflammatory cytokine TGF-β level in CSF, which showed a positive correlation with a higher risk of disease progression from MCI to AD [103]. The concentration of cytokine I-309 level was found to be increased in CSF and suggested as a possible predictor of progression from MCI to AD patients [104]. It has been suggested that the presence of cytokines elevated steadily or reached the highest level upon progression from MCI to AD individuals, including IL-1β, IL-6, TNF-α, IL-18, monocyte chemotactic protein (MCP)-1 and IL-10 can be used as a predicting biomarker for early diagnosis [102].

Microglial activation involved in the stimulation of astrocytic expression of YKL-40 (also known as chitinase-3-like protein-1 (CHI3L1)), which was observed in significantly higher levels in the CSF of AD patients compared to the cognitively normal individuals [105]. Most of the studies have investigated the elevated effect of YKL-40 in CSF; however, less studies have been able to detect YKL-40 in blood, showing a similar finding of increased YKL-40 level in plasma [106].

7.4. Assessment of Inflammatory Biomarkers in AD

Despite the elevation of the inflammatory biomarker TREM-2 in AD, few studies have reported conflicting results with no significant change in CSF TREM-2 levels in MCI and AD patients compared to the controls [107]. In addition, to recognize TREM-2 as a potential inflammatory biomarker in AD diagnosis, their physiological function has been questioned whether it has a constructive or a harmful effect in human body. Due to non-specific diagnosis of TREM-2 in other neuroinflammatory diseases, the biomarkers have faced challenges and required further studies to answer these questions on the molecular basis. The other biomarker YKL-40 investigation in AD have shown a limited diagnostic value due to their non-specific findings in neurological disease other than AD. However, it has been suggested that YKL-40 has a potential role in astroglial activation and the assessment of neuroinflammation treatment, which required further investigation with a specified sensitive method and an inflammatory biomarker in AD.

The majority of studies investigated inflammatory cytokines or chemokines as biomarkers insufficiently sensitive in plasma and could not be reproduced. In addition, there was a lack in the conduction of study in a large cohort using imaging or CSF samples of individuals with MCI and AD for the detection of inflammatory biomarkers. Therefore, it is warranted to investigate and confirm inflammatory biomarkers targeting individuals for early intervention in future studies.

7.5. Oral, Ocular and Olfactory Fluid Biomarkers in AD

Body fluid other than CSF and blood, including oral, ocular and olfactory have received attention for detecting the biomarkers of AD because of their easily available, noninvasive nature and inexpensive sample collection methods. A decade ago, one pilot study reported a significant rise in saliva $A\beta_{42}$ levels in patients with mild AD compared to the control, while saliva $A\beta_{40}$ level was detected unchanged [108]. Further study reported a two-folds increase in salivary $A\beta_{42}$ concentration in AD patients compared to the controls, which have identical levels of salivary $A\beta_{42}$ regardless of sex or age [109]. Further pilot study using the 1H NMR metabolomics technique for detecting salivary $A\beta_{42}$ found a significant rise in salivary $A\beta_{42}$ concentration in MCI and AD patients compared to controls [110]. In the line of previous results showing the elevated level of salivary $A\beta_{42}$, a study based on enzyme-linked immunosorbent-type assays methods reported an increased $A\beta_{42}$ level in patients with AD compared to controls [111].

In order to attempt early diagnosis and the development of a non-invasive method for AD, studies have reported the presence of significant Aβ plaque concentration deposited in the retina [112]. A quantitative and histological study showed a two-fold increase in retinal Aβ deposition in the form of protofibrils and fibrils among AD patients versus controls [113]. A similar study has detected retinal Aβ plaque deposition two months prior to their presence in the hippocampus and cortices of AD murine models and suggested the appearance of Aβ in the retina is an early event in the pathogenesis of AD [113]. The emerging single visit, label-free, cost-effective eye scan along with the emergence of mobile imaging modalities for the early detection of Aβ plaques in retina through the polarization imaging of retinal Aβ and retinal fluorescence lifetime imaging ophthalmoscopy have been suggested as early diagnostic tools [114].

The olfactory dysfunction has been associated with tau pathology from early to advanced AD and is well recognized. A study based on the Braak stage of AD showed the presence of tau pathology 90% and Aβ 9% in stage 4 followed by 44.6% of tau pathology and Aβ 9% in stage 3 [115]. The olfactory tau pathology in stage 2 represented by 36.4% without Aβ deposition; however, Braak stages 0 and 1 do not show any positive association of tau pathology [115]. Further study showed significant elevation in t-tau protein and p-tau tau protein levels in the patients with AD suffering from loss of smell, compared to the healthy controls [116]. The results of a recent meta-analysis suggested that the identification of olfactory dysfunction was more profound in AD patients compared to MCI patients [117].

7.6. Assessment of Oral, Ocular and Olfactory Fluid Biomarkers in AD

The oral, ocular and olfactory biofluid as potential biomarkers in AD diagnosis are still in the preliminary stage of research, requiring further investigation to overcome the methodological heterogeneity and discrepancy in accuracy. Thus, there is a need to develop a reliable quantitative method among consecutive or random samples to determine these biomarkers as an effective tool for diagnosing AD.

8. Conclusions

AD is a multifactorial disease without a confirmatory biomarker; however, based on the NIA-AA guideline, the currently available biomarkers may provide a positive direction to identify individuals who are on risk of AD, and need of routine screening for early diagnosis. The most studied and practiced biomarkers for AD diagnosis are CSF $A\beta_{42}$, CSF $A\beta_{42}/A\beta_{40}$, CSF p-tau, amyloid PET, tau PET, structural MRI and fMRI. The accumulated evidences have been established that $A\beta_{42}$ and tau levels were found quite lower (~30 to 100 times) in plasma compared to CSF. Furthermore, because plasma and serum already enriched with immense level of several proteins (~50–70 g/L) which interferes in detection and face challenges in poor outcome of NIA-AA suggested biomarkers in blood compared to CSF. Therefore, there is no doubt that the investigation of biomarkers in blood face inconsistency in findings due to their low appearance (concentration) in blood (plasma or serum) than in the CSF. To date, there are weak evidences supporting the dominance of biomarker over the other (CSF/imaging) for diagnostic tools in AD. Thus, in terms of availability or diagnosis, CSF have less challenges in the A/T/N framework-based biomarkers compared to blood-based biomarkers (Figure 2). Despite of challenges in blood-based biomarkers, the early detection of biomarkers (plasma NfL) could be a promising diagnostic tool in body fluid blood which can be routinely investigate in the individual reaching the age of 60 years. In a nut-shell, blood-based biomarkers should pay more attention in order to support the patient's comfort, highly sensitive, least invasive and cost-effective inexpensive technologies for biomarker detection are required for detection and analysis in the range of 10^{-15} to 10^{-12} M in individuals before entering MCI stage.

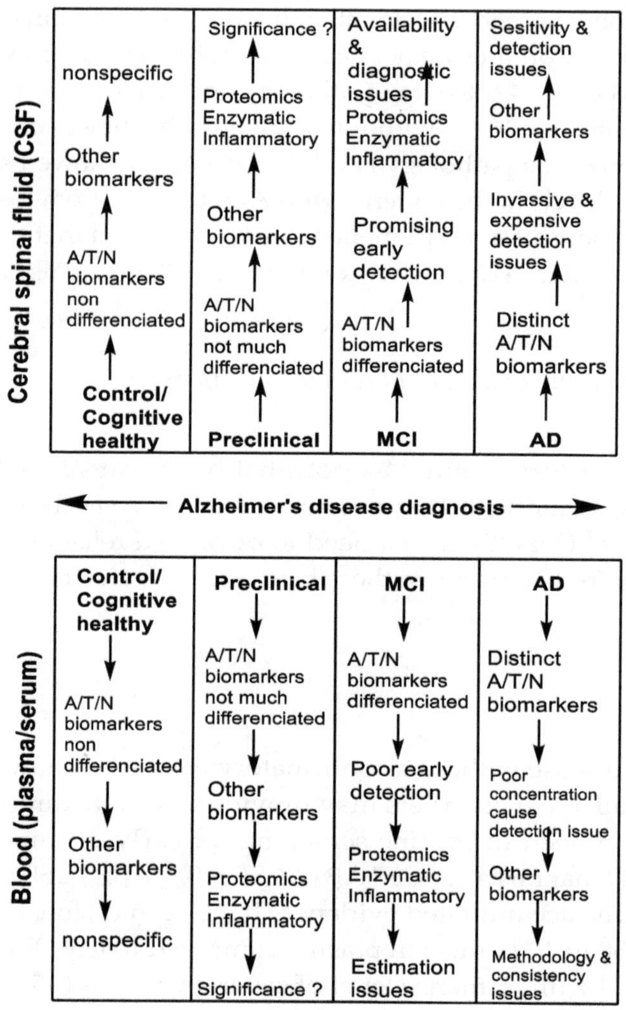

Figure 2. Overview of investigation and development CSF and blood-based biomarkers in Alzheimer's disease diagnosis.

Author Contributions: S.H.O. has created idea, designed and wrote the manuscript; J.P. has assisted in drafting the manuscript. All authors have read and agreed to the published version of the manuscript.

Acknowledgments: Rural Clinical School, Faculty of Medicine, University of New South Wales, Wagga Wagga, NSW, Australia & *Murrumbidgee Local Health District*, NSW Health, Wagga Wagga, NSW 2650.

References

1. Scheltens, P.; Blennow, K.; Breteler, M.M.; de Strooper, B.; Frisoni, G.B.; Salloway, S.; Van der Flier, W.M. Alzheimer's disease. *Lancet* **2016**, *388*, 505–517. [CrossRef]
2. Alzheimer's, A. 2016 Alzheimer's disease facts and figures. *Alzheimers Dement.* **2016**, *12*, 459–509. [CrossRef] [PubMed]
3. Pozueta, J.; Lefort, R.; Shelanski, M.L. Synaptic changes in Alzheimer's disease and its models. *Neuroscience* **2013**, *251*, 51–65. [CrossRef]
4. Sharma, P.; Srivastava, P.; Seth, A.; Tripathi, P.N.; Banerjee, A.G.; Shrivastava, S.K. Comprehensive review of mechanisms of pathogenesis involved in Alzheimer's disease and potential therapeutic strategies. *Prog. Neurobiol.* **2019**, *174*, 53–89. [CrossRef]
5. Selkoe, D.J.; Hardy, J. The amyloid hypothesis of Alzheimer's disease at 25 years. *EMBO Mol. Med.* **2016**, *8*, 595–608. [CrossRef]

6. Sadigh-Eteghad, S.; Sabermarouf, B.; Majdi, A.; Talebi, M.; Farhoudi, M.; Mahmoudi, J. Amyloid-beta: A crucial factor in Alzheimer's disease. *Med. Princ. Pract.* **2015**, *24*, 1–10. [CrossRef]
7. Braak, H.; Del Tredici, K. Alzheimer's pathogenesis: Is there neuron-to-neuron propagation? *Acta Neuropathol.* **2011**, *121*, 589–595. [CrossRef] [PubMed]
8. Omar, S.H.; Scott, C.J.; Hamlin, A.S.; Obied, H.K. The protective role of plant biophenols in mechanisms of Alzheimer's disease. *J. Nutr. Biochem.* **2017**, *47*, 1–20. [CrossRef] [PubMed]
9. Omar, S.H.; Scott, C.J.; Hamlin, A.S.; Obied, H.K. Biophenols: Enzymes (beta-secretase, Cholinesterases, histone deacetylase and tyrosinase) inhibitors from olive (Olea europaea L.). *Fitoterapia* **2018**, *128*, 118–129. [CrossRef]
10. Omar, S.H.; Scott, C.J.; Hamlin, A.S.; Obied, H.K. Olive Biophenols Reduces Alzheimer's Pathology in SH-SY5Y Cells and APPswe Mice. *Int. J. Mol. Sci.* **2018**, *20*, 125. [CrossRef]
11. Omar, S.H. Biophenols pharmacology against the amyloidogenic activity in Alzheimer's disease. *Biomed. Pharm.* **2017**, *89*, 396–413. [CrossRef] [PubMed]
12. Omar, S.H. Oleuropein in olive and its pharmacological effects. *Sci. Pharm.* **2010**, *78*, 133–154. [CrossRef] [PubMed]
13. Omar, S.H. Ginkgolides and Neuroprotective Effects. In *Natural Products: Phytochemistry, Botany and Metabolism of Alkaloids, Phenolics and Terpenes*; Ramawat, K.G., Mérillon, J.-M., Eds.; Springer: Berlin/Heidelberg, Germany, 2013; pp. 3697–3741. [CrossRef]
14. Omar, S.H. Mediterranean and MIND Diets Containing Olive Biophenols Reduces the Prevalence of Alzheimer's Disease. *Int. J. Mol. Sci.* **2019**, *20*, 2797. [CrossRef] [PubMed]
15. McKhann, G.M.; Knopman, D.S.; Chertkow, H.; Hyman, B.T.; Jack, C.R., Jr.; Kawas, C.H.; Klunk, W.E.; Koroshetz, W.J.; Manly, J.J.; Mayeux, R.; et al. The diagnosis of dementia due to Alzheimer's disease: Recommendations from the National Institute on Aging-Alzheimer's Association workgroups on diagnostic guidelines for Alzheimer's disease. *Alzheimers Dement.* **2011**, *7*, 263–269. [CrossRef]
16. Reitz, C.; Brayne, C.; Mayeux, R. Epidemiology of Alzheimer disease. *Nat. Rev. Neurol.* **2011**, *7*, 137–152. [CrossRef]
17. Jack, C.R., Jr.; Bennett, D.A.; Blennow, K.; Carrillo, M.C.; Dunn, B.; Haeberlein, S.B.; Holtzman, D.M.; Jagust, W.; Jessen, F.; Karlawish, J.; et al. NIA-AA Research Framework: Toward a biological definition of Alzheimer's disease. *Alzheimers Dement.* **2018**, *14*, 535–562. [CrossRef]
18. Food, U.; Administration, D. Early Alzheimer's Disease: Developing Drugs for Treatment–Guidance for Industry. 2018. Available online: https://www.fda.gov/downloads/Drugs/GuidanceComplianceRegulatoryInformation/Guidances/UCM596728.pdf (accessed on 25 May 2020).
19. Hansson, O.; Zetterberg, H.; Buchhave, P.; Londos, E.; Blennow, K.; Minthon, L. Association between CSF biomarkers and incipient Alzheimer's disease in patients with mild cognitive impairment: A follow-up study. *Lancet Neurol.* **2006**, *5*, 228–234. [CrossRef]
20. Humpel, C. Identifying and validating biomarkers for Alzheimer's disease. *Trends Biotechnol.* **2011**, *29*, 26–32. [CrossRef]
21. Mattsson, N.; Rosen, E.; Hansson, O.; Andreasen, N.; Parnetti, L.; Jonsson, M.; Herukka, S.K.; van der Flier, W.M.; Blankenstein, M.A.; Ewers, M.; et al. Age and diagnostic performance of Alzheimer disease CSF biomarkers. *Neurology* **2012**, *78*, 468–476. [CrossRef]
22. Potter, R.; Patterson, B.W.; Elbert, D.L.; Ovod, V.; Kasten, T.; Sigurdson, W.; Mawuenyega, K.; Blazey, T.; Goate, A.; Chott, R.; et al. Increased in vivo amyloid-beta42 production, exchange, and loss in presenilin mutation carriers. *Sci. Transl. Med.* **2013**, *5*, 189ra177. [CrossRef]
23. Blennow, K. A Review of Fluid Biomarkers for Alzheimer's Disease: Moving from CSF to Blood. *Neurol. Ther.* **2017**, *6*, 15–24. [CrossRef] [PubMed]
24. Grimmer, T.; Riemenschneider, M.; Forstl, H.; Henriksen, G.; Klunk, W.E.; Mathis, C.A.; Shiga, T.; Wester, H.J.; Kurz, A.; Drzezga, A. Beta amyloid in Alzheimer's disease: Increased deposition in brain is reflected in reduced concentration in cerebrospinal fluid. *Biol. Psychiatry* **2009**, *65*, 927–934. [CrossRef] [PubMed]
25. Hansson, O.; Lehmann, S.; Otto, M.; Zetterberg, H.; Lewczuk, P. Advantages and disadvantages of the use of the CSF Amyloid beta (Abeta) 42/40 ratio in the diagnosis of Alzheimer's Disease. *Alzheimers Res. Ther.* **2019**, *11*, 34. [CrossRef] [PubMed]

26. Tapiola, T.; Pirttila, T.; Mikkonen, M.; Mehta, P.D.; Alafuzoff, I.; Koivisto, K.; Soininen, H. Three-year follow-up of cerebrospinal fluid tau, beta-amyloid 42 and 40 concentrations in Alzheimer's disease. *Neurosci. Lett.* **2000**, *280*, 119–122. [CrossRef]
27. Blennow, K.; Dubois, B.; Fagan, A.M.; Lewczuk, P.; de Leon, M.J.; Hampel, H. Clinical utility of cerebrospinal fluid biomarkers in the diagnosis of early Alzheimer's disease. *Alzheimers Dement.* **2015**, *11*, 58–69. [CrossRef]
28. Andreasen, N.; Hesse, C.; Davidsson, P.; Minthon, L.; Wallin, A.; Winblad, B.; Vanderstichele, H.; Vanmechelen, E.; Blennow, K. Cerebrospinal fluid beta-amyloid(1-42) in Alzheimer disease: Differences between early- and late-onset Alzheimer disease and stability during the course of disease. *Arch. Neurol.* **1999**, *56*, 673–680. [CrossRef] [PubMed]
29. Spies, P.E.; Verbeek, M.M.; van Groen, T.; Claassen, J.A. Reviewing reasons for the decreased CSF Abeta42 concentration in Alzheimer disease. *Front. Biosci.* **2012**, *17*, 2024–2034. [CrossRef]
30. Janelidze, S.; Zetterberg, H.; Mattsson, N.; Palmqvist, S.; Vanderstichele, H.; Lindberg, O.; van Westen, D.; Stomrud, E.; Minthon, L.; Blennow, K.; et al. CSF Abeta42/Abeta40 and Abeta42/Abeta38 ratios: Better diagnostic markers of Alzheimer disease. *Ann. Clin. Transl. Neurol.* **2016**, *3*, 154–165. [CrossRef]
31. Koychev, I.; Galna, B.; Zetterberg, H.; Lawson, J.; Zamboni, G.; Ridha, B.H.; Rowe, J.B.; Thomas, A.; Howard, R.; Malhotra, P.; et al. Abeta42/Abeta40 and Abeta42/Abeta38 Ratios Are Associated with Measures of Gait Variability and Activities of Daily Living in Mild Alzheimer's Disease: A Pilot Study. *J. Alzheimers Dis.* **2018**, *65*, 1377–1383. [CrossRef]
32. Mehta, P.D.; Pirttila, T.; Mehta, S.P.; Sersen, E.A.; Aisen, P.S.; Wisniewski, H.M. Plasma and cerebrospinal fluid levels of amyloid beta proteins 1-40 and 1-42 in Alzheimer disease. *Arch. Neurol.* **2000**, *57*, 100–105. [CrossRef]
33. Baldeiras, I.; Santana, I.; Leitao, M.J.; Gens, H.; Pascoal, R.; Tabuas-Pereira, M.; Beato-Coelho, J.; Duro, D.; Almeida, M.R.; Oliveira, C.R. Addition of the Abeta42/40 ratio to the cerebrospinal fluid biomarker profile increases the predictive value for underlying Alzheimer's disease dementia in mild cognitive impairment. *Alzheimers Res. Ther.* **2018**, *10*, 33. [CrossRef] [PubMed]
34. Shaw, L.M.; Korecka, M.; Clark, C.M.; Lee, V.M.; Trojanowski, J.Q. Biomarkers of neurodegeneration for diagnosis and monitoring therapeutics. *Nat. Rev. Drug Discov.* **2007**, *6*, 295–303. [CrossRef] [PubMed]
35. Southwick, P.C.; Yamagata, S.K.; Echols, C.L., Jr.; Higson, G.J.; Neynaber, S.A.; Parson, R.E.; Munroe, W.A. Assessment of amyloid beta protein in cerebrospinal fluid as an aid in the diagnosis of Alzheimer's disease. *J. Neurochem.* **1996**, *66*, 259–265. [CrossRef] [PubMed]
36. Bouwman, F.H.; van der Flier, W.M.; Schoonenboom, N.S.; van Elk, E.J.; Kok, A.; Rijmen, F.; Blankenstein, M.A.; Scheltens, P. Longitudinal changes of CSF biomarkers in memory clinic patients. *Neurology* **2007**, *69*, 1006–1011. [CrossRef]
37. Ittner, L.M.; Gotz, J. Amyloid-beta and tau–a toxic pas de deux in Alzheimer's disease. *Nat. Rev. Neurosci.* **2011**, *12*, 65–72. [CrossRef]
38. Bloom, G.S. Amyloid-beta and tau: The trigger and bullet in Alzheimer disease pathogenesis. *JAMA Neurol.* **2014**, *71*, 505–508. [CrossRef]
39. Tapiola, T.; Alafuzoff, I.; Herukka, S.K.; Parkkinen, L.; Hartikainen, P.; Soininen, H.; Pirttila, T. Cerebrospinal fluid {beta}-amyloid 42 and tau proteins as biomarkers of Alzheimer-type pathologic changes in the brain. *Arch. Neurol.* **2009**, *66*, 382–389. [CrossRef]
40. Buerger, K.; Ewers, M.; Pirttila, T.; Zinkowski, R.; Alafuzoff, I.; Teipel, S.J.; DeBernardis, J.; Kerkman, D.; McCulloch, C.; Soininen, H.; et al. CSF phosphorylated tau protein correlates with neocortical neurofibrillary pathology in Alzheimer's disease. *Brain* **2006**, *129*, 3035–3041. [CrossRef]
41. Buerger, K.; Teipel, S.J.; Zinkowski, R.; Blennow, K.; Arai, H.; Engel, R.; Hofmann-Kiefer, K.; McCulloch, C.; Ptok, U.; Heun, R.; et al. CSF tau protein phosphorylated at threonine 231 correlates with cognitive decline in MCI subjects. *Neurology* **2002**, *59*, 627–629. [CrossRef]
42. Sjogren, M.; Vanderstichele, H.; Agren, H.; Zachrisson, O.; Edsbagge, M.; Wikkelso, C.; Skoog, I.; Wallin, A.; Wahlund, L.O.; Marcusson, J.; et al. Tau and Abeta42 in cerebrospinal fluid from healthy adults 21-93 years of age: Establishment of reference values. *Clin. Chem.* **2001**, *47*, 1776–1781. [CrossRef]
43. Sunderland, T.; Linker, G.; Mirza, N.; Putnam, K.T.; Friedman, D.L.; Kimmel, L.H.; Bergeson, J.; Manetti, G.J.; Zimmermann, M.; Tang, B.; et al. Decreased beta-amyloid1-42 and increased tau levels in cerebrospinal fluid of patients with Alzheimer disease. *JAMA* **2003**, *289*, 2094–2103. [CrossRef]

44. Burger nee Buch, K.; Padberg, F.; Nolde, T.; Teipel, S.J.; Stubner, S.; Haslinger, A.; Schwarz, M.J.; Sunderland, T.; Arai, H.; Rapoport, S.I.; et al. Cerebrospinal fluid tau protein shows a better discrimination in young old (<70 years) than in old old patients with Alzheimer's disease compared with controls. *Neurosci. Lett.* **1999**, *277*, 21–24. [CrossRef]
45. Ost, M.; Nylen, K.; Csajbok, L.; Ohrfelt, A.O.; Tullberg, M.; Wikkelso, C.; Nellgard, P.; Rosengren, L.; Blennow, K.; Nellgard, B. Initial CSF total tau correlates with 1-year outcome in patients with traumatic brain injury. *Neurology* **2006**, *67*, 1600–1604. [CrossRef] [PubMed]
46. Skillback, T.; Zetterberg, H.; Blennow, K.; Mattsson, N. Cerebrospinal fluid biomarkers for Alzheimer disease and subcortical axonal damage in 5,542 clinical samples. *Alzheimers Res. Ther.* **2013**, *5*, 47. [CrossRef] [PubMed]
47. Ritchie, C.; Smailagic, N.; Noel-Storr, A.H.; Ukoumunne, O.; Ladds, E.C.; Martin, S. CSF tau and the CSF tau/ABeta ratio for the diagnosis of Alzheimer's disease dementia and other dementias in people with mild cognitive impairment (MCI). *Cochrane Database Syst. Rev.* **2017**, *3*, CD010803. [CrossRef] [PubMed]
48. Kern, S.; Syrjanen, J.A.; Blennow, K.; Zetterberg, H.; Skoog, I.; Waern, M.; Hagen, C.E.; van Harten, A.C.; Knopman, D.S.; Jack, C.R., Jr.; et al. Association of Cerebrospinal Fluid Neurofilament Light Protein With Risk of Mild Cognitive Impairment Among Individuals Without Cognitive Impairment. *JAMA Neurol.* **2019**, *76*, 187–193. [CrossRef] [PubMed]
49. Olsson, B.; Portelius, E.; Cullen, N.C.; Sandelius, A.; Zetterberg, H.; Andreasson, U.; Hoglund, K.; Irwin, D.J.; Grossman, M.; Weintraub, D.; et al. Association of Cerebrospinal Fluid Neurofilament Light Protein Levels With Cognition in Patients With Dementia, Motor Neuron Disease, and Movement Disorders. *JAMA Neurol.* **2019**, *76*, 318–325. [CrossRef]
50. Brys, M.; Pirraglia, E.; Rich, K.; Rolstad, S.; Mosconi, L.; Switalski, R.; Glodzik-Sobanska, L.; De Santi, S.; Zinkowski, R.; Mehta, P.; et al. Prediction and longitudinal study of CSF biomarkers in mild cognitive impairment. *Neurobiol. Aging* **2009**, *30*, 682–690. [CrossRef] [PubMed]
51. Castellani, R.J.; Nunomura, A.; Lee, H.G.; Perry, G.; Smith, M.A. Phosphorylated tau: Toxic, protective, or none of the above. *J. Alzheimers Dis.* **2008**, *14*, 377–383. [CrossRef]
52. O'Bryant, S.E.; Mielke, M.M.; Rissman, R.A.; Lista, S.; Vanderstichele, H.; Zetterberg, H.; Lewczuk, P.; Posner, H.; Hall, J.; Johnson, L.; et al. Blood-based biomarkers in Alzheimer disease: Current state of the science and a novel collaborative paradigm for advancing from discovery to clinic. *Alzheimers Dement.* **2017**, *13*, 45–58. [CrossRef]
53. Mawuenyega, K.G.; Sigurdson, W.; Ovod, V.; Munsell, L.; Kasten, T.; Morris, J.C.; Yarasheski, K.E.; Bateman, R.J. Decreased clearance of CNS beta-amyloid in Alzheimer's disease. *Science* **2010**, *330*, 1774. [CrossRef] [PubMed]
54. van Oijen, M.; Hofman, A.; Soares, H.D.; Koudstaal, P.J.; Breteler, M.M. Plasma Abeta(1-40) and Abeta(1-42) and the risk of dementia: A prospective case-cohort study. *Lancet Neurol.* **2006**, *5*, 655–660. [CrossRef]
55. Mayeux, R.; Honig, L.S.; Tang, M.X.; Manly, J.; Stern, Y.; Schupf, N.; Mehta, P.D. Plasma A[beta]40 and A[beta]42 and Alzheimer's disease: Relation to age, mortality, and risk. *Neurology* **2003**, *61*, 1185–1190. [CrossRef]
56. Sundelof, J.; Giedraitis, V.; Irizarry, M.C.; Sundstrom, J.; Ingelsson, E.; Ronnemaa, E.; Arnlov, J.; Gunnarsson, M.D.; Hyman, B.T.; Basun, H.; et al. Plasma beta amyloid and the risk of Alzheimer disease and dementia in elderly men: A prospective, population-based cohort study. *Arch. Neurol.* **2008**, *65*, 256–263. [CrossRef] [PubMed]
57. Pomara, N.; Willoughby, L.M.; Sidtis, J.J.; Mehta, P.D. Selective reductions in plasma Abeta 1-42 in healthy elderly subjects during longitudinal follow-up: A preliminary report. *Am. J. Geriatr. Psychiatry* **2005**, *13*, 914–917. [CrossRef]
58. Hansson, O.; Zetterberg, H.; Vanmechelen, E.; Vanderstichele, H.; Andreasson, U.; Londos, E.; Wallin, A.; Minthon, L.; Blennow, K. Evaluation of plasma Abeta(40) and Abeta(42) as predictors of conversion to Alzheimer's disease in patients with mild cognitive impairment. *Neurobiol. Aging* **2010**, *31*, 357–367. [CrossRef]
59. Olsson, B.; Lautner, R.; Andreasson, U.; Ohrfelt, A.; Portelius, E.; Bjerke, M.; Holtta, M.; Rosen, C.; Olsson, C.; Strobel, G.; et al. CSF and blood biomarkers for the diagnosis of Alzheimer's disease: A systematic review and meta-analysis. *Lancet Neurol.* **2016**, *15*, 673–684. [CrossRef]
60. Nakamura, A.; Kaneko, N.; Villemagne, V.L.; Kato, T.; Doecke, J.; Dore, V.; Fowler, C.; Li, Q.X.; Martins, R.; Rowe, C.; et al. High performance plasma amyloid-beta biomarkers for Alzheimer's disease. *Nature* **2018**, *554*, 249–254. [CrossRef]

61. Ovod, V.; Ramsey, K.N.; Mawuenyega, K.G.; Bollinger, J.G.; Hicks, T.; Schneider, T.; Sullivan, M.; Paumier, K.; Holtzman, D.M.; Morris, J.C.; et al. Amyloid beta concentrations and stable isotope labeling kinetics of human plasma specific to central nervous system amyloidosis. *Alzheimers Dement.* **2017**, *13*, 841–849. [CrossRef]
62. Li, Q.X.; Berndt, M.C.; Bush, A.I.; Rumble, B.; Mackenzie, I.; Friedhuber, A.; Beyreuther, K.; Masters, C.L. Membrane-associated forms of the beta A4 amyloid protein precursor of Alzheimer's disease in human platelet and brain: Surface expression on the activated human platelet. *Blood* **1994**, *84*, 133–142. [CrossRef]
63. Zetterberg, H.; Wilson, D.; Andreasson, U.; Minthon, L.; Blennow, K.; Randall, J.; Hansson, O. Plasma tau levels in Alzheimer's disease. *Alzheimers Res. Ther.* **2013**, *5*, 9. [CrossRef] [PubMed]
64. Mattsson, N.; Zetterberg, H.; Janelidze, S.; Insel, P.S.; Andreasson, U.; Stomrud, E.; Palmqvist, S.; Baker, D.; Tan Hehir, C.A.; Jeromin, A.; et al. Plasma tau in Alzheimer disease. *Neurology* **2016**, *87*, 1827–1835. [CrossRef] [PubMed]
65. Mielke, M.M.; Hagen, C.E.; Xu, J.; Chai, X.; Vemuri, P.; Lowe, V.J.; Airey, D.C.; Knopman, D.S.; Roberts, R.O.; Machulda, M.M.; et al. Plasma phospho-tau181 increases with Alzheimer's disease clinical severity and is associated with tau- and amyloid-positron emission tomography. *Alzheimers Dement.* **2018**, *14*, 989–997. [CrossRef]
66. Yang, C.C.; Chiu, M.J.; Chen, T.F.; Chang, H.L.; Liu, B.H.; Yang, S.Y. Assay of Plasma Phosphorylated Tau Protein (Threonine 181) and Total Tau Protein in Early-Stage Alzheimer's Disease. *J. Alzheimers Dis.* **2018**, *61*, 1323–1332. [CrossRef] [PubMed]
67. Tatebe, H.; Kasai, T.; Ohmichi, T.; Kishi, Y.; Kakeya, T.; Waragai, M.; Kondo, M.; Allsop, D.; Tokuda, T. Quantification of plasma phosphorylated tau to use as a biomarker for brain Alzheimer pathology: Pilot case-control studies including patients with Alzheimer's disease and down syndrome. *Mol. Neurodegener.* **2017**, *12*, 63. [CrossRef]
68. Fossati, S.; Ramos Cejudo, J.; Debure, L.; Pirraglia, E.; Sone, J.Y.; Li, Y.; Chen, J.; Butler, T.; Zetterberg, H.; Blennow, K.; et al. Plasma tau complements CSF tau and P-tau in the diagnosis of Alzheimer's disease. *Alzheimers Dement.* **2019**, *11*, 483–492. [CrossRef]
69. Khalil, M.; Teunissen, C.E.; Otto, M.; Piehl, F.; Sormani, M.P.; Gattringer, T.; Barro, C.; Kappos, L.; Comabella, M.; Fazekas, F.; et al. Neurofilaments as biomarkers in neurological disorders. *Nat. Rev. Neurol.* **2018**, *14*, 577–589. [CrossRef]
70. Weston, P.S.J.; Poole, T.; Ryan, N.S.; Nair, A.; Liang, Y.; Macpherson, K.; Druyeh, R.; Malone, I.B.; Ahsan, R.L.; Pemberton, H.; et al. Serum neurofilament light in familial Alzheimer disease: A marker of early neurodegeneration. *Neurology* **2017**, *89*, 2167–2175. [CrossRef]
71. Weston, P.S.J.; Poole, T.; O'Connor, A.; Heslegrave, A.; Ryan, N.S.; Liang, Y.; Druyeh, R.; Mead, S.; Blennow, K.; Schott, J.M.; et al. Longitudinal measurement of serum neurofilament light in presymptomatic familial Alzheimer's disease. *Alzheimers Res. Ther.* **2019**, *11*, 19. [CrossRef]
72. Mattsson, N.; Andreasson, U.; Zetterberg, H.; Blennow, K.; Alzheimer's Disease Neuroimaging, I. Association of Plasma Neurofilament Light With Neurodegeneration in Patients With Alzheimer Disease. *JAMA Neurol.* **2017**, *74*, 557–566. [CrossRef]
73. Preische, O.; Schultz, S.A.; Apel, A.; Kuhle, J.; Kaeser, S.A.; Barro, C.; Graber, S.; Kuder-Buletta, E.; LaFougere, C.; Laske, C.; et al. Serum neurofilament dynamics predicts neurodegeneration and clinical progression in presymptomatic Alzheimer's disease. *Nat. Med.* **2019**, *25*, 277–283. [CrossRef] [PubMed]
74. Lopez, O.L.; McDade, E.; Riverol, M.; Becker, J.T. Evolution of the diagnostic criteria for degenerative and cognitive disorders. *Curr. Opin. Neurol.* **2011**, *24*, 532–541. [CrossRef] [PubMed]
75. Folstein, M.F.; Folstein, S.E.; McHugh, P.R. "Mini-mental state". A practical method for grading the cognitive state of patients for the clinician. *J. Psychiatr. Res.* **1975**, *12*, 189–198. [CrossRef]
76. Creavin, S.T.; Wisniewski, S.; Noel-Storr, A.H.; Trevelyan, C.M.; Hampton, T.; Rayment, D.; Thom, V.M.; Nash, K.J.; Elhamoui, H.; Milligan, R.; et al. Mini-Mental State Examination (MMSE) for the detection of dementia in clinically unevaluated people aged 65 and over in community and primary care populations. *Cochrane Database Syst. Rev.* **2016**, CD011145. [CrossRef] [PubMed]
77. Chapman, K.R.; Bing-Canar, H.; Alosco, M.L.; Steinberg, E.G.; Martin, B.; Chaisson, C.; Kowall, N.; Tripodis, Y.; Stern, R.A. Mini Mental State Examination and Logical Memory scores for entry into Alzheimer's disease trials. *Alzheimers Res. Ther.* **2016**, *8*, 9. [CrossRef]
78. Li, M.; Ng, T.P.; Kua, E.H.; Ko, S.M. Brief informant screening test for mild cognitive impairment and early Alzheimer's disease. *Dement. Geriatr. Cogn. Disord.* **2006**, *21*, 392–402. [CrossRef]

79. Sheikh-Bahaei, N.; Sajjadi, S.A.; Manavaki, R.; Gillard, J.H. Imaging Biomarkers in Alzheimer's Disease: A Practical Guide for Clinicians. *J. Alzheimers Dis. Rep.* **2017**, *1*, 71–88. [CrossRef]
80. Scheltens, P.; Leys, D.; Barkhof, F.; Huglo, D.; Weinstein, H.C.; Vermersch, P.; Kuiper, M.; Steinling, M.; Wolters, E.C.; Valk, J. Atrophy of medial temporal lobes on MRI in "probable" Alzheimer's disease and normal ageing: Diagnostic value and neuropsychological correlates. *J. Neurol. Neurosurg. Psychiatry* **1992**, *55*, 967–972. [CrossRef]
81. Wang, L.; Zang, Y.; He, Y.; Liang, M.; Zhang, X.; Tian, L.; Wu, T.; Jiang, T.; Li, K. Changes in hippocampal connectivity in the early stages of Alzheimer's disease: Evidence from resting state fMRI. *Neuroimage* **2006**, *31*, 496–504. [CrossRef]
82. Kadir, A.; Almkvist, O.; Forsberg, A.; Wall, A.; Engler, H.; Langstrom, B.; Nordberg, A. Dynamic changes in PET amyloid and FDG imaging at different stages of Alzheimer's disease. *Neurobiol. Aging* **2012**, *33*, 198.e1–198.e4. [CrossRef]
83. Cohen, A.D.; Klunk, W.E. Early detection of Alzheimer's disease using PiB and FDG PET. *Neurobiol. Dis.* **2014**, *72 Pt A*, 117–122. [CrossRef]
84. Chiotis, K.; Saint-Aubert, L.; Boccardi, M.; Gietl, A.; Picco, A.; Varrone, A.; Garibotto, V.; Herholz, K.; Nobili, F.; Nordberg, A.; et al. Clinical validity of increased cortical uptake of amyloid ligands on PET as a biomarker for Alzheimer's disease in the context of a structured 5-phase development framework. *Neurobiol. Aging* **2017**, *52*, 214–227. [CrossRef] [PubMed]
85. Grill, J.D.; Apostolova, L.G.; Bullain, S.; Burns, J.M.; Cox, C.G.; Dick, M.; Hartley, D.; Kawas, C.; Kremen, S.; Lingler, J.; et al. Communicating mild cognitive impairment diagnoses with and without amyloid imaging. *Alzheimers Res. Ther.* **2017**, *9*, 35. [CrossRef] [PubMed]
86. Ray, S.; Britschgi, M.; Herbert, C.; Takeda-Uchimura, Y.; Boxer, A.; Blennow, K.; Friedman, L.F.; Galasko, D.R.; Jutel, M.; Karydas, A.; et al. Classification and prediction of clinical Alzheimer's diagnosis based on plasma signaling proteins. *Nat. Med.* **2007**, *13*, 1359–1362. [CrossRef] [PubMed]
87. Yao, F.; Zhang, K.; Zhang, Y.; Guo, Y.; Li, A.; Xiao, S.; Liu, Q.; Shen, L.; Ni, J. Identification of Blood Biomarkers for Alzheimer's Disease Through Computational Prediction and Experimental Validation. *Front. Neurol.* **2018**, *9*, 1158. [CrossRef]
88. Brinkmalm, A.; Brinkmalm, G.; Honer, W.G.; Frolich, L.; Hausner, L.; Minthon, L.; Hansson, O.; Wallin, A.; Zetterberg, H.; Blennow, K.; et al. SNAP-25 is a promising novel cerebrospinal fluid biomarker for synapse degeneration in Alzheimer's disease. *Mol. Neurodegener.* **2014**, *9*, 53. [CrossRef]
89. Ohrfelt, A.; Brinkmalm, A.; Dumurgier, J.; Brinkmalm, G.; Hansson, O.; Zetterberg, H.; Bouaziz-Amar, E.; Hugon, J.; Paquet, C.; Blennow, K. The pre-synaptic vesicle protein synaptotagmin is a novel biomarker for Alzheimer's disease. *Alzheimers Res. Ther.* **2016**, *8*, 41. [CrossRef] [PubMed]
90. Kitamura, Y.; Usami, R.; Ichihara, S.; Kida, H.; Satoh, M.; Tomimoto, H.; Murata, M.; Oikawa, S. Plasma protein profiling for potential biomarkers in the early diagnosis of Alzheimer's disease. *Neurol. Res.* **2017**, *39*, 231–238. [CrossRef]
91. Ewers, M.; Cheng, X.; Zhong, Z.; Nural, H.F.; Walsh, C.; Meindl, T.; Teipel, S.J.; Buerger, K.; He, P.; Shen, Y.; et al. Increased CSF-BACE1 activity associated with decreased hippocampus volume in Alzheimer's disease. *J. Alzheimers Dis.* **2011**, *25*, 373–381. [CrossRef]
92. Zhong, Z.; Ewers, M.; Teipel, S.; Burger, K.; Wallin, A.; Blennow, K.; He, P.; McAllister, C.; Hampel, H.; Shen, Y. Levels of beta-secretase (BACE1) in cerebrospinal fluid as a predictor of risk in mild cognitive impairment. *Arch. Gen. Psychiatry* **2007**, *64*, 718–726. [CrossRef]
93. Shen, Y.; Wang, H.; Sun, Q.; Yao, H.; Keegan, A.P.; Mullan, M.; Wilson, J.; Lista, S.; Leyhe, T.; Laske, C.; et al. Increased Plasma Beta-Secretase 1 May Predict Conversion to Alzheimer's Disease Dementia in Individuals With Mild Cognitive Impairment. *Biol. Psychiatry* **2018**, *83*, 447–455. [CrossRef] [PubMed]
94. Wu, G.; Sankaranarayanan, S.; Wong, J.; Tugusheva, K.; Michener, M.S.; Shi, X.; Cook, J.J.; Simon, A.J.; Savage, M.J. Characterization of plasma beta-secretase (BACE1) activity and soluble amyloid precursor proteins as potential biomarkers for Alzheimer's disease. *J. Neurosci. Res.* **2012**, *90*, 2247–2258. [CrossRef] [PubMed]
95. Veitinger, M.; Varga, B.; Guterres, S.B.; Zellner, M. Platelets, a reliable source for peripheral Alzheimer's disease biomarkers? *Acta Neuropathol. Commun.* **2014**, *2*, 65. [CrossRef] [PubMed]
96. Lista, S.; O'Bryant, S.E.; Blennow, K.; Dubois, B.; Hugon, J.; Zetterberg, H.; Hampel, H. Biomarkers in Sporadic and Familial Alzheimer's Disease. *J. Alzheimers Dis* **2015**, *47*, 291–317. [CrossRef] [PubMed]

97. Hye, A.; Kerr, F.; Archer, N.; Foy, C.; Poppe, M.; Brown, R.; Hamilton, G.; Powell, J.; Anderton, B.; Lovestone, S. Glycogen synthase kinase-3 is increased in white cells early in Alzheimer's disease. *Neurosci. Lett.* **2005**, *373*, 1–4. [CrossRef]

98. Brosseron, F.; Traschutz, A.; Widmann, C.N.; Kummer, M.P.; Tacik, P.; Santarelli, F.; Jessen, F.; Heneka, M.T. Characterization and clinical use of inflammatory cerebrospinal fluid protein markers in Alzheimer's disease. *Alzheimers Res. Ther.* **2018**, *10*, 25. [CrossRef]

99. Yarchoan, M.; Louneva, N.; Xie, S.X.; Swenson, F.J.; Hu, W.; Soares, H.; Trojanowski, J.Q.; Lee, V.M.; Kling, M.A.; Shaw, L.M.; et al. Association of plasma C-reactive protein levels with the diagnosis of Alzheimer's disease. *J. Neurol. Sci.* **2013**, *333*, 9–12. [CrossRef]

100. Rauchmann, B.S.; Schneider-Axmann, T.; Alexopoulos, P.; Perneczky, R.; Alzheimer's Disease Neuroimaging, I. CSF soluble TREM2 as a measure of immune response along the Alzheimer's disease continuum. *Neurobiol. Aging* **2019**, *74*, 182–190. [CrossRef]

101. Piccio, L.; Deming, Y.; Del-Aguila, J.L.; Ghezzi, L.; Holtzman, D.M.; Fagan, A.M.; Fenoglio, C.; Galimberti, D.; Borroni, B.; Cruchaga, C. Cerebrospinal fluid soluble TREM2 is higher in Alzheimer disease and associated with mutation status. *Acta Neuropathol.* **2016**, *131*, 925–933. [CrossRef]

102. Brosseron, F.; Krauthausen, M.; Kummer, M.; Heneka, M.T. Body fluid cytokine levels in mild cognitive impairment and Alzheimer's disease: A comparative overview. *Mol. Neurobiol.* **2014**, *50*, 534–544. [CrossRef]

103. Heneka, M.T.; Carson, M.J.; El Khoury, J.; Landreth, G.E.; Brosseron, F.; Feinstein, D.L.; Jacobs, A.H.; Wyss-Coray, T.; Vitorica, J.; Ransohoff, R.M.; et al. Neuroinflammation in Alzheimer's disease. *Lancet Neurol.* **2015**, *14*, 388–405. [CrossRef]

104. Hu, W.T.; Chen-Plotkin, A.; Arnold, S.E.; Grossman, M.; Clark, C.M.; Shaw, L.M.; Pickering, E.; Kuhn, M.; Chen, Y.; McCluskey, L.; et al. Novel CSF biomarkers for Alzheimer's disease and mild cognitive impairment. *Acta Neuropathol.* **2010**, *119*, 669–678. [CrossRef] [PubMed]

105. Muszynski, P.; Groblewska, M.; Kulczynska-Przybik, A.; Kulakowska, A.; Mroczko, B. YKL-40 as a Potential Biomarker and a Possible Target in Therapeutic Strategies of Alzheimer's Disease. *Curr. Neuropharmacol.* **2017**, *15*, 906–917. [CrossRef] [PubMed]

106. Craig-Schapiro, R.; Perrin, R.J.; Roe, C.M.; Xiong, C.; Carter, D.; Cairns, N.J.; Mintun, M.A.; Peskind, E.R.; Li, G.; Galasko, D.R.; et al. YKL-40: A novel prognostic fluid biomarker for preclinical Alzheimer's disease. *Biol. Psychiatry* **2010**, *68*, 903–912. [CrossRef] [PubMed]

107. Henjum, K.; Almdahl, I.S.; Arskog, V.; Minthon, L.; Hansson, O.; Fladby, T.; Nilsson, L.N. Cerebrospinal fluid soluble TREM2 in aging and Alzheimer's disease. *Alzheimers Res. Ther.* **2016**, *8*, 17. [CrossRef]

108. Bermejo-Pareja, F.; Antequera, D.; Vargas, T.; Molina, J.A.; Carro, E. Saliva levels of Abeta1-42 as potential biomarker of Alzheimer's disease: A pilot study. *BMC Neurol.* **2010**, *10*, 108. [CrossRef]

109. Lee, M.; Guo, J.P.; Kennedy, K.; McGeer, E.G.; McGeer, P.L. A Method for Diagnosing Alzheimer's Disease Based on Salivary Amyloid-beta Protein 42 Levels. *J. Alzheimers Dis.* **2017**, *55*, 1175–1182. [CrossRef]

110. Yilmaz, A.; Geddes, T.; Han, B.; Bahado-Singh, R.O.; Wilson, G.D.; Imam, K.; Maddens, M.; Graham, S.F. Diagnostic Biomarkers of Alzheimer's Disease as Identified in Saliva using 1H NMR-Based Metabolomics. *J. Alzheimers Dis.* **2017**, *58*, 355–359. [CrossRef]

111. Sabbagh, M.N.; Shi, J.; Lee, M.; Arnold, L.; Al-Hasan, Y.; Heim, J.; McGeer, P. Salivary beta amyloid protein levels are detectable and differentiate patients with Alzheimer's disease dementia from normal controls: Preliminary findings. *BMC Neurol.* **2018**, *18*, 155. [CrossRef]

112. Koronyo, Y.; Salumbides, B.C.; Black, K.L.; Koronyo-Hamaoui, M. Alzheimer's disease in the retina: Imaging retinal abeta plaques for early diagnosis and therapy assessment. *Neurodegener. Dis.* **2012**, *10*, 285–293. [CrossRef]

113. Koronyo, Y.; Biggs, D.; Barron, E.; Boyer, D.S.; Pearlman, J.A.; Au, W.J.; Kile, S.J.; Blanco, A.; Fuchs, D.T.; Ashfaq, A.; et al. Retinal amyloid pathology and proof-of-concept imaging trial in Alzheimer's disease. *JCI Insight* **2017**, *2*. [CrossRef] [PubMed]

114. Shah, T.M.; Gupta, S.M.; Chatterjee, P.; Campbell, M.; Martins, R.N. Beta-amyloid sequelae in the eye: A critical review on its diagnostic significance and clinical relevance in Alzheimer's disease. *Mol. Psychiatry* **2017**, *22*, 353–363. [CrossRef]

115. Attems, J.; Jellinger, K.A. Olfactory tau pathology in Alzheimer disease and mild cognitive impairment. *Clin. Neuropathol.* **2006**, *25*, 265–271. [PubMed]

116. Passali, G.C.; Politi, L.; Crisanti, A.; Loglisci, M.; Anzivino, R.; Passali, D. Tau Protein Detection in Anosmic Alzheimer's Disease Patient's Nasal Secretions. *Chemosens. Percept.* **2015**, *8*, 201–206. [CrossRef]
117. Jung, H.J.; Shin, I.S.; Lee, J.E. Olfactory function in mild cognitive impairment and Alzheimer's disease: A meta-analysis. *Laryngoscope* **2019**, *129*, 362–369. [CrossRef] [PubMed]

4

Behavioral and Psychological Symptoms of Dementia (BPSD): Clinical Characterization and Genetic Correlates in an Italian Alzheimer's Disease Cohort

Catia Scassellati [1,2,†], Miriam Ciani [3,†], Carlo Maj [1,4], Cristina Geroldi [5], Orazio Zanetti [5], Massimo Gennarelli [1,6] and Cristian Bonvicini [3,*]

1 Genetics Unit, IRCCS Istituto Centro San Giovanni di Dio Fatebenefratelli, 25123 Brescia, Italy; c.scassellati@fatebenefratelli.eu (C.S.); cmaj@uni-bonn.de (C.M.); gennarelli@fatebenefratelli.eu (M.G.)
2 Biological Psychiatry Unit, IRCCS Istituto Centro San Giovanni di Dio Fatebenefratelli, 25123 Brescia, Italy
3 Molecular Markers Laboratory, IRCCS Istituto Centro San Giovanni di Dio Fatebenefratelli, 25123 Brescia, Italy; mciani@fatebenefratelli.eu
4 Institute of Genomic Statistics and Bioinformatics, University of Bonn, 53127 Bonn, Germany
5 Alzheimer's Research Unit-Memory Clinic, IRCCS Istituto Centro San Giovanni di Dio Fatebenefratelli, 25123 Brescia, Italy; cgeroldi@fatebenefratelli.eu (C.G.); ozanetti@fatebenefratelli.eu (O.Z.)
6 Section of Biology and Genetic, Department of Molecular and Translational Medicine, University of Brescia, 25123 Brescia, Italy
* Correspondence: cbonvicini@fatebenefratelli.eu
† These authors contributed equally to this work.

Abstract: Background: The occurrence of Behavioral and Psychological Symptoms of Dementia (BPSD) in Alzheimer's Disease (AD) patients hampers the clinical management and exacerbates the burden for caregivers. The definition of the clinical distribution of BPSD symptoms, and the extent to which symptoms are genetically determined, are still open to debate. Moreover, genetic factors that underline BPSD symptoms still need to be identified. Purpose. To characterize our Italian AD cohort according to specific BPSD symptoms as well as to endophenotypes. To evaluate the associations between the considered BPSD traits and *COMT, MTHFR,* and *APOE* genetic variants. Methods. AD patients (n = 362) underwent neuropsychological examination and genotyping. BPSD were assessed with the Neuropsychiatric Inventory scale. Results. *APOE* and *MTHFR* variants were significantly associated with specific single BPSD symptoms. Furthermore, "Psychosis" and "Hyperactivity" resulted in the most severe endophenotypes, with *APOE* and *MTHFR* implicated as both single risk factors and "gene×gene" interactions. Conclusions. We strongly suggest the combined use of both BPSD single symptoms/endophenotypes and the "gene×gene" interactions as valid strategies for expanding the knowledge about the BPSD aetiopathogenetic mechanisms.

Keywords: behavioral and psychological symptoms of dementia (BPSD); Alzheimer's disease (AD); neuropsychiatry inventory scale (NPI); endophenotypes; CART analysis; *MTHFR; APOE; COMT;* genetic variants

1. Introduction

The core clinical criteria for Alzheimer's Disease (AD), the most common neurodegenerative dementing illness, focus on the presence of memory disturbance or other cognitive symptoms that interfere with the ability to function at work or in usual daily activities [1].

Although cognitive symptoms are the actual hallmark of disease, patients often show also a broad range of "non-cognitive" disturbances, more commonly known with the term "Behavioral and Psychological Symptoms of Dementia (BPSD)". Highlighting the importance of these symptoms is pivotal because BPSD represents the leading reason for loss of independence and institutionalization for AD *patients* [2–4]. About up to 90% of people with AD can present neuropsychiatric disturbances including agitation, aggression, irritation, disinhibition, anxiety, depression, apathy, delusions, and hallucinations at onset or later in the course of the disease [5,6].

Furthermore, BPSD can be recognized individually, but more often they occur in association. Indeed, 50% of subjects with AD show at least four neuropsychiatric symptoms simultaneously [7]. Their clusterization into distinct domains based on their frequency of co-occurrence allowed the definition of distinct behavioral endophenotypes [8]. In systematic reviews of studies that applied unbiased approaches to cluster BPSD, the following domains were identified: Affective (anxiety and depression), Disinhibition/Hyperactivity (aggression, impulsivity, and motor hyperactivity), Apathy and Psychosis (hallucinations, delusions, and paranoia) [3,8,9]. However, the debate about the definition of an appropriate clusterization in dementia is still ongoing [3]. More importantly, the studies available to date are characterized by a high heterogeneity, also because a certain number of symptoms (i.e., apathy, sleep disorders, eating disturbances) are not adequately grouped [3].

The susceptibility to BPSD is somewhat unclear as well as the molecular link between BPSD and AD. Within this complex of aetiological interplay, genetic background has been considered one of the key players involved in predisposing patients to specific behavioral and psychological manifestations in AD [10]. Multiple genes, prevalently involved in the processes of neurotransmission/neurodevelopment, have been assessed for their putative influence on BPSD risk, whose findings have been often inconsistent (for review [10]). For instance, the Catechol-O-Methyltransferase (*COMT*) gene was investigated in five published papers, four of which were conducted by the same authors [11–14], and the association found with "frontal"/cognitive and "psychosis" endophenotypes was weak. COMT protein is one of the major enzymes involved in the synaptic dopamine catabolism and, thus, has a crucial role in the prefrontal cortex. The well-known functional single nucleotide polymorphism (SNP) is characterized by a G to A transition at codon 108/158 (soluble/membrane-bound COMT) resulting in a valine-to-methionine substitution, giving rise to a significant, three-to-four-fold reduction in its enzymatic activity. The presence of valine (H allele = high activity) in the coding sequence corresponds dose-dependently with reduced prefrontal dopamine levels, leading subsequently to the upregulation of striatal dopamine activity [15].

On the other hand, the Apolipoprotein E (*APOE*) gene, the main recognized genetic risk factor for late-onset AD (LOAD) (allele ε4) [16], seems to give more consistent results, with the well-known alleles ε4 and ε2 associated with specific BPSD symptoms (for review [10]).

Thus, further new biological and molecular mechanisms could be involved in BPSD genetics architecture. For instance, *COMT* also regulates the folate pathway [17]. Folate is a cofactor in one-carbon metabolism, where it promotes the remethylation of homocysteine (Hcy). Numerous studies associate the folate deficiency and the resultant increase of Hcy levels with AD [18]. Interestingly, circulating Hcy levels in AD patients with and without BPSD were higher compared to the control subjects, and the plasma Hcy concentration in AD patients with BPSD was the highest among the three considered groups [19]. Hyperhomocysteinemia has been also correlated with psychosis and depression [20–22]. The Methylene tetrahydrofolate reductase (*MTHFR*) gene, whose genetic defects lead to hyperhomocysteinemia, could be a good and new candidate in the aetiopathogenetic mechanisms of BPSD. Within this gene, the two most commonly studied SNPs are the C677T (rs1801133) and the A1298C (rs1801131). The T allele of the C677T polymorphism provokes the synthesis of an athermolabile variant of the enzyme leading to a reduced enzymatic activity, which in turn produce an increase in the blood Hcy levels [23,24]. Recent findings supported that this allele was associated with an increased risk of LOAD [25,26], and correlated with a significant increase of Hcy levels [27,28]. Concerning the A1298C, the C allele results in a reduced enzymatic activity, but does not influence its thermolability [29,30].

Based on this rationale, in this study we analyzed an Italian cohort of AD patients in order to:

1. define the clinical distribution of BPSD symptoms through the characterization of single BPSD

symptoms as well as of endophenotype clusters; 2. confirm and clarify the aetiopathogenetic effect of *APOE* and *COMT* variants in relation to both single symptoms and behavioral endophenotypes, selecting functional polymorphisms such as rs429358 (Cys130Arg) and rs7412 (Arg176Cys) and Val108/158Met, respectively [15,16]; 3. evaluate for the first time the putative involvement of *MTHFR* in single BPSD symptoms and likewise behavioral endophenotypes, selecting functional polymorphisms such as C677T (rs1801133) and the A1298C (rs1801131) [23,24,29,30]; 4. highlight for individual symptoms and endophenotypes a "single gene" involvement and/or a "gene*x*gene" interaction of *APOE*, *COMT*, and *MTHFR*.

2. Materials and Methods

2.1. Sample and Clinical Evaluation

The study was approved by the Local Ethics Committee (IRCCS Istituto Centro San Giovanni di Dio Fatebenefratelli, Brescia, Italy, n. 6/2006) and conducted in accordance with local clinical research regulations. Written informed consent was obtained from all participants.

AD subjects (n = 362) were recruited from the Alzheimer Unit of the IRCCS Istituto Centro San Giovanni di Dio Fatebenefratelli, Brescia, Italy. All patients were unrelated Caucasian subjects residing in Northern Italy with an Italian origin descent for at least two generations. All of them were assessed at their admittance with a complete sociodemographic and clinical data collection (cognitive, behavioral, neurological, functional, and physical abilities). A multidisciplinary clinical examination was performed and the diagnosis of probable AD was established based on criteria of the "National Institute of Neurological and Communicative Disorders" and the "Stroke-Alzheimer's disease and Related Disorders Association" [31]. To assess cognitive decline, the Mini Mental State Examination (MMSE) test was used [32], in addition to the Cumulative Illness Rating Scale for Geriatrics (CIRS-G) [33]; function abilities were evaluated with the Basic Activity Daily Living (BADL), and the Instrumental Activity Daily Living (IADL) scales [34,35].

BPSD were assessed with the Neuropsychiatric Inventory (NPI) scale [36], a fully structured interview exploring 12 behavioral and neuropsychiatric domains (i.e., delusions, hallucinations, agitation/aggression, disphoria/depression, anxiety, apathy, irritability, euphoria, disinhibition, aberrant motor behavior, sleep behavior disturbances, besides appetite and eating abnormalities). It specifically provides an individual score for each explored cognitive domain specifically obtained by multiplying the severity of symptoms (1 = mild; 2 = moderate; 3 = severe) with their frequencies (4-point scale from 1 = occasionally to 4 = very frequently, more than once a day). The NPI then yields a domain rating of frequency times severity (range = 0–12). In agreement with a group of expert clinicians, each of the 12 behavioral/neuropsychiatric symptoms was classified in three groups, according to the "severity*frequency" score: 1—symptom-free (NPI = 0); 2—with low "severity*frequencies" score (NPI from 1 to 4); 3—with high "severity*frequencies" score (NPI from 6 to 12). Moreover, NPI provides a total score that globally evaluates the 12 domains for a complete clinical picture given by the sum of the individual scores (defining a range from 0 to 144).

The adopted exclusionary criteria for subjects were: (a) A history of schizophrenia, schizoaffective disorder, delusional disorder, mood disorder with psychotic features, major depressive disorder, substance use disorder, or mental retardation according to The Diagnostic and Statistical Manual of Mental Disorders (DSM-IV) criteria; (b) severe cerebrovascular disorders, hydrocephalus and intra-cranial mass, documented by *Computed Tomography* or *Magnetic Resonance Imaging* within the past 12 months; (c) abnormalities in serum folate and Vitamin B12, syphilis serology or altered thyroid hormone levels; (d) a history of traumatic brain injury or other neurological diseases (e.g., Parkinson's Disease, Huntington Disease, seizure disorders); (e) current acute or poorly controlled medical problems (e.g., poorly controlled diabetes or hypertension; cancer within the past five years; clinically significant hepatic, renal, cardiac or pulmonary disorders); (f) absence of knowledgeable informant who could properly report information regarding the patient's behavior.

2.2. Genetic Analysis

Genomic DNA (gDNA) was extracted from peripheral blood with the PureGene genomic DNA isolation kit (Gentra Systems, Minneapolis, MN, USA). The obtained gDNA was quantified by spectrophotometric quantification using the NanoDrop microvolume sample retention system (Thermo Fisher Scientific, Waltham, MA, USA) [37]. In order to verify the possible degradation, all samples were analyzed on a 0.8% agarose gel electrophoresis and a long *Polymerase Chain Reaction* (PCR) protocol was developed for exploring genetic variability in *MTHFR, COMT,* and *APOE.*

In all samples, the *MTHFR* [rs1801133 (C677T) and rs1801131 (A1298C)], *COMT* [rs4680 (Val158Met)], and *APOE* [rs429358 (Cys130Arg) and rs7412 (Arg176Cys)] polymorphisms were genotyped by using the SNaPshot assay [38]. Briefly, 100 ng of gDNA of each sample were amplified in the GeneAmp PCR System 9700 (Applied Biosystems, Foster City, CA, USA), and the PCR-amplification products were used as a template in a SNaPshot Multiplex assay performed according to the manufacturer's instructions. Finally, samples were analyzed, and the allele peak determination was performed on an ABI 3130xl Genetic Analyzer. Electrophoresis results were analyzed using the GeneMapper ID software v4.0 (Applied Biosystems, Foster City, CA, USA).

2.3. Statistical Analyses

All statistical analyses were conducted by using the SPSS version 23.0 (SPSS Inc., Chicago, IL, USA). The Hardy-Weinberg equilibrium (HWE) was calculated using an online calculator (http://www.husdyr.kvl.dk/htm/kc/popgen/genetik/applets/kitest.htm) for the presence of multiallelic genotypes.

2.3.1. Principal Component Analysis (PCA)

In the first exploratory phase, the set of symptoms from the NPI scale was factorially analyzed to identify possible underlying latent variables. The Principal Component Analysis (PCA) method and Varimax rotation were performed. The number of factors was determined on the basis of eigenvalues greater than one of the Pearson's correlation matrix, and by sharp breaks in the size of the eigenvalues using a scree plot [39]. Symptom-factor correlations, (i.e., factor loading) being greater than 0.40 in absolute value were chosen to identify a simple factor structure (i.e., factors with non-overlapping clusters of symptoms).

2.3.2. Classification and Regression Tree (CART) Analysis for Single BPSD Symptoms and Endophenotypes

The Classification and Regression Tree (CART) analysis using the exhaustive Chi-squared Automatic Interaction Detector (CHAID) algorithm was performed to explore the interaction between single BPSD symptoms as well as endophenotypes and all polymorphisms in *APOE, MTHFR,* and *COMT* genes in the BPSD cohort [40,41]. Specifically, we performed the analyses considering ε4 carriers (ε2ε4 + ε3ε4 + ε4ε4 genotypes) versus the others indicated as *APOE* ε4 non-carriers (ε2ε3 + ε3ε3 genotypes). *APOE* allele ε4 carriers, the carriers of both alleles in 677C/T *MTHFR,* in 1298A/C *MTHFR,* and in Val108/158Met *COMT* genes polymorphisms were used as a dominant model of inheritance. Moreover, the comparisons were performed incorporating "Free group" (NPI 0) along with "Low group" (NPI 1–4) versus "High group" (NPI 6–12). This is due to the evidence that "Low group" is present in our population with a frequency < 20%. As this study does not have a longitudinal design, we assumed causality in our CART model [https://www.epa.gov/caddis-vol4/caddis-volume-4-data-analysis-classification-and-regression-tree-cart-analysis].

The exhaustive CHAID data mining algorithm is a nonparametric procedure that makes no assumptions of the underlying data. In the CHAID analysis, nominal, ordinal, and continuous data can be used, where continuous predictors are split into categories with approximately an equal number of observations. CHAID creates all possible cross tabulations for each categorical predictor until the best outcome is achieved and no further splitting can be performed [42]. In the CHAID technique, we can visually see the relationships between the split variables and the associated related factor within the tree. The development of the decision, or classification tree, starts with identifying the target variable or dependent variable, which would be considered the root. CHAID analysis splits the target into two or more categories that are called the initial, or parent nodes, and then the nodes are split using statistical algorithms into child nodes.

The exhaustive CHAID data mining algorithm automatically pruning insignificant nodes in a decision tree was constructed through the IBM SPSS 23 statistical package program. It works on the basis of F test if a continuous dependent variable is used as in our study (endophenotypes), whereas, if the predictor variable has only two categories (single items), the χ^2-test for independence is performed for each pair of categories of the predictor variable in relation to the binary target variable. For non-significant outcomes, those paired categories are merged.

Minimum subject numbers for the parent and child nodes were fixed at 20 and 10 for constructing an optimal decision tree structure and improving the predictive performance of the algorithms. A ten-fold cross validation was activated in the study.

Since the analyses were conducted by using decision tree models, it was not needed to have transformed data.

SPSS automatically made a Bonferroni adjustment to calculate the adjusted p-values for the merged categories to control for the Type I error rate.

To exclude the influence of age and gender, we performed the univariate analyses (ANOVA) related to BPSD endophenotypes, including the variables age or gender. Selecting ENDOPHENOTYPES ("Psychosis", "Hyperactivity", "Mood", "Frontal") as a dependent variable, AGE as covariate, SEX as an independent variable, we did not find any significant association in separate analyses (Table S1—gender and Table S2—age, Supplementary Materials). The only significant association was observed in the "Mood" endophenotype (Table S1, $F = 4.7$; $p = 0.032$); data not confirmed by the exhaustive CHAID data mining algorithm. Thus, given the non-significant analyses, age and sex were not included in the calculations. Medications as well as comorbidity were not included in our analyses.

The Hosmer-Lemeshow goodness of fit test was used to confirm the suitability of the trees. The interactions were given by calculating the sum of the scores relative to "severity*frequencies" of the single BSPD symptoms components as a mean risk ± SD.

The stepwise multiple logistic regression was used to confirm the classification trees.

3. Results

Socio-demographic and clinical features of our Italian AD cohort, as well as the alleles, genotypes, and carriers frequencies of the all polymorphisms in *APOE*, *MTHFR*, and *COMT* genes are shown in Tables 1 and 2. Table 1 describes also the clinical features according to stratification for gender; whereas in Table 2 we reported the HWE results where no HWE deviation was observed.

3.1. Clinical Characterization according to Single NPI Scores

Three hundred and eight patients were characterized by the NPI scale. Considering the NPI scores and the relative proposed ranges (Table 3), our population was mainly characterized by agitation, irritability, night-time behavior disturbances, and aberrant motor behavior. Within each group, we found that: 52% of AD patients showed higher severity in agitation symptomatology, 48% in irritability, 42% in night-time behavior disturbances and, finally, 39% showed higher severity in aberrant motor behavior.

Slightly less representative in our sample, there were: Apathy (28% higher severity), delusions (29% higher severity), anxiety (25% higher severity), depression (22% higher severity), and hallucinations (21% higher severity).

On the contrary, appetite and eating disturbances were referred in only a minority of patients, while no one presented disinhibition or euphoria according to their caregivers' reports.

Table 1. Clinical features of our Alzheimer's Disease Italian cohort, stratified according to gender.

Gender (F/M)	241/121	Female	Male
Age (years)	80.5 ± 7.0	80.9 ± 7.1	79.7 ± 6.7
Schooling (years)	6.0 ± 3.6	5.4 ± 2.9	7.4 ± 4.4
MMSE, total score	11.7 ± 7.3	12.0 ± 6.9	10.9 ± 8.1
Onset (years)	76.1 ± 7.9	76.5 ± 8.1	75.4 ± 7.6
Illness Duration (years)	4.5 ± 2.9	4.4 ± 2.6	4.5 ± 3.5
BMI	22.3 ± 4.1	22.2 ± 4.2	22.5 ± 3.8
IADL	7.2 ± 1.5	7.4 ± 1.2	6.8 ± 1.9
BADL	3.7 ± 1.9	3.6 ± 1.9	3.8 ± 1.8
Tinetti	19.8 ± 5.4	19.8 ± 5.2	19.6 ± 5.9
CIRS	12.7 ± 9.7	12.2 ± 9.5	13.8 ± 10.0
Hypertension	27.9%	29.5%	24.8%
Cardiopathy	28.7%	26.1%	33.9%
Hypercholesterolemia	4.7%	5.8%	2.5%
Diabetes	6.6%	5.4%	9.1%
Psychiatric diseases	26.0%	27.4%	23.1%
AChEIs	20.2%	21.6%	17.4%
Neuroleptics	45.5%	41.1%	51.2%
Antidepressants	45.6%	46.9%	43.0%
Benzodiazepines/hypnotics	41.4%	46.1%	32.2%

Note: The measurement data are expressed as mean ± standard deviation (mean ± SD) or in percentual (%). MMSE: Mini-Mental State Examination; BMI: Body max index; IADL: Instrumental activities daily living; BADL: Basic activities of daily living; Tinetti; CIRS: Cumulative illness rating scales; AChEIs: Acetylcholinesterase inhibitors.

Table 2. Genetic distribution of our Alzheimer's Disease Italian cohort for *APOE*, *MTHFR*, and *COMT* genes polymorphisms.

***APOE* Haplotypes (rs429358 and rs7412)**			***MTHFR* (rs1801133: C677T)**			***MTHFR* (rs1801131: A1298C)**			***COMT* (rs4680: V158M)**		
HWE	$\chi^2 = 0.91$	$p = 0.92$	HWE	$\chi^2 = 1.70$	$p = 0.19$	HWE	$\chi^2 = 0.53$	$p = 0.47$	HWE	$\chi^2 = 1.22$	$p = 0.27$
Alleles	N	freq	*Alleles*	N	freq	*Alleles*	N	freq	*Alleles*	N	freq
ε2	20	0.03	T	314	0.43	A	499	0.69	A	330	0.46
ε3	510	0.70	C	410	0.57	C	225	0.31	G	394	0.54
ε4	194	0.27									
total	724	1.00	total	724	1.00	total	724	1.00	total	724	1.00
Genotypes	N	freq	*Genotypes*	N	freq	*Genotypes*	N	freq	*Genotypes*	N	freq
ε2 ε3	16	0.04	TT	62	0.17	AA	169	0.47	AA	70	0.19
ε2 ε4	4	0.01	TC	190	0.52	AC	161	0.44	AG	190	0.52
ε3 ε3	178	0.49	CC	110	0.30	CC	32	0.09	GG	102	0.28
ε3 ε4	138	0.38									
ε4 ε4	26	0.07									
total	362	1.00	total	362	1.00	total	362	1.00	total	362	1.00
ε2 carriers	20	0.06	T carriers	252	0.70	A carriers	330	0.91	A carriers	260	0.72
ε3 carriers	332	0.92	C carriers	300	0.83	C carriers	193	0.53	G carriers	292	0.81
ε4 carriers	168	0.46									

Note: *APOE*: Apolipoprotein E; *MTHFR*: Methylenetetrahydrofolate Reductase; *COMT*: Catechol-O-Methyltransferase; HWE: Hardy-Weinberg equilibrium.

Table 3. Clinical distributions of single Behavioral and Psychological Symptoms of Dementia (BPSD) in our Italian Alzheimer's Disease cohort.

Symptoms ("Severity*Frequencies" = 0–12)	Mean ± SD §	"Severity*Frequencies" Groups N Subjects (%) &		
		Free (NPI 0)	Low (NPI 1–4)	High (NPI 6–12)
Agitation	4.96 ± 4.32	102 (33.0)	47 (15.2)	160 (51.8)
Irritability	4.57 ± 4.25	109 (35.4)	52 (16.9)	147 (47.7)
Night-time behavior disturbances	4.22 ± 4.55	136 (44.0)	44 (14.2)	129 (41.7)
Aberrant motor behavior	4.12 ± 4.72	148 (48.2)	39 (12.7)	120 (39.1)
Apathy	3.03 ± 4.19	178 (58.0)	42 (13.7)	87 (28.3)
Delusions	3.00 ± 4.00	166 (54.1)	52 (16.9)	89 (29.0)
Anxiety	2.53 ± 4.10	200 (65.4)	30 (9.8)	76 (24.8)
Depression	2.50 ± 3.90	185 (60.3)	53 (17.3)	69 (22.5)
Hallucination	2.30 ± 3.55	187 (60.9)	55 (17.9)	65 (21.2)
Appetite and eating disturbances	1.94 ± 3.59	223 (72.2)	28 (9.1)	58 (18.8)
Disinhibition	0.93 ± 2.44	253 (82.4)	28 (9.1)	26 (8.5)
Euphoria	0.12 ± 0.86	299 (97.4)	6 (2.0)	2 (0.7)
NPI, total score (0–144)	34.1 ± 22.6			
NPI, n symptoms	4.9 ± 2.4			

Note: § Mean ± standard deviation (SD) of the scores relative to "severity*frequencies" of the single items. & Number (N) and percentage (%) of subjects present in each group (Free, Low, and High) compared to individual symptoms. Free: "severity*frequencies" score (NPI 0) for all the individual symptoms; Low: "severity*frequencies" score (NPI 1–4) for all the individual symptoms; High: "severity*frequencies" score (NPI 6–12) for all the individual symptoms.

3.2. Clinical Characterization according to Behavioral Endophenotypes

The results of the exploratory factor analysis on BPSD in AD, conducted by PCA and Varimax rotation, are shown in Table 4. Using the criterion of eigenvalues greater than 1 and the scree plot, PCA allowed grouping the 12 explored BPSD symptoms in four endophenotypes. These factors explained the 56% of the total variance of data. Specifically, thanks to this approach, the following clinical categories were established in our cohort: (a) "Psychosis" characterized by delusions, hallucinations, agitation, aberrant motor behavior, and night-time behavioral symptoms; (b) "Hyperactivity" with agitation, irritability, appetite and eating disturbances; (c) "Mood" associated with high loadings on anxiety, depression, and apathy; (d) "Frontal" including disinhibition and euphoria.

The endophenotypes more representative in our population were "Psychosis" (37% higher severity), and "Hyperactivity" (39% higher severity). These were followed by the "Mood" and "Frontal" endophenotypes (Table 5).

3.3. APOE, MTHFR, and COMT Genetic Correlates in Endophenotype Clusterization and in Single BPSD Symptoms

All polymorphisms investigated in this study within the *APOE*, *MTHFR*, and *COMT* genes showed a prevalence comparable to that reported in https://www.alzforum.org/, considering Caucasian Populations (Table 2). Globally, the prevalence of ε2, ε3, and ε4 alleles for the *APOE* gene was estimated to be 8%, 78%, and 14%, respectively; for rs1801133 *MTHFR* gene to be 39% (allele T) and 61% (allele C); for rs1801131 *MTHFR* gene to be 34% (allele C) and 66% (allele A); for Val108/158Met *COMT* gene to be 49% (allele A) and 51% (allele G).

In order to explore the genetic correlates in both approaches, we exploited the potential of genetic analysis by using the exhaustive CHAID data mining algorithm to reveal "gene×gene" interaction as aetiopathogenetic mechanisms in BPSD. The Hosmer-Lemeshow goodness of fit test confirmed the suitability of the trees (Table S3 Supplementary Materials). Moreover, the stepwise multiple logistic regression validated the classification trees (Tables S4 and S5 Supplementary Materials).

Table 4. Principal component analysis (PCA) of the Behavioral and Psychological Symptoms of Dementia (BPSD) in our Italian Alzheimer's Disease cohort.

Symptoms	Endophenotype Components			
	Factor 1	**Factor 2**	**Factor 3**	**Factor 4**
	Mood	**Hyperactivity**	**Psychosis**	**Frontal**
Delusions	0.276	0.372	*0.463*	0.144
Hallucination	0.022	0.011	*0.690*	0.248
Agitation	0.058	*0.654*	*0.468*	0.068
Depression	*0.855*	0.058	0.166	0.089
Anxiety	*0.820*	0.062	0.156	0.075
Euphoria	−0.040	−0.109	0.186	*0.766*
Apathy	*0.579*	0.292	−0.212	−0.184
Disinhibition	0.131	0.376	−0.166	*0.687*
Irritability	0.028	*0.645*	0.367	0.119
Aberrant motor behavior	0.104	0.373	*0.402*	−0.157
Night-time behavior disturbances	0.029	0.056	*0.621*	−0.087
Appetite and eating disturbances	0.191	*0.671*	−0.157	0.014

Note: Extraction method: Principal component analysis. Rotation Method: Varimax with Kaiser normalization. Coefficients with values over 0.4 are italicized and in bold.

Table 5. Clinical distributions of behavioral endophenotypes in our Italian Alzheimer's Disease cohort.

Endophenotypes (Components; "Severity*Frequencies" Range)	Mean ± SD §	Mean of N Subjects ± SD £ (% Mean of N Subjects ± SD) $		
		Free	**Low**	**High**
Psychosis (Delusions, Hallucination, Agitation, Aberrant motor behavior, Night-time behavior disturbances; 0–60)	18.5 ± 13.3	148 ± 32 (48.0 ± 10.5)	47 ± 6 (15.4 ± 2.1)	113 ± 37 (36.6 ± 11.8)
Hyperactivity (Agitation, Irritability, Appetite and eating disturbances; 0–36)	11.4 ± 9.2	145 ± 68 (46.9 ± 22.0)	42 ± 13 (13.7 ± 4.1)	122 ± 56 (39.4 ± 18.0)
Mood (Depression, Anxiety, Apathy; 0–36)	8.1 ± 9.4	188 ± 11 (61.2 ± 3.8)	42 ± 12 (13.6 ± 3.7)	77 ± 9 (25.0 ± 3.0)
Frontal (Euphoria, Disinhibition; 0–24)	1.0 ± 2.7	276 ± 33 (89.9 ± 10.6)	17 ± 16 (5.5 ± 5.1)	14 ± 17 (4.6 ± 5.5)

Note: § Mean ± standard deviation (SD) of the scores relative to "severity*frequencies" of the endophenotype components. Free: NPI = 0 for all the individual components involved in the endophenotype; Low: Sum of the "severity*frequencies" score (NPI 1–4) for all the individual components involved in the endophenotype; High: Sum of the "severity*frequencies" score (NPI 6–12) for all the individual components involved in the endophenotype. £ Mean number of subjects N ± SD present in each group (Free, Low, and High) compared to individual endophenotypes. $ Percentage (%) of the mean of the number of subjects (N ± SD) present in each group (Free, Low, and High) compared to individual endophenotypes.

3.3.1. "Genexgene" Interactions in "Psychosis" Endophenotype and the Relative Single BPSD Symptoms

Table 6 reports the main significant results obtained in the genetic analyses performed on single BPSD symptoms. Starting by the agitation, we found that the *APOE* ε4 allele carriers showed a high risk to develop more severe symptoms (odd ratio (OR) = 1.87, 95% CI: 1.19–2.95). Concerning the aberrant motor behavior, we evidenced similar results with *APOE* ε4 allele carriers showing higher risk to develop high severity in this symptomatology (OR = 1.91, 95% CI: 1.20–3.04). In relation to *MTHFR*, we found that the homozygotes CC (C677T) showed a high risk to develop more severe delusions symptoms (OR = 1.75, 95% CI: 1.04–2.94).

Table 6. Genetic correlates related to single BPSD symptoms in our Italian Alzheimer's Disease cohort according to different values of "severity*frequencies" (exhaustive CHAID data mining algorithm).

	Gene	Free + Low [&] N (Freq.)	High [&] N (Freq.)	
Agitation	*APOE*			$\chi^2 = 7.435$, $p_{adjusted} = 0.006$ OR = 1.87; 95% CI: 1.19–2.95
	ε4-carriers	58 (0.39)	86 (0.54)	
	ε4-non-carriers	91 (0.61)	72(0.46)	
	total	149 (1.00)	158 (1.00)	
Aberrant motor behavior	*APOE*			$\chi^2 = 7.553$, $p_{adjusted} = 0.006$ OR = 1.91; 95% CI: 1.20–3.04
	4-carriers	76 (0.41)	68 (0.57)	
	ε4-non-carriers	111 (0.59)	52 (0.43)	
	total	187 (1.00)	120 (1.00)	
Delusions	*MTHFR*			$\chi^2 = 4.363$, $p_{adjusted} = 0.037$ OR = 1.75; 95% CI: 1.04–2.94
	CC	59 (0.27)	35 (0.39)	
	Genotypes_C677T	159 (0.73)	54 (0.61)	
	T-carriers_C677T	218 (1.00)	89 (1.00)	
Appetite/eating abnormalities	*APOE*			$\chi^2 = 5.922$, $p_{adjusted} = 0.015$ OR = 2.06; 95% CI: 1.14–3.71
	ε4-carriers	109 (0.44)	35 (0.60)	
	ε4-non-carriers	141 (0.56)	22 (0.40)	
	total	250 (1.00)	57 (1.00)	

Note: [&] Free + Low: "severity*frequencies" scores (NPI 0–4) for all individual symptoms; High: "severity*frequencies" scores (NPI 6–12) for all the individual symptoms. OR: Odd ratio.

On the contrary, no genetic correlates were observed for night-time behavior disturbances.

These results were further represented as decision model trees in Figure S1 (Supplementary Materials).

When we considered the "Psychosis" endophenotype as whole, we confirmed the effect of *APOE* ε4 allele alone (risk mean = 20.7, 95% CI: 18.5–22.9), but also a "genexgene" interaction with *MTHFR* for both polymorphisms. In particular, *APOE* ε4 non-carriers along with the homozygotes CC (C677T) showed a high risk to develop psychosis (risk mean = 20.2, 95% CI: 18.9–29.3), but also with the homozygotes CC (C677T) and with the 1298A allele carriers (risk mean = 23.1, 95% CI: 18.7–27.6) (Figure 1A).

3.3.2. "Genexgene" Interactions in "Hyperactivity" Endophenotype and the Relative Single BPSD Symptoms

For irritability symptoms, no genetic correlates were observed, whereas for agitation, the results are reported above. Although in an unrepresentative sample, a risk role of *APOE* ε4 allele was found with higher severity in appetite/eating abnormalities (OR = 2.06, 95% CI: 1.14–3.71) (Table 6). These results were further represented in Figure S1 (Supplementary Materials) as decision model trees.

When we consider the "Hyperactivity" endophenotype as a whole, the most significant result is represented by the risk role of *APOE* ε4 allele (risk mean = 13.2, 95% CI: 11.8–14.7). Moreover, an interaction with the *MTHFR* C677T CC genotype and *APOE* ε4 non-carriers was observed (risk mean = 12.1, 95% CI: 9.7–14.4) (Figure 1B).

3.3.3. "Genexgene" Interactions in "Mood"/"Frontal" Endophenotypes and the Relative Single BPSD Symptoms

No significant results were found for these endophenotype as well as for the relative single BPSD symptoms.

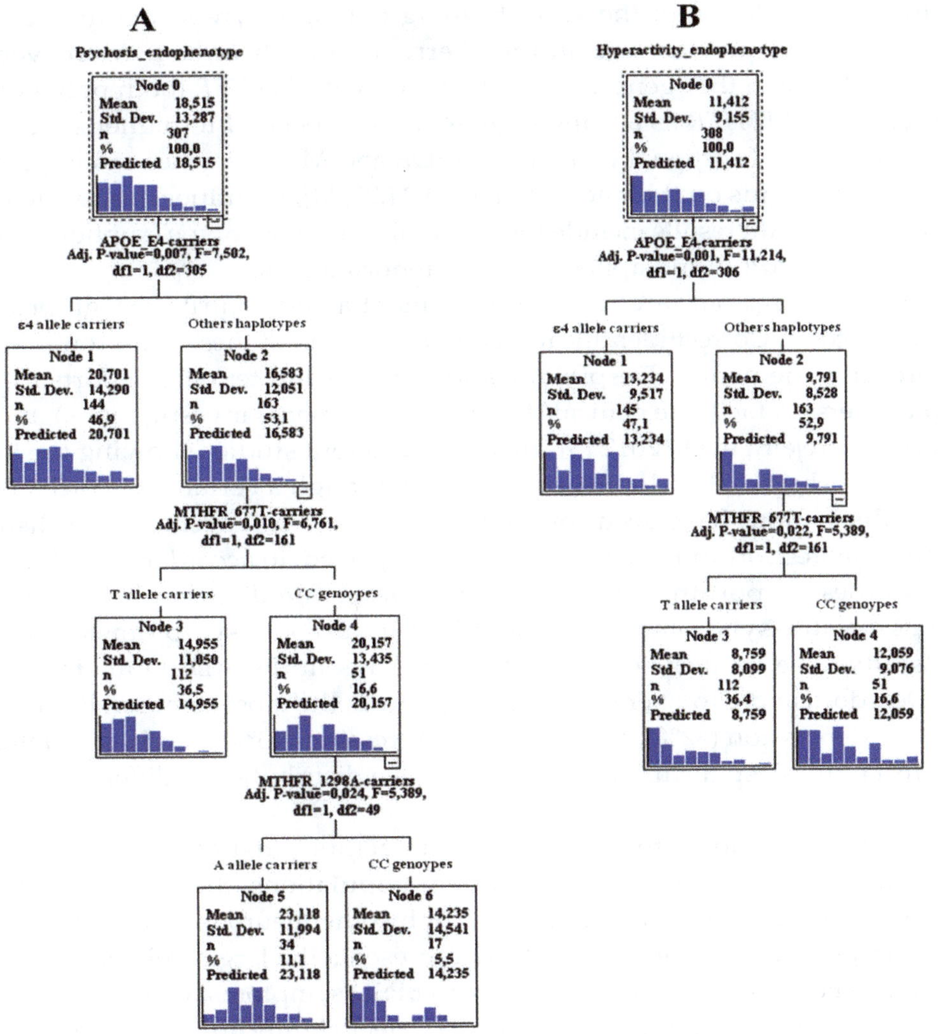

Figure 1. Exhaustive Chi-squared Automatic Interaction Detector (CHAID) data mining algorithm analysis results ("genexgene" interaction) for "Psychosis" (**A**) and "Hyperactivity" (**B**) endophenotypes. Note: Mean ± SD is given by the sum of the scores relative to "severity*frequencies" of the endophenotype components. For other haplotypes, we meant "*APOE* ε4 non-carriers".

4. Discussion

This study wants to deeply define the clinical distribution of BPSD symptoms in an Italian cohort of AD patients by the NPI scale. To the best of our knowledge, this is the largest BPSD cohort investigated until now. In this population, "Psychosis" and "Hyperactivity" endophenotypes as well as "agitation" as single symptoms were revealed to be associated with a high severity in symptomatology. In addition, "Mood" was associated to lower mean values, and, for last there was the "Frontal" endophenotype. As major clinical information, we suggest two combinatorial approaches to characterize a BPSD cohort: through 12 individual symptoms as well as four specific behavioral and neuropsychiatric endophenotypes. This choice allows us to overcome the limitations linked to a single methodological approach, bringing to light the interconnected aspects of the complex pathogenic mechanisms of BPSD. Moreover, we strongly propose analyzing the genetic correlates also in relation to single BPSD symptoms as well as to BPSD endophenotypes. This represents a valid strategy for expanding the knowledge about the aetiopathogenetic mechanisms of BPSD. There is more. We strongly suggest the use of both strategies also in relation to the genetic approach "single gene" involvement/"gene*x*gene" interaction, because this contributes to clarifying deeply the complex genetic architecture underlying BPSD. The main results obtained in this work are represented by the involvement of *APOE* as a "single gene" in the modulation of the severity in agitation, also reflected in "Psychosis" as well as in "Hyperactivity" endophenotypes, and in aberrant motor behavior. Moreover, we found the involvement of *APOE* also in the "gene$\times$gene" interaction with *MTHFR* (both polymorphisms) as risk factors for "Psychosis". *MTHFR* as a "single gene" was associated to higher severity of delusions. This implicates that specific functional variants in *APOE* and *MTHFR* genes can impact on the relative proteins' translation and thus on their activity [16,23,24,29,30], to influence specific BPSD traits. No associations or minor relevant results include the "Frontal" endophenotype (euphoria and disinhibition) and the relation between *APOE* and appetite/eating abnormalities.

Neuropsychiatric symptoms are frequent in dementia and contribute significantly for burden caregiver and illness costs. Correct identification and evaluation of these symptoms is a crucial part of the clinical approach to dementia. Despite the added value and tentative efforts to group different symptoms into clusters (to facilitate clinical/diagnostic/treatments investigations), there is not yet an established model. Cerejeira et al., 2012 [3] reviewed different studies showing the heterogeneity in the clusterization of behavioral endophenotypes, even though a certain concordance can be found. Delusions and hallucinations have been consistently grouped in "Psychosis". A distinct "Mood" or "Affective" cluster (depression and anxiety) has been suggested, in accordance with our study. On the contrary, some studies support that apathy and depression are distinct phenomena and belong to different neuropsychiatric syndromes, whereas others group both symptoms in the same factor [3], as in our case study. The frequencies of BPSD symptoms in the AD population can change [43]. As reported in Deardorff and Grossberg, 2019 [43], apathy is the most common BPSD symptom in AD (49%), followed by depression (42%), agitation and aggression (40%), psychosis (delusions, 31% and hallucinations, 16%), and sleep disturbances (39%). Such a distribution is different as compared to our BPSD/AD cohort.

These discrepancies could be related to different factors. First of all, the distribution of BPSD symptoms is strongly linked to differences in patient populations, their ethnicity, and composition (for instance whether the patients are affected by AD or by other neurodegenerative disorders). A small sample size is an important limitation. This study represents the larger cohort available to date, that permits performing a better stratification according to BPSD symptoms, where the range of symptoms has been precisely defined, besides being crucial to detect significant genetic associations. Indeed, genome-wide association studies and studies examining copy number variations performed in AD and psychosis have detected only suggestive underpowered associations in intronic SNPs (review in [44,45]). Moreover, individual symptoms evolve differently over the course of dementia. Notwithstanding the general impression that the overall level of psychopathology increases with dementia severity, they have a tendency to wax and wane, their severity fluctuating over time. For this reason, longitudinal studies are required to achieve significant insights into the evolution of BPSD during the course of disease [3]. Finally, the choice of setting for patient recruitment is a further important selection bias: Nursing home dwellers, inpatients, or patients treated in an ambulatory setting. The most inclusive population-based studies recruit "real-life" patients, making the results much more practical, although at a price of numerous medical, environmental, and drug-related confounders [10]. In our case, we have recruited patients from the department of our hospital, who in the majority of cases, enter for a control of BPSD. Thus, for definition, they are affected by disorders with a more prevalent "agitated" symptomatology rather than "apathy".

If age is the greatest risk factor for AD, the ε4 allele of the *APOE* is the greatest genetic risk factor for LOAD [16]. ε4 carriers showed higher severity in agitation symptoms, grouping in "Hyperactivity"/"Psychosis" endophenotypes. The single association with agitation is confirmed in different studies, including recent reviews [10,46,47]. Based on neuroimaging studies, agitation is associated with volume loss in the frontal cortex, circulate cortex, insula, amygdala, and hippocampus [48]. Neurochemically, agitation is associated with decreased cholinergic activity in the frontal and temporal cortex. Interestingly, AD patients carrying the *APOE* ε4 allele show a more profound loss in cholinergic activity in the hippocampus and the cortex, and in neuroimaging studies the presence of the *APOE* ε4 allele was associated with a greater rate of hippocampal, cortical, and whole-brain atrophy [10]. On the other hand, there are also negative studies, reporting no associations of this gene with agitation [49]. These findings, thus, further emphasize the importance of sub-grouping BPSD in distinct neuropsychiatric syndromes. In fact, we found an association of *APOE* also within "Hyperactivity"/"Psychosis" endophenotypes. We therefore support the evidence on the role played by the allele ε4 as a risk factor in these endophenotypes, along with the importance of the BPSD clusterization.

The ε4 carriers showed also higher severity in aberrant motor behavior, the finding was confirmed also in other different studies [50–52], where they demonstrated that the *APOE* ε4 status increased the tendency toward this symptom.

Another more significant result of this work regarding the "gene*x*gene" interactions between *APOE* and *MTHFR* (both polymorphisms) as risk factors for higher severity in the "Psychosis" endophenotype, underlies the important role played by *MTHFR* as a single gene in delusions (genotype CC of C677T). This interaction was observed also in "Hyperactivity". What is highlighted from the CART analysis, is that also the other *APOE* ε4 non carriers can play a role, and this is performed through the interactions with the CC genotype (C677T) and/or 1298A allele carriers. Different studies supported the epistatic effect between *MTHFR* and *APOE* on cognitive performance in the elderly but also in AD [53–55]. Moreover, plasma homocysteine concentrations are associated with increased amyloid-β (Aβ) deposition in the brain [28]. Although this effect was supported, no studies are available to confirm this interaction also in the psychosis/hyperactivity dimension. The most probable hypotheses behind this result could be that *MTHFR* contributes to the regulation of relin [56], whose expression is decreased in the hippocampus of subjects suffering from schizophrenia and major depressive disorder (MDD) [57]. Relin binds to the receptor for APOE, and might thus similarly modulate glutamatergic neurotransmission, altered in psychosis. Moreover, a significant positive correlation of serum homocysteine levels was found with delusions [58].

In relation to *COMT* as a "single gene", we did not confirm the results reported by Borroni et al., 2006 [12,13]. Further studies are needed to clarify the role of this gene, that seems to be less relevant as compared to the findings found for *APOE* and *MTHFR* genes, also in their interaction.

If we select in PubMed the following keywords "BPSD-gene-Alzheimer", we found 32 results where the studies have been actively published until 2013, from 2013 to 2020 there are only seven works performed on the genetics of BPSD. To date, the classic limitations linked to genetic studies remain and there is still the necessity of: larger cohorts with appropriate assessment tools and statistical methods with correction for multiple testing. There are limitations regarding inconsistent data in genome-wide association studies with prevalently intronic SNPs detection and presence of confounders influencing the associations. In this study, appropriate statistical tools such as the exhaustive CHAID data mining algorithm were used allowing to obtain the adjusted *p*-values for multiple testing, and where age and sex did not influence the calculations. The only variable not included in our analyses was "Medications". Medications as well as comorbidity are clinical information extremely heterogeneous in a BPSD population, including our cohort (Table 1). To include "Medications" or "Comorbidity" as variables in the statistical analyses would result in being overly complex, especially in a sample of sample sizes such as ours. Thus, we suggest that future studies should consider these variables, but starting from homogeneous groups for medications and for comorbidity, on which then to investigate the genetic correlates.

Although aware that further studies are still needed, we want to ignite the enthusiasm and encourage more research to deepen the etiopathogenetic mechanisms of BPSD in AD, starting by a well-defined BPSD population, appropriate statistical methods with multiple corrections, larger sample, and "gene*x*gene" and possibly "gene*x*environment" interactions. This permits not only to facilitate a clinical/diagnostic assessment, but also and mainly to define appropriate treatments chosen that, to date, represent the major concern for the clinicals.

5. Conclusions

We strongly suggest the combined use of both BPSD single symptoms/endophenotypes and the "gene*x*gene" interactions as valid strategies for expanding the knowledge about the BPSD aetiopathogenetic mechanisms.

Supplementary Materials:
Table S1: Univariate Analysis of Variance in our BPSD cohort: Tests of Between-Subjects Effects for Gender variable and BPSD endophenotypes, Table S2: Univariate Analysis of Variance in our BPSD cohort: Tests of Between-Subjects Effects for Age variable and BPSD endophenotypes, Table S3: Hosmer-Lemeshow goodness of fit test in single BSPD symptoms. Table S4: Stepwise multiple logistic regression for "Psychosis" endophenotype, Table S5: Stepwise multiple logistic regression for "Hyperactivity" endophenotype, Figure S1: Exaustive CHAID data mining algorithm analysis results ("gene × gene" interaction) for single BPSD symptoms according to different values of "severity*frequencies".

Author Contributions: Conceptualization, C.S., M.C., and C.B.; data curation, M.C. and C.B.; formal analysis, M.C., C.M., and C.B.; investigation, C.B.; project administration, C.B.; validation, C.S. and C.B.; writing—review and editing, C.S., M.C., C.M., C.G., O.Z., M.G., and C.B. All authors have read and agreed to the published version of the manuscript.

References

1. McKhann, G.M.; Knopman, D.S.; Chertkow, H.; Hyman, B.T.; Jack, C.R., Jr.; Kawas, C.H.; Klunk, W.E.; Koroshetz, W.J.; Manly, J.J.; Mayeux, R.; et al. The diagnosis of dementia due to Alzheimer's disease: Recommendations from the National Institute on Aging-Alzheimer's Association workgroups on diagnostic guidelines for Alzheimer's disease. *Alzheimers Dement.* **2011**, *7*, 263–269. [CrossRef]
2. Haupt, M.; Kurz, A.; Janner, M. A 2-year follow-up of behavioural and psychological symptoms in Alzheimer's disease. *Dement. Geriatr. Cogn. Disord.* **2000**, *11*, 147–152. [CrossRef] [PubMed]
3. Cerejeira, J.; Lagarto, L.; Mukaetova-Ladinska, E.B. Behavioral and psychological symptoms of dementia. *Front. Neurol.* **2012**, *3*, 73. [CrossRef] [PubMed]
4. Cloak, N.; Al Khalili, Y. *Behavioral and Psychological Symptoms in Dementia (BPSD)*; StatPearls Publishing LLC: Treasure Island, FL, USA, 2020.
5. Angelucci, F.; Spalletta, G.; di Iulio, F.; Ciaramella, A.; Salani, F.; Colantoni, L.; Varsi, A.E.; Gianni, W.; Sancesario, G.; Caltagirone, C.; et al. Alzheimer's disease (AD) and Mild Cognitive Impairment (MCI) patients are characterized by increased BDNF serum levels. *Curr. Alzheimer Res.* **2010**, *7*, 15–20. [CrossRef] [PubMed]
6. Finkel, S.I.; Costa e Silva, J.; Cohen, G.; Miller, S.; Sartorius, N. Behavioral and psychological signs and symptoms of dementia: A consensus statement on current knowledge and implications for research and treatment. *Int. Psychogeriatr.* **1996**, *8*, 497–500. [CrossRef] [PubMed]
7. Frisoni, G.B.; Rozzini, L.; Gozzetti, A.; Binetti, G.; Zanetti, O.; Bianchetti, A.; Trabucchi, M.; Cummings, J.L. Behavioral syndromes in Alzheimer's disease: Description and correlates. *Dement. Geriatr. Cogn. Disord.* **1999**, *10*, 130–138. [CrossRef]
8. van der Linde, R.M.; Dening, T.; Matthews, F.E.; Brayne, C. Grouping of behavioural and psychological symptoms of dementia. *Int. J. Geriatr. Psychiatry* **2014**, *29*, 562–568. [CrossRef]
9. Mushtaq, R.; Pinto, C.; Tarfarosh, S.F.; Hussain, A.; Shoib, S.; Shah, T.; Shah, S.; Manzoor, M.; Bhat, M.; Arif, T. A Comparison of the Behavioral and Psychological Symptoms of Dementia (BPSD) in Early-Onset and Late-Onset Alzheimer's Disease-A Study from South East Asia (Kashmir, India). *Cureus* **2016**, *8*, e625. [CrossRef]
10. Flirski, M.; Sobow, T.; Kloszewska, I. Behavioural genetics of Alzheimer's disease: A comprehensive review. *Arch. Med. Sci.* **2011**, *7*, 195–210. [CrossRef]
11. Borroni, B.; Agosti, C.; Archetti, S.; Costanzi, C.; Bonomi, S.; Ghianda, D.; Lenzi, G.L.; Caimi, L.; Di Luca, M.; Padovani, A. Catechol-O-methyltransferase gene polymorphism is associated with risk of psychosis in Alzheimer Disease. *Neurosci. Lett.* **2004**, *370*, 127–129. [CrossRef]

12. Borroni, B.; Grassi, M.; Agosti, C.; Archetti, S.; Costanzi, C.; Cornali, C.; Caltagirone, C.; Caimi, L.; Di Luca, M.; Padovani, A. Cumulative effect of COMT and 5-HTTLPR polymorphisms and their interaction with disease severity and comorbidities on the risk of psychosis in Alzheimer disease. *Am. J. Geriatr. Psychiatry* **2006**, *14*, 343–351. [CrossRef] [PubMed]
13. Borroni, B.; Grassi, M.; Agosti, C.; Costanzi, C.; Archetti, S.; Franzoni, S.; Caltagirone, C.; Di Luca, M.; Caimi, L.; Padovani, A. Genetic correlates of behavioral endophenotypes in Alzheimer disease: Role of COMT, 5-HTTLPR and APOE polymorphisms. *Neurobiol. Aging* **2006**, *27*, 1595–1603. [CrossRef] [PubMed]
14. Borroni, B.; Grassi, M.; Costanzi, C.; Zanetti, M.; Archetti, S.; Franzoni, S.; Caimi, L.; Padovani, A. Haplotypes in cathechol-O-methyltransferase gene confer increased risk for psychosis in Alzheimer disease. *Neurobiol. Aging* **2007**, *28*, 1231–1238. [CrossRef] [PubMed]
15. Akil, M.; Kolachana, B.S.; Rothmond, D.A.; Hyde, T.M.; Weinberger, D.R.; Kleinman, J.E. Catechol-O-methyltransferase genotype and dopamine regulation in the human brain. *J. Neurosci.* **2003**, *23*, 2008–2013. [CrossRef]
16. Lewandowski, C.T.; Maldonado Weng, J.; LaDu, M.J. Alzheimer's disease pathology in APOE transgenic mouse models: The Who, What, When, Where, Why, and How. *Neurobiol. Dis.* **2020**, *139*, 104811. [CrossRef]
17. Muller, T. Catechol-O-methyltransferase enzyme: Cofactor S-adenosyl-L-methionine and related mechanisms. *Int. Rev. Neurobiol.* **2010**, *95*, 49–71.
18. Seshadri, S.; Beiser, A.; Selhub, J.; Jacques, P.F.; Rosenberg, I.H.; D'Agostino, R.B.; Wilson, P.W.; Wolf, P.A. Plasma homocysteine as a risk factor for dementia and Alzheimer's disease. *N. Engl. J. Med.* **2002**, *346*, 476–483. [CrossRef]
19. Zheng, Z.; Wang, J.; Yi, L.; Yu, H.; Kong, L.; Cui, W.; Chen, H.; Wang, C. Correlation between behavioural and psychological symptoms of Alzheimer type dementia and plasma homocysteine concentration. *BioMed Res. Int.* **2014**, *2014*, 383494. [CrossRef]
20. Reif, A.; Pfuhlmann, B.; Lesch, K.P. Homocysteinemia as well as methylenetetrahydrofolate reductase polymorphism are associated with affective psychoses. *Prog. Neuro-psychopharmacol. Biol. Psychiatry* **2005**, *29*, 1162–1168. [CrossRef]
21. Monji, A.; Yanagimoto, K.; Maekawa, T.; Sumida, Y.; Yamazaki, K.; Kojima, K. Plasma folate and homocysteine levels may be related to interictal "schizophrenia-like" psychosis in patients with epilepsy. *J. Clin. Psychopharmacol.* **2005**, *25*, 3–5. [CrossRef]
22. Vogel, T.; Dali-Youcef, N.; Kaltenbach, G.; Andres, E. Homocysteine, vitamin B12, folate and cognitive functions: A systematic and critical review of the literature. *Int. J. Clin. Pract.* **2009**, *63*, 1061–1067. [CrossRef] [PubMed]
23. Frosst, P.; Blom, H.J.; Milos, R.; Goyette, P.; Sheppard, C.A.; Matthews, R.G.; Boers, G.J.; den Heijer, M.; Kluijtmans, L.A.; van den Heuvel, L.P. A candidate genetic risk factor for vascular disease: A common mutation in methylenetetrahydrofolate reductase. *Nat. Genet.* **1995**, *10*, 111–113. [CrossRef] [PubMed]
24. Rozen, R. Genetic predisposition to hyperhomocysteinemia: Deficiency of methylenetetrahydrofolate reductase (MTHFR). *Thromb. Haemost.* **1997**, *78*, 523–526. [CrossRef] [PubMed]
25. Rai, V. Methylenetetrahydrofolate Reductase (MTHFR) C677T Polymorphism and Alzheimer Disease Risk: A Meta-Analysis. *Mol. Neurobiol.* **2017**, *54*, 1173–1186. [CrossRef]
26. Stoccoro, A.; Tannorella, P.; Salluzzo, M.G.; Ferri, R.; Romano, C.; Nacmias, B.; Siciliano, G.; Migliore, L.; Coppede, F. The Methylenetetrahydrofolate Reductase C677T Polymorphism and Risk for Late-Onset Alzheimer's disease: Further Evidence in an Italian Multicenter Study. *J. Alzheimers Dis.* **2017**, *56*, 1451–1457. [CrossRef]
27. Hu, Q.; Teng, W.; Li, J.; Hao, F.; Wang, N. Homocysteine and Alzheimer's Disease: Evidence for a Causal Link from Mendelian Randomization. *J. Alzheimers Dis.* **2016**, *52*, 747–756. [CrossRef]
28. Roussotte, F.F.; Hua, X.; Narr, K.L.; Small, G.W.; Thompson, P.M. Alzheimer's Disease Neuroimaging Initiative The C677T variant in MTHFR modulates associations between brain integrity, mood, and cognitive functioning in old age. *Biol. Psychiatry Cogn. Neurosci. Neuroimaging* **2017**, *2*, 280–288.
29. van der Put, N.M.; Gabreels, F.; Stevens, E.M.; Smeitink, J.A.; Trijbels, F.J.; Eskes, T.K.; van den Heuvel, L.P.; Blom, H.J. A second common mutation in the methylenetetrahydrofolate reductase gene: An additional risk factor for neural-tube defects? *Am. J. Hum. Genet.* **1998**, *62*, 1044–1051. [CrossRef]
30. Weisberg, I.; Tran, P.; Christensen, B.; Sibani, S.; Rozen, R. A second genetic polymorphism in methylenetetrahydrofolate reductase (MTHFR) associated with decreased enzyme activity. *Mol. Genet. Metab.* **1998**, *64*, 169–172. [CrossRef]

31. McKhann, G.; Drachman, D.; Folstein, M.; Katzman, R.; Price, D.; Stadlan, E.M. Clinical diagnosis of Alzheimer's disease: Report of the NINCDS-ADRDA Work Group under the auspices of Department of Health and Human Services Task Force on Alzheimer's Disease. *Neurology* **1984**, *34*, 939–944. [CrossRef]
32. Folstein, M.F.; Folstein, S.E.; McHugh, P.R. "Mini-mental state". A practical method for grading the cognitive state of patients for the clinician. *J. Psychiatr. Res.* **1975**, *12*, 189–198. [CrossRef]
33. Miller, M.D.; Paradis, C.F.; Houck, P.R.; Mazumdar, S.; Stack, J.A.; Rifai, A.H.; Mulsant, B.; Reynolds, C.F., 3rd. Rating chronic medical illness burden in geropsychiatric practice and research: Application of the Cumulative Illness Rating Scale. *Psychiatry Res.* **1992**, *41*, 237–248. [CrossRef]
34. Katz, S.; Downs, T.D.; Cash, H.R.; Grotz, R.C. Progress in development of the index of ADL. *Gerontologist* **1970**, *10*, 20–30. [CrossRef] [PubMed]
35. Lawton, M.P.; Brody, E.M. Assessment of older people: Self-maintaining and instrumental activities of daily living. *Gerontologist* **1969**, *9*, 179–186. [CrossRef] [PubMed]
36. Cummings, J.L.; Mega, M.; Gray, K.; Rosenberg-Thompson, S.; Carusi, D.A.; Gornbein, J. The Neuropsychiatric Inventory: Comprehensive assessment of psychopathology in dementia. *Neurology* **1994**, *44*, 2308–2314. [CrossRef] [PubMed]
37. Desjardins, P.; Conklin, D. NanoDrop microvolume quantitation of nucleic acids. *J. Vis. Exp.* **2010**, *45*, 2565. [CrossRef]
38. Ingelsson, M.; Shin, Y.; Irizarry, M.C.; Hyman, B.T.; Lilius, L.; Forsell, C.; Graff, C. Genotyping of apolipoprotein E: Comparative evaluation of different protocols. *Curr. Protoc. Hum. Genet.* **2003**, *38*, 9–14. [CrossRef]
39. Gorsuch, R. *Factor Analysis*; Erlbaum: Hillsdale, NJ, USA, 1983.
40. Breiman, L.; Friedman, J.; Stone, C.J.; Olshen, R.A. *Classification and Regression Trees*; CRC Press: Boca Raton, FL, USA, 1984.
41. Zhang, H.; Bonney, G. Use of classification trees for association studies. *Genet. Epidemiol.* **2000**, *19*, 323–332. [CrossRef]
42. Biggs, D.; De Ville, B.; Suen, E. A method of choosing multiway partitions for classification and decision trees. *J. Appl. Stat.* **1991**, *18*, 49–62. [CrossRef]
43. Deardorff, W.J.; Grossberg, G.T. Behavioral and psychological symptoms in Alzheimer's dementia and vascular dementia. *Handb. Clin. Neurol.* **2019**, *165*, 5–32.
44. Shah, C.; DeMichele-Sweet, M.A.; Sweet, R.A. Genetics of psychosis of Alzheimer disease. *Am. J. Med. Genet. B Neuropsychiatr. Genet.* **2017**, *174*, 27–35. [CrossRef] [PubMed]
45. DeMichele-Sweet, M.A.A.; Weamer, E.A.; Klei, L.; Vrana, D.T.; Hollingshead, D.J.; Seltman, H.J.; Sims, R.; Foroud, T.; Hernandez, I.; Moreno-Grau, S.; et al. Genetic risk for schizophrenia and psychosis in Alzheimer disease. *Mol. Psychiatry* **2018**, *23*, 963–972. [CrossRef] [PubMed]
46. Panza, F.; Frisardi, V.; Seripa, D.; D'Onofrio, G.; Santamato, A.; Masullo, C.; Logroscino, G.; Solfrizzi, V.; Pilotto, A. Apolipoprotein E genotypes and neuropsychiatric symptoms and syndromes in late-onset Alzheimer's disease. *Ageing Res. Rev.* **2012**, *11*, 87–103. [CrossRef] [PubMed]
47. Ruthirakuhan, M.; Lanctot, K.L.; Di Scipio, M.; Ahmed, M.; Herrmann, N. Biomarkers of agitation and aggression in Alzheimer's disease: A systematic review. *Alzheimers Dement.* **2018**, *14*, 1344–1376. [CrossRef]
48. Rosenberg, P.B.; Nowrangi, M.A.; Lyketsos, C.G. Neuropsychiatric symptoms in Alzheimer's disease: What might be associated brain circuits? *Mol. Asp. Med.* **2015**, *43–44*, 25–37. [CrossRef]
49. Banning, L.C.P.; Janssen, E.P.C.J.; Hamel, R.E.G.; de Vugt, M.; Kohler, S.; Wolfs, C.A.G.; Oosterveld, S.M.; Melis, R.J.F.; Olde Rikkert, M.G.M.; Kessels, R.P.C.; et al. Determinants of Cross-Sectional and Longitudinal Health-Related Quality of Life in Memory Clinic Patients Without Dementia. *J. Geriatr. Psychiatry Neurol.* **2019**, *33*, 256–264. [CrossRef]
50. Garcia-Segura, M.E.; Fischer, C.E.; Schweizer, T.A.; Munoz, D.G. APOE varepsilon4/varepsilon4 Is Associated with Aberrant Motor Behavior Through Both Lewy Body and Cerebral Amyloid Angiopathy Pathology in High Alzheimer's Disease Pathological Load. *J. Alzheimers Dis.* **2019**, *72*, 1077–1087. [CrossRef]
51. Oliveira, F.F.; Chen, E.S.; Smith, M.C.; Bertolucci, P.H. Associations of cerebrovascular metabolism genotypes with neuropsychiatric symptoms and age at onset of Alzheimer's disease dementia. *Braz. J. Psychiatry.* **2017**, *39*, 95–103. [CrossRef]
52. Steinberg, M.; Corcoran, C.; Tschanz, J.T.; Huber, C.; Welsh-Bohmer, K.; Norton, M.C.; Zandi, P.; Breitner, J.C.; Steffens, D.C.; Lyketsos, C.G. Risk factors for neuropsychiatric symptoms in dementia: The Cache County Study. *Int. J. Geriatr. Psychiatry* **2006**, *21*, 824–830. [CrossRef]

53. Polito, L.; Poloni, T.E.; Vaccaro, R.; Abbondanza, S.; Mangieri, M.; Davin, A.; Villani, S.; Guaita, A. High homocysteine and epistasis between MTHFR and APOE: Association with cognitive performance in the elderly. *Exp. Gerontol.* **2016**, *76*, 9–16. [CrossRef]
54. Durmaz, A.; Kumral, E.; Durmaz, B.; Onay, H.; Aslan, G.I.; Ozkinay, F.; Pehlivan, S.; Orman, M.; Cogulu, O. Genetic factors associated with the predisposition to late onset Alzheimer's disease. *Gene* **2019**, *707*, 212–215. [CrossRef] [PubMed]
55. Yi, J.; Xiao, L.; Zhou, S.Q.; Zhang, W.J.; Liu, B.Y. The C677T Polymorphism of the Methylenetetrahydrofolate Reductase Gene and Susceptibility to Late-onset Alzheimer's Disease. *Open Med.* **2019**, *14*, 32–40. [CrossRef] [PubMed]
56. Chen, Z.; Schwahn, B.C.; Wu, Q.; He, X.; Rozen, R. Postnatal cerebellar defects in mice deficient in methylenetetrahydrofolate reductase. *Int. J. Dev. Neurosci.* **2005**, *23*, 465–474. [CrossRef] [PubMed]
57. Fatemi, S.H.; Earle, J.A.; McMenomy, T. Reduction in Reelin immunoreactivity in hippocampus of subjects with schizophrenia, bipolar disorder and major depression. *Mol. Psychiatry* **2000**, *5*, 654–663. [CrossRef] [PubMed]
58. Soni, R.M.; Tiwari, S.C.; Mahdi, A.A.; Kohli, N. Serum Homocysteine and Behavioral and Psychological Symptoms of Dementia: Is There Any Correlation in Alzheimer's Disease? *Ann. Neurosci.* **2019**, *25*, 152–159. [CrossRef]

5

Biomarkers for Alzheimer's Disease (AD) and the Application of Precision Medicine

Walter J. Lukiw [1,2,3,4,*], Andrea Vergallo [5], Simone Lista [5,6,7], Harald Hampel [5] and Yuhai Zhao [1,2]

1 LSU Neuroscience Center, Louisiana State University Health Science Center, New Orleans, LA 70112, USA; yzhao4@lsuhsc.edu
2 Department of Cell Biology and Anatomy, LSU-HSC, New Orleans, LA 70112, USA
3 Department of Ophthalmology, LSU Neuroscience Center, LSU-HSC, New Orleans, LA 70112, USA
4 Department Neurology, LSU Neuroscience Center, LSU-HSC, New Orleans, LA 70112, USA
5 Sorbonne University, GRC no 21, Alzheimer Precision Medicine (APM), AP-HP, Pitié-Salpêtrière hospital, F-75013 Paris, France; a_vergallo@yahoo.com (A.V.); slista@libero.it (S.L.); harald.hampel@med.uni-muenchen.de (H.H.)
6 Brain & Spine Institute (ICM), INSERM U 1127, CNRS UMR 7225, Boulevard de l'Hôpital, F-75013 Paris, France
7 Department of Neurology, Institute of Memory and Alzheimer's Disease (IM2A), Pitié-Salpêtrière Hospital, AP-HP, F-75013 Paris, France
* Correspondence: wlukiw@lsuhsc.edu

Abstract: An accurate diagnosis of Alzheimer's disease (AD) currently stands as one of the most difficult and challenging in all of clinical neurology. AD is typically diagnosed using an integrated knowledge and assessment of multiple biomarkers and interrelated factors. These include the patient's age, gender and lifestyle, medical and genetic history (both clinical- and family-derived), cognitive, physical, behavioral and geriatric assessment, laboratory examination of multiple AD patient biofluids, especially within the systemic circulation (blood serum) and cerebrospinal fluid (CSF), multiple neuroimaging-modalities of the brain's limbic system and/or retina, followed up in many cases by post-mortem neuropathological examination to finally corroborate the diagnosis. More often than not, prospective AD cases are accompanied by other progressive, age-related dementing neuropathologies including, predominantly, a neurovascular and/or cardiovascular component, multiple-infarct dementia (MID), frontotemporal dementia (FTD) and/or strokes or 'mini-strokes' often integrated with other age-related neurological and non-neurological disorders including cardiovascular disease and cancer. Especially over the last 40 years, enormous research efforts have been undertaken to discover, characterize, and quantify more effectual and reliable biological markers for AD, especially during the pre-clinical or prodromal stages of AD so that pre-emptive therapeutic treatment strategies may be initiated. While a wealth of genetic, neurobiological, neurochemical, neuropathological, neuroimaging and other diagnostic information obtainable for a single AD patient can be immense: (**i**) it is currently challenging to integrate and formulate a definitive diagnosis for AD from this multifaceted and multidimensional information; and (**ii**) these data are unfortunately not directly comparable with the etiopathological patterns of other AD patients even when carefully matched for age, gender, familial genetics, and drug history. Four decades of AD research have repeatedly indicated that diagnostic profiles for AD are reflective of an extremely heterogeneous neurological disorder. This commentary will illuminate the heterogeneity of biomarkers for AD, comment on emerging investigative approaches and discuss why ***'precision medicine'*** is emerging as our best paradigm yet for the most accurate and definitive prediction, diagnosis, and prognosis of this insidious and lethal brain disorder.

Keywords: Alzheimer's disease (AD); biomarkers; diagnostics; messenger RNA; microRNA; neuroimaging; neurotropic microbes; precision medicine; prognostics

---

1. Overview

Senile dementia is the progressive, age-related loss of memory and cognition sufficiently severe to irreversibly affect social, behavioral, perceptual, occupational, and functional capabilities. Recent statistics indicate that globally, about ~50 million people live with dementia, now costing an estimated one trillion dollars in annual healthcare. By 2050, the number of people with dementia is projected to increase to ~130 million. In the United States, Alzheimer disease (AD), the leading cause of senile dementia in the elderly, currently affects about ~6 million people age 65 and older; by 2050, the number of people aged 65 and older with AD will grow to a projected ~15 million if no medical breakthroughs occur to prevent, slow, or cure this incapacitating disorder of the human mind [1–3]. One hundred and fourteen years since its original description, despite immense research efforts and clinical trials employing multiple strategic therapeutic approaches, there is currently no adequate treatment or cure for this widely expanding socioeconomic and healthcare concern [2–8].

The discovery, characterization, and quantification of biomarkers as measurable substances or cognitive disruptions in the ***'prospective AD patient'***, whose presence are indicative of disease, are urgently needed so that: (**i**) AD may be more accurately diagnosed, especially at an earlier ***'prodromal'*** stage and with the goal of preventive and or targeted therapeutic strategies that may be implemented at the earliest signs of AD onset; and (**ii**) more effective and reliable integration of multi-modal biomarkers for AD that can streamline, support, and strengthen the diagnostic and therapeutic decision-making. Remarkably, peer-reviewed publications on biomarkers for AD have yielded almost ~53,000 original research reports and reviews since 1983 crossing the words ***'Alzheimer's disease'*** and ***'biomarkers'***; [2,3,8–10]. These include observations on the classical and established AD biomarkers [11–14], including altered genetics (incorporating genome-wide association studies or GWAS), genetic mutations and gene modifications (including methylation and post-transcriptional modifications), end-stage neurotoxic and pathogenic metabolic products that accumulate in AD brains, such as multiple forms of tau aggregates and amyloid-beta (Aβ) aggregation species and plaques. AD biomarkers also include protein, lipid, proteolipid, inflammatory cytokine, chemokine, carbohydrate, microRNA (miRNA), and messenger RNA (mRNA) abundance, speciation, and complexity, as well as an evolving assortment of neuro-radiological and neuroimaging technologies (Table 1). AD biomarkers are certainly useful in the detection of dementing illness during its progressive course, and their appearance and magnitude correlate with cognitive loss in a dynamic way, allowing clinicians to monitor responses to therapeutic intervention across a background of aging of the AD patient.

Table 1. Multiple interrelated factors contribute to AD. The considerable heterogeneity of Alzheimer's disease (AD) appears to be mediated in part by a highly interconnected network of biological factors, and each of these can be used as diagnostic biomarkers which appear to each have a variable potential to contribute to AD-type change. There is abundant evidence that all 23 of these biomarkers and/or factors (listed alphabetically) contribute to AD initiation, onset, or propagation, and there may be other important biological factors and other elements that may contribute to this complex neurological disease that we have not yet recognized or even considered. Data derived from each of these multiple biomarkers and factors combined is amenable to systems and network analysis, information integration, and the application of ***precision medicine*** that should ultimately yield a more accurate diagnosis of AD at any stage of the disease (see text for references; specific references to the biomarkers listed in Table 1 can be found in [15–29]. Abbreviations: BACE = β-amyloid cleavage enzyme; CRP = C-reactive protein (a blood-serum-based inflammatory biomarker); lncRNA = long non-coding RNA; PSI, PS2 = presenilin 1, presenilin 2; rRNA = ribosomal RNA; sncRNA = sall non-coding RNA.

age and age-related effects; amyloid (Aβ40 and Aβ42 peptides); compartmentalization of biomarkers [brain tissue, extracellular fluid (ECF), CSF, blood serum, urine]; cytokine storm (cytokines and chemokines); environment and environmental effects; epigenetics (methylation, mRNA and miRNA editing); exosomes and extracellular micro-vesicles (EXs and EMVs); gender and gender-related effects; genetics (mutations in BACE, PS1, PS2, etc.,); gastrointestinal (GI) tract microbiome; innate immunity; Neuro-inflammatory markers (CRP); inter-current illness (cardiovascular disease); lifestyle (diet, smoking); messenger RNA (mRNA); microbial contribution (viral, bacterial, fungal, other); microbiome (oral, other); microRNA (miRNA); miRNA-mRNA linking patterns; misdiagnosis; oral microbiome and dental hygiene; other RNA (sncRNA, lncRNA); overlapping neurological disorders: [Downs syndrome (Trisomy 21), frontotemporal dementia (FTD), multi-infarct dementia (MID), neuro-vascular disease, prion disease (PrD), etc.,].

As improvements in AD diagnostics are based on advances in both AD biomarker acquisition and the technologies used to gain these data, below we briefly discuss some of the most recent advances contributing in a major way to the more accurate and comprehensive accrual of important AD biomarker data.

2. Novel, Emerging, and Advanced Diagnostic Biomarkers for AD

2.1. Analysis of Exosomes (EXs), Extracellular Microvesicles (EMVs), and Their Molecular Cargos

Currently, the complex molecular cargos of exosomes and extracellular microvesicles (EXs and EMVs) have emerged as one of the most representative, significant, dependable, and trustworthy of all AD biomarkers. Typically, EX and EMV cargos consist of various mixtures of protein, lipid, proteolipid, cytokine, chemokine, carbohydrate, microRNA (miRNA) and messenger RNA (mRNA), and other constituents including end-stage neurotoxic and pathogenic metabolic products. These in part, consist of tau proteins, amyloid beta (Aβ) peptides, alpha-synuclein, TAR DNA-binding protein 43 (TDP-43) and others. EXs and EMVs (**i**) have been analyzed in the cerebrospinal fluid (CSF), blood serum, and post-mortem tissues of AD patients; (**ii**) are derived from their cells of origin and typically contain hundreds of different signaling molecules, many of which are potentially pathogenic and may be involved in the horizontal spread of neurological disease from one brain region to another; (**iii**) may represent a defined class of plasma membrane-derived nanovesicles released by all cell lineages of the human central nervous system (CNS); and (**iv**) as potential biomarkers, may contribute to an additional element of certainty into the diagnostic assessment of AD [20,21,26,30–32].

2.2. The Evaluation of Neurotropic Microbes in AD as Potential Diagnostic Biomarkers

There is a wealth of data indicating that neurotropic microbes including both DNA and RNA viruses (such as *Herpes simplex 1* or *SARS-CoV-2*) or bacterial Phyla such as *Proteobacteria, Verrucomicrobia, Fusobacteria, Cyanobacteria, Actinobacteria*, and *Spirochetes* or microbe-derived viral, fungal, or prokaryotic cellular components or microbial neurotoxins have high affinity for neural cells of the human brain and CNS [24,33–41]. Multiple independent laboratories continue to report the detection of viral, bacterial, fungal, protozoal, or other microbially-derived nucleic acid sequences or neurotoxins, such as highly inflammatory bacterial amyloid peptides, lipopolysaccharide (LPS), and many microbe-derived endotoxins within AD affected brain tissues [24,29,34,36,39,40]. Microbial biomarkers and systems biology approaches to understand host–microbiome interactions have been suggested by multiple AD researchers that both: (**i**) predict the risk of developing AD well before the onset of cognitive decline; and (**ii**) stimulate and/or accelerate the development of classical AD neuropathology [24,34,39,41–44].

Whether these viral, bacterial, or other microbial DNA- or RNA-based nucleic acids or associated lipoproteins, liposaccharides, peptidoglycans, bacterial-derived amyloids, and/or neurotoxins originate from the gastrointestinal (GI) tract microbiome, a potential brain microbiome, or some dormant pathological microbiome is currently not well understood [24,35,36,40,43,45]. Since 1978, at least ~4400 peer-reviewed research articles provide convincing evidence that multiple species of microbes, including viruses, bacteria (especially Gram-negative bacteria), and other microorganisms or their secreted components are strongly associated with the onset and/or the development of AD-type change [24,29,33,34,41–43,46]. If microbial presence in the brain is involved in the early initiation or propagation of AD, as currently suspected, then specialized RNA-sequencing applications or nucleic acid-containing gene chips, electrochemical biosensors, or panels of microbial-derived 16S ribosomal RNA (rRNA) interrogated with nucleic acid probes derived from AD biofluids might be useful as novel AD biomarkers in the detection of microbial patterns of expression from human brain tissues at any stage or degree of AD neuropathology.

2.3. Linking microRNA-messenger RNA (miRNA-mRNA) Signaling Patterns in AD

DNA microfluidic array technologies, quantitative reverse transcription PCR (RT-qPCR), RNA sequencing, LED-Northern, Western immunoassay, and electrochemical biosensors, integrated by advanced bioinformatics tools have uncovered families of up-regulated human brain enriched microRNAs (miRNAs) and their down-regulated messenger RNA (mRNA) targets. These have been found in short post-mortem interval (PMI) sporadic AD brain, in transgenic animal models of AD (TgAD), in brain biopsies, and in biofluids from AD patients. Genome-wide association studies (GWAS), epigenetic evaluations, such as miRNA-mRNA linkage or association mapping for AD-relevant neurological pathways, should provide useful diagnostic approaches since it has recently become apparent that miRNA-mediated mRNA-targeted regulatory mechanisms involve a large number of pathogenic and highly integrated gene expression pathways in the CNS [25,32,45–48]. To cite one very recent example, the human-brain-resident, nuclear factor kappa B p50/p65 (NF-κB p50/p65)-regulated microRNA-146a (miRNA-146a) is an inducible, 22-nucleotide, single-stranded non-coding RNA (sncRNA) easily detected in CNS neurons and immunological cell types. An inducible miRNA-146a: (**i**) is significantly up-regulated in AD brain tissues, CSF, and blood serum [25,48]; (**ii**) is an important epigenetic modulator of inflammatory signaling and the innate-immune response in several neurological disorders; and (**iii**) is essential in the down-regulation of the innate-immune regulator complement factor H (CFH; [10,20,23,25,40,46,49]).

LPS- and NF-kB (p50/p65)-inducible microRNAs, such as miRNA-146a and miRNA-125b, appear to contribute to neuropathological, neuro-inflammatory, and altered neuro-immunological aspects of both AD and prion disease (PrD; [25,32,40,46,48–50]). Interestingly, NF-κB-sensitive up-regulated miRNAs and their down-regulated mRNA targets appear to constitute an integrated NF-κB-miRNA-mRNA signaling network implicated in multiple AD pathophysiological processes [10,40,45,48,50,51]. Hence, potential signaling pathways to the acquisition of the AD phenotype appear to occur in part via an integrated and highly complex system of multiple miRNA-mRNA interactions that define many key pathogenic and pro-inflammatory gene expression pathways. Genetic and epigenetic signaling via miRNA-mRNA networks in the brain may be one of the most useful as potential biomarkers for early AD detection as they can detect subtle failure in multiple AD-relevant brain signaling systems and metabolic pathways [10,25,45,49,51].

2.4. *Recent Advances in Neuro-Radiological and Neuroimaging Technologies*

A number of neuro-radiological and neuroimaging technologies are currently being used to view physical atrophy and structural change in specific anatomical regions of the human brain, such as the hippocampus, neocortex (gray matter), white matter, ventricles, and other brain regions for the purpose of acquiring real time data for the diagnosis of AD [19,28,52–61]. These neuroimaging technologies and structural and functional imaging techniques include computerized tomography (CT; including dual-energy CT), positron emission tomography (PET), scintigraphic neuroimaging (PET-SN), diffuse optical imaging (DOT), structural and functional magnetic resonance imaging (MRI), including ultra-high field MRI (UHF-MRI), magnetoencephalography (MEG), single-photon emission computed tomography (SPECT), cranial ultrasound, and functional ultrasound imaging (fUS) in the search for anatomically-based diagnostic biomarkers for AD with high accuracy and sensitivity [19,28,57–62]. Neuroimaging techniques, hardware and software design, and imaging resolution are being constantly improved, updated, and refined [28,60–62]. For example, with high signal-to-noise (S/N) ratios, improved contrast and unparalleled spatial resolution, ultra-high field MRI of $\geq$7 tesla (T) has been highly successful in imaging the neuroanatomy of highly focused brain regions targeted by AD pathophysiology while providing additional information on morphological, quantitative, and subtle metabolic changes associated with early AD-type pathological alterations [57,61]. In vivo biomarkers for AD performed by recently implemented scintigraphic neuroimaging and employing amyloid binding PET agents along with non-scintigraphic biomarkers from blood (plasma/serum) and CSF have provided unique and novel opportunities to investigate the pathogenesis, prodromal changes, and time course of the disease in living individuals across the AD continuum [19,28,61–63]. Imaging technologies have indicated that AD changes in brain tissues begin as much as ~25 years prior to the onset of clinical symptomatology [28,61,63,64]. The opportunities afforded by *in vivo* biomarkers of AD, whether by blood (plasma/serum) or CSF examination or imaging technologies, are beginning to transform the strategic design of AD therapeutic trials by shifting the focus to the preclinical stages of the disease and massively integrating both molecular-based and neuroimaging data [60,61,63–67].

3. AD Biomarkers and Post-Mortem Neuropathological Examination of the AD Brain

Classically, the diagnosis of AD was a clinic-pathological one and there was a considerable error rate in the clinical diagnosis, especially early in the course of the disease. The differential diagnosis for AD by exclusion was confounded by a great many clinically overlapping neurological disorders including, mainly, MID, FTD, prion disease, tumors, subdural hematomas, neurovascular disruption and disease, and others [4–6]. Early neurophysiological diagnostic observations of AD included a diffusely slow electroencephalogram (EEG) and reduced cerebral blood flow [4,5,7]. Early PET studies demonstrated that oxygen extraction in the AD brain was relatively normal, thus tentatively excluding ischemia as a potential pathogenic factor [4,5,64]. Morphological pathological changes including the appearance of amyloid-enriched senile plaques (SP) and neurofibrillary tangles (NFT), widely distributed in neocortex but excluded from the basal ganglia, thalamus, and substantia nigra, and a severe loss of large neocortical neurons, were 'classical' diagnostic characteristics of the AD patient [4–8].

Usually at the family or care-giver's request, post-mortem neuropathological examinations of the deceased AD patient's brain were routinely performed by qualified AD-trained specialists and neuropathologists and brain tissues were often subsequently provided to AD researchers for further molecular-genetic and biomarker research including the examination for the presence of AD-relevant brain lesions. Light microscopy, NFT and SP amyloid dyes (such as Congo red, Thioflavin S, Thioflavin T and methylene yellow), and antibody-based staining (such as 6E10 and 10G4), the evaluation, density, composition, and quantitation of NFT and SP amyloid, and the examination of blood (plasma/serum) or CSF amyloid were additional indicators of immune- or inflammatory-neuropathology in the individual AD patient, which often contributed to the confirmation of AD in the ***'prospective AD patient'***. Currently, in many medical schools in the US and Canada, the post-mortem examination of the AD brain still remains the classical exercise to certify and verify the existence of AD. It is generally appreciated that the application of ***'precision medicine'***, involving massively integrated data sets of multi-faceted AD biomarkers, data-driven analytical methodologies, and the application of systems theory, will challenge and may eventually supersede the need for the classical post-mortem neuropathological examination of the brain in order to verify and confirm the diagnosis of AD [10–16,22,59,64,65,68].

3.1. Challenges in the Validation of AD Biomarkers

There are inherent problems in current approaches to AD biomarker research: (**i**) as most early reports emphasized just one or at most a few AD molecular-genetic biomarkers, biophysical, and neuroimaging modalities without consideration of the other hundreds or thousands of proteins, peptides, carbohydrates, lipids, or DNA and multiple species of RNA that have been previously implicated as being 'probable' diagnostic markers for AD; (**ii**) very often the nature of the acquisition of AD biomarkers represented a ***'snapshot in time'*** of one specific portion of the AD continuum that does not take into consideration the time course of changes observed in AD and/or the progressive nature of the disorder; (**iii**) because easily accessible and non-invasive AD biomarkers are often limited in their diagnostic applicability because of their overlap with other neurological diseases related to AD, such as Down's syndrome, Parkinson's and Lewy body disease, prion disease, FTD, hippocampal sclerosis, and MID and stroke; and (**iv**) no single newly generated ***de novo*** biomarker has ever been found to be associated with AD; that is, fluctuations in the abundance of pre-existing AD biomarkers reflect significant and absolute differences in the quantity, speciation, and stoichiometric relationships of AD-related biomolecules, including indicators of pro-inflammatory and immune system dysfunction. Put another way, no 'specific' AD biomarker 'suddenly appears' at the earliest onset, or propagation, or throughout any time-point during the course of AD, or at any stage of cognitive failure for that matter. Rather, it is usually a quantifiable up-regulation or down-regulation of an already existing biomarker in a specific anatomical region or biofluid compartment that has been the most consistently observed in the progressively degenerating brain. To cite a recent example, over 50 susceptibility genes and gene loci have been associated with late-onset AD and multiple models have been proposed [27], however, these associations are relatively rare and non-penetrant, occur in a few but not all AD cases, adding to the complexity and heterogeneity in the diagnosis of AD [15,56,58,63,64,69,70]. To further confound the establishment of definitive AD biomarkers, AD is commonly associated with more than one single neuropathology, in the case of AD usually with cerebrovascular and/or neurovascular involvement, and every one of these ancillary neurological disorders can carry their own set of complex and often overlapping disease biomarkers [10,63,64,69,70].

Especially over the last 10 years, the progressive and steadily increasing accumulation of molecular, genetic, epigenetic, neuroimaging, clinical, and geriatric data acquired from multiple AD cohorts has significantly increased our appreciation and understanding of the intrinsic variability and heterogeneity of AD biomarkers associated with the continuum of AD and other forms of progressive age-related neurodegenerative disease. The generation of massive datasets integrating multiple genetic-, epigenetic-, molecular-, and neuroimaging-derived biomarkers is enabling the application of clustering techniques and the identification and stratification of AD subtypes that may further categorize the multiple aspects of AD heterogeneity [10–18,67–70]. These approaches hold great potential: **(i)** for improving both the diagnosis and prognosis of AD; **(ii)** for projecting the clinical and neurological evolution of AD for planning suitable directions in therapeutic mediation; **(iii)** in providing multiple opportunities for the more directed analysis of AD heterogeneity in a data driven manner; **(iv)** in providing strategic guidelines for more decisive therapeutic intervention and the more efficacious clinical management of AD; and **(v)** for advancing ***'precision medicine'*** not only for the individual AD patient, but also for other cases of inflammatory neurodegeneration and neurological disease.

3.2. Using Precision Medicine in the Diagnosis of AD

Multiple analytical molecular-genetic approaches, advances in geriatric psychiatry and clinical evaluation, advancements in neuro-radiological labelling techniques and neuroimaging technologies, integrated diagnostic and predictive strategies and methodological improvements, discoveries of the comprehensive pathophysiological profiles of complex multi-factorial neurodegenerative diseases: **(i)** are presently well within the capabilities and scope of contemporary clinical, medical, and diagnostic neurology; **(ii)** are currently yielding increasingly large volumes of biomarker data for both individual AD patients, large populations of AD cases and age- and gender-matched controls; and **(iii)** are providing a data-driven basis for the paradigm shift of using the ***'precision medicine'*** approach in AD prevention, diagnostics, prognostics, and therapeutics [10,13,14,16,22,27,64]. Less common clinical presentations of AD are becoming increasingly recognized, adding to the increasing volume of AD biomarker data [10,14,17,19,64]. Since one of the pillars of ***'precision medicine'*** is supported by biomarker-derived medical data, further improvements in the acquisition, integration, interpretation, and bioinformatics aspects of clinical data and the coordination and analysis of clinical, laboratory, molecular-genetic, and neuroimaging data, geriatric and psychological information and related healthcare resources should obtain significantly increased accuracy in the diagnostic synopsis for the ***"prospective AD patient"***. The significant heterogeneity of the AD condition: **(i)** will certainly benefit from an equally wide variety of AD biomarker-derived ***'precision medicine'***-oriented treatment approaches and/or data-driven pharmacological strategies; and **(ii)** whose biomarker-based therapeutic design will greatly improve the current situation regarding the healthcare, more effective and successful treatment, and the development of disease-modifying drugs for AD patients at any stage of the disease [10,22,65,68,71].

4. Summary

The ongoing search for valid biomarkers for AD is being carried out globally in at least a dozen major geriatric, bioinformatic, neurobiological, neuro-genetic and neurological bioscience arenas: **(i)** those involving the age, gender, and geriatrics of the ***'prospectiveAD patient'***; **(ii)** in the genetics and epigenetics of the AD patient including messenger RNA (mRNA) and microRNA (miRNA) signaling patterns, complexity and genomic methylation research; **(iii)** in multiple biofluids from AD patients including the blood (plasma/serum) of the systemic circulation, the glymphatic system, the cerebrospinal fluid (CSF) and/or urine; **(iv)**; through the detailed analysis of molecular cargos from both biofluids and tissue-compartmentalized exosomes and extracellular microvesicles (EXs and EMVs); **(v)** throughout the peripheral nervous system (PNS; typically using skin biopsies); **(vi)** via clinically-based geriatric, psychiatric, and neurological assessment and testing; **(vii)** via advances in neuro-radiological labeling techniques and neuroimaging technologies including CAT, PET, PET-SN,

MRI, fMRI; UHF-MRI, DOT, MEG, SPECT, cranial ultrasound, functional ultrasound (fUS) imaging, and immunohistochemistry involving confocal laser scanning microscopy and other advanced microscopic and neuroimaging techniques; (**viii**) from the quantitation and characterization of the load of microbial and microbial-derived components in the AD-affected brain; (**ix**) via the identification, quantitation, and characterization of AD-specific lesions including amyloid peptide-enriched SPs and NFTs; (**x**) after post-mortem examination and biopsies of AD cases, again matched up against those same biomarkers in age- and gender-matched neurologically normal controls to corroborate the prospective diagnosis of AD; (**xi**) via the comprehensive analysis of the potential contribution of overlapping progressive, age-related neurological disorders to AD-type change; and lastly (**xii**), through the assessment of the socioeconomic, environmental, and lifestyle factors of the ***'prospectiveAD patient'*** (Table 1). The recent application of highly integrated data sets of these multiple AD biomarkers and analytical techniques on large cohorts of AD patients and involving systems-biology and ***'precision medicine'*** may well serve to unravel many of the more intricate aspects of AD heterogeneity and expand and build on current therapeutic strategies to more effectively address both the diagnosis and clinical management of this devastating neurological disease.

Author Contributions: Conceptualization, W.J.L. and H.H.; writing original draft preparation, W.J.L. and Y.Z.; Validation/formal analysis/writing review and editing/visualization/supervision/project administration/funding acquisitions W.J.L., H.H., A.V., S.L., Y.Z. All authors have read and agreed to the published version of the manuscript.

Acknowledgments: A.V. is an employee of Eisai Inc. This work has been performed during his previous position at Sorbonne University, Paris, France. H.H. is an employee of Eisai Inc. This work has been performed during his previous position at Sorbonne University, Paris, France. At Sorbonne University he was supported by the AXA Research Fund, the "*Fondation partenariale Sorbonne Université*" and the "*Fondation pour la Recherche sur Alzheimer*", Paris, France. This work was presented in part at the Society for Neuroscience (SFN) Annual Meeting 19–23 October 2019 Chicago IL, USA. Sincere thanks are extended to L. Carver, E. Head, W. Poon, H. LeBlanc, F. Culicchia, C. Eicken and C. Hebel for short post-mortem interval (PMI) human brain and/or retinal tissues or extracts, miRNA array work and initial data interpretation, and to D Guillot and AI Pogue for expert technical assistance. Thanks are also extended to the many neuropathologists, physicians and researchers of Canada and the US who have provided high quality, short post-mortem interval (PMI), human CNS, retinal tissues or extracted total brain and retinal RNA and biofluids (ECF, CSF and blood serum sample) for scientific studies.

Appendix A

H.H. is an employee of Eisai Inc. and serves as Senior Associate Editor for the Journal Alzheimer's & Dementia and does not receive any fees or honoraria since May 2019; before May 2019 he had received lecture fees from Servier, Biogen and Roche, research grants from Pfizer, Avid, and MSD Avenir (paid to the institution), travel funding from Functional Neuromodulation, Axovant, Eli Lilly and company, Takeda and Zinfandel, GE-Healthcare and Oryzon Genomics, consultancy fees from Qynapse, Jung Diagnostics, Cytox Ltd., Axovant, Anavex, Takeda and Zinfandel, GE Healthcare and Oryzon Genomics, and Functional Neuromodulation, and participated in scientific advisory boards of Functional Neuromodulation, Axovant, Eisai, Eli Lilly and company, Cytox Ltd., GE Healthcare, Takeda and Zinfandel, Oryzon Genomics and Roche Diagnostics. H.H. is co-inventor in the following patents as a scientific expert and has received no royalties: In Vitro Multiparameter Determination Method for The Diagnosis and Early Diagnosis of Neurodegenerative Disorders Patent Number: 8916388; In Vitro Procedure for Diagnosis and Early Diagnosis of Neurodegenerative Diseases Patent Number: 8298784; Neurodegenerative Markers for Psychiatric Conditions Publication Number: 20120196300; In Vitro Multiparameter Determination Method for The Diagnosis and Early Diagnosis of Neurodegenerative Disorders Publication Number: 20100062463; In Vitro Method for The Diagnosis and Early Diagnosis of Neurodegenerative Disorders Publication Number: 20100035286; In Vitro Procedure for Diagnosis and Early Diagnosis of Neurodegenerative Diseases Publication Number: 20090263822; In Vitro Method for The Diagnosis of Neurodegenerative Diseases Patent Number: 7547553; CSF Diagnostic in Vitro Method for Diagnosis of Dementias and Neuroinflammatory Diseases Publication Number: 20080206797; In Vitro Method for The Diagnosis of Neurodegenerative Diseases

Publication Number: 20080199966; Neurodegenerative Markers for Psychiatric Conditions Publication Number: 20080131921; A.V. is an employee of Eisai Inc. He does not receive any fees or honoraria since November 2019. Before November 2019 he had received lecture honoraria from Roche, MagQu LLC, and Servier. S.L. has received lecture honoraria from Roche and Servier. W.J.L. is the Bollinger Professor of Alzheimer's disease (AD) at the LSU School of Medicine and Health Sciences Center. He serves on 36 journal editorial boards and study sections and is senior academic editor for the journals *Frontiers in Genetics, Neurochemical Research, Folia Neuropathologica* and *PLoS One.* Research on miRNA and mRNA in the Lukiw laboratory involving biomarkers in AD and in other forms of neurological or retinal disease, prion disease, amyloidogenesis, synaptogenesis, neuro-inflammation and environmental neurotoxicology was supported through an unrestricted grant to the LSU Eye Center from Research to Prevent Blindness (RPB); the Louisiana Biotechnology Research Network (LBRN) and NIH grants NEI EY006311, NIA AG18031 and NIA AG038834 (W.J.L.).

References

1. Available online: https://www.alz.org/alzheimers-dementia/facts (accessed on 17 September 2020).
2. Arvanitakis, Z.; Shah, R.C.; Bennett, D.A. Diagnosis and management of dementia: Review. *JAMA* **2019**, *322*, 1589–1599. [CrossRef]
3. Patnode, C.D.; Perdue, L.A.; Rossom, R.C.; Rushkin, M.C.; Redmond, N.; Thomas, R.G.; Lin, J.S. *Screening for Cognitive Impairment in Older Adults: An Evidence Update for the U.S. Preventive Services Task Force*; Rockville, M.D., Ed.; Agency for Healthcare Research and Quality (US): Rockville, MD, USA, 2020.
4. Terry, R.D.; Katzman, R. Senile dementia of the Alzheimer type. *Ann. Neurol.* **1983**, *14*, 497–506. [CrossRef]
5. Thienhaus, O.J.; Hartford, J.T.; Skelly, M.F.; Bosmann, H.B. Biologic markers in Alzheimer's disease. *J. Am. Geriatr. Soc.* **1985**, *33*, 715–726. [CrossRef]
6. Alzheimer, A.; Stelzmann, R.A.; Schnitzlein, H.N.; Murtagh, F.R. An English translation of Alzheimer's 1907 paper, "Uber eine eigenartige Erkankung der Hirnrinde". *Clin. Anat.* **1995**, *8*, 429–431. [CrossRef] [PubMed]
7. Lukiw, W.J. 100 years of Alzheimer's disease research: Are we any closer to a cure? *Aging Health* **2007**, *3*. [CrossRef]
8. Available online: https://www.alz.org/alzheimers-dementia (accessed on 17 September 2020).
9. Available online: www.ncbi.nlm.nih.gov/pmc (accessed on 17 September 2020).
10. Zhao, Y.; Jaber, V.; Alexandrov, P.N.; Vergallo, A.; Lista, S.; Hampel, H.; Lukiw, W.J. microRNA-Based Biomarkers and Alzheimer's disease (AD) Frontiers in Neuroscience—Neurodegeneration—Special Research Topic 'Deciphering the Biomarkers of Alzheimer's disease'. **2020**, in press.
11. Blennow, K.; Hampel, H.; Weiner, M.; Zetterberg, H. Cerebrospinal fluid and plasma biomarkers in Alzheimer disease. *Nat. Rev. Neurol.* **2010**, *6*, 131–144. [CrossRef] [PubMed]
12. Hampel, H.; Frank, R.; Broich, K.; Teipel, S.J.; Katz, R.G.; Hardy, J.; Herholz, K.; Bokde, A.L.; Jessen, F.; Hoessler, Y.C.; et al. Biomarkers for Alzheimer's disease: Academic, industry and regulatory perspectives. *Nat. Rev. Drug Discov.* **2010**, *9*, 560–574. [CrossRef] [PubMed]
13. Hampel, H.; O'Bryant, S.E.; Molinuevo, J.L.; Zetterberg, H.; Masters, C.L.; Lista, S.; Kiddle, S.J.; Batrla, R.; Blennow, K. Blood-based biomarkers for Alzheimer disease: Mapping the road to the clinic. *Nat. Rev. Neurol.* **2018**, *14*, 639–652. [CrossRef] [PubMed]
14. Hampel, H.; Vergallo, A.; Afshar, M.; Akman-Anderson, L.; Arenas, J.; Benda, N.; Batrla, R.; Broich, K.; Caraci, F.; Claudio Cuello, A.; et al. Blood-based systems biology biomarkers for next-generation clinical trials in Alzheimer's disease. *Dialogues Clin Neurosci.* **2019**, *21*, 177–191. [CrossRef]
15. Kim, D.H.; Yeo, S.H.; Park, J.M.; Choi, J.Y.; Lee, T.H.; Park, S.Y.; Ock, M.S.; Eo, J.; Kim, H.S.; Cha, H.J. Genetic markers for diagnosis and pathogenesis of Alzheimer's disease. *Gene* **2014**, *545*, 185–193. [CrossRef] [PubMed]
16. Lista, S.; Khachaturian, Z.S.; Rujescu, D.; Garaci, F.; Dubois, B.; Hampel, H. Application of systems theory in longitudinal studies on the origin and progression of Alzheimer's disease. *Methods Mol. Biol.* **2016**, *1303*, 49–67. [CrossRef] [PubMed]
17. DeTure, M.A.; Dickson, D.W. The neuropathological diagnosis of Alzheimer's disease. *Mol. Neurodegener.* **2019** *14*, 32. [CrossRef] [PubMed]

18. Toschi, N.; Lista, S.; Baldacci, F.; Cavedo, E.; Zetterberg, H.; Blennow, K.; Kilimann, I.; Teipel, S.J.; dos Santos, A.M.; Epelbaum, S.; et al. INSIGHT-preAD study group; Alzheimer Precision Medicine Initiative (APMI); Biomarker-guided clustering of Alzheimer's disease clinical syndromes. *Neurobiol. Aging* **2019**, *83*, 42–53. [CrossRef] [PubMed]
19. Veitch, D.P.; Weiner, M.W.; Aisen, P.S.; Beckett, L.A.; Cairns, N.J.; Green, R.C.; Harvey, D.; Jack Jr, C.R.; Jagust, W.; Morris, J.C.; et al. Understanding disease progression and improving Alzheimer's disease clinical trials: Recent highlights from the Alzheimer's Disease Neuroimaging Initiative. *Alzheimers Dement.* **2019**, *15*, 106–152. [CrossRef]
20. Aharon, A.; Spector, P.; Ahmad, R.S.; Horrany, N.; Sabbach, A.; Brenner, B.; Aharon-Peretz, J. Extracellular vesicles of Alzheimer's disease patients as a biomarker for disease progression. *Mol. Neurobiol.* **2020**. [CrossRef]
21. Ellegaard Nielsen, J.; Sofie Pedersen, K.; Vestergård, K.; Georgiana Maltesen, R.; Christiansen, G.; Lundbye-Christensen, S.; Moos, T.; Risom Kristensen, S.; Pedersen, S. Novel blood-derived extracellular vesicle-based biomarkers in Alzheimer's disease identified by proximity extension assay. *Biomedicines* **2020**, *8*, 199. [CrossRef]
22. Hampel, H.; Vergallo, A.; Caraci, F.; Cuello, A.C.; Lemercier, P.; Vellas, B.; Giudici, K.V.; Baldacci, F.; Hänisch, B.; Haberkamp, M.; et al. Alzheimer precision medicine initiative (APMI). Future avenues for Alzheimer's disease detection and therapy: Liquid biopsy, intracellular signaling modulation, systems pharmacology drug discovery. *Neuropharmacology* **2020**, 108081. [CrossRef]
23. Lu, G.; Liu, W.; Huang, X.; Zhao, Y. Complement factor H levels are decreased and correlated with serum C-reactive protein in late-onset Alzheimer's disease. *Arq. Neuropsiquiatr.* **2020**, *78*, 76–80. [CrossRef]
24. Lukiw, W.J. Gastrointestinal (GI) tract microbiome-derived neurotoxins-potent neuro-inflammatory signals from the GI tract via the systemic circulation into the brain. *Front. Cell Infect. Microbiol.* **2020**, *10*, 22. [CrossRef]
25. Lukiw, W.J. microRNA-146a Signaling in Alzheimer's disease (AD) and prion disease (PrD). *Front. Neurol.* **2020**, *11*, 462. [CrossRef] [PubMed]
26. Lukiw, W.J.; Pogue, A.I. Vesicular transport of encapsulated microRNA between glial and neuronal cells. *Int. J. Mol. Sci.* **2020**, *21*, 5078. [CrossRef] [PubMed]
27. Sims, R.; Hill, M.; Williams, J. The multiplex model of the genetics of Alzheimer's disease. *Nat. Neurosci.* **2020**, *23*, 311–322. [CrossRef] [PubMed]
28. Vernooij, M.W.; van Buchem, M.A. Neuroimaging in Dementia. In *Diseases of the Brain, Head and Neck, Spine 2020–2023: Diagnostic Imaging*; Hodler, J., Kubik-Huch, R.A., von Schulthess, G.K., Eds.; Springer: Cham, Switzerland, 2020; pp. 131–142.
29. Zhao, Y.; Lukiw, W.J. Bacteroidetes neurotoxins and inflammatory neurodegeneration. *Mol. Neurobiol.* **2018**, *55*, 9100–9107. [CrossRef] [PubMed]
30. Ruan, Z.; Ikezu, T. Tau Secretion. *Adv. Exp. Med. Biol.* **2019**, *1184*, 123–134. [CrossRef]
31. Sheng, L.; Stewart, T.; Yang, D.; Thorland, E.; Soltys, D.; Aro, P.; Khrisat, T.; Xie, Z.; Li, N.; Liu, Z.; et al. Erythrocytic α-synuclein contained in microvesicles regulates astrocytic glutamate homeostasis: A new perspective on Parkinson's disease pathogenesis. *Acta Neuropathol. Commun.* **2020**, *8*, 102. [CrossRef]
32. Zhao, Y.; Jaber, V.; Lukiw, W.J. Over-expressed pathogenic miRNAs in Alzheimer's disease (AD) and prion disease (PrD) drive deficits in TREM2-mediated Aβ42 peptide clearance. *Front. Aging Neurosci.* **2016**, *6*, 140. [CrossRef]
33. Bhattacharjee, S.; Lukiw, W.J. Alzheimer's disease and the microbiome. *Front. Cell Neurosci.* **2013**, *7*, 153. [CrossRef]
34. Emery, D.C.; Shoemark, D.K.; Batstone, T.E.; Waterfall, C.M.; Coghill, J.A.; Cerajewska, T.L.; Davies, M.; West, N.X.; Allen, S.J. 16S rRNA next generation sequencing analysis shows bacteria in Alzheimer's post-mortem brain. *Front. Aging Neurosci.* **2017**, *9*, 195. [CrossRef]
35. Pisa, D.; Alonso, R.; Fernández-Fernández, A.M.; Rábano, A.; Carrasco, L. Polymicrobial infections in brain tissue from Alzheimer's disease patients. *Sci. Rep.* **2017**, *7*, 5559. [CrossRef]
36. Zhan, X.; Stamova, B.; Sharp, F.R. Lipopolysaccharide associates with amyloid plaques, neurons and oligodendrocytes in Alzheimer's disease brain: A Review. *Front. Aging Neurosci.* **2018**, *10*, 42. [CrossRef] [PubMed]

37. Ceppa, F.A.; Izzo, L.; Sardelli, L.; Raimondi, I.; Tunesi, M.; Albani, D.; Giordano, C. Human gut-microbiota interaction in neurodegenerative disorders and current engineered tools for its modeling. *Front. Cell Infect. Microbiol.* **2020**, *10*, 297. [CrossRef] [PubMed]
38. Lukiw, W.J.; Pogue, A.I.; Hill, J.M. SARS-CoV-2 infectivity and neurological targets in the brain. *Cell. Mol. Neurobiol.* **2020**. [CrossRef] [PubMed]
39. Itzhaki, R.F. Corroboration of a major role for herpes simplex virus Type 1 in Alzheimer's disease. *Front. Aging Neurosci.* **2018**, *10*, 324. [CrossRef] [PubMed]
40. Alexandrov, P.; Zhao, Y.; Li, W.; Lukiw, W.J. Lipopolysaccharide-stimulated, NF-kB-, miRNA-146a- and miRNA-155-mediated molecular-genetic communication between the human gastrointestinal tract microbiome and the brain. *Folia Neuropathol.* **2019**, *57*, 211–219. [CrossRef] [PubMed]
41. Johnson, R.T.; ter Meulen, V. Slow infections of the nervous system. *Adv. Intern. Med.* **1978**, *23*, 353–383.
42. Hill, J.M.; Bhattacharjee, S.; Pogue, A.I.; Lukiw, W.J. The gastrointestinal tract microbiome and potential link to Alzheimer's disease. *Front. Neurol.* **2014**, *5*, 43. [CrossRef]
43. Naughton, S.X.; Raval, U.; Pasinetti, G.M. The viral hypothesis in Alzheimer's disease: Novel insights and pathogen-based biomarkers. *J. Pers. Med.* **2020**, *10*, 74. [CrossRef]
44. Rosario, D.; Boren, J.; Uhlen, M.; Proctor, G.; Aarsland, D.; Mardinoglu, A.; Shoaie, S. Systems biology approaches to understand the host-microbiome interactions in neurodegenerative diseases. *Front. Neurosci.* **2020**, *14*, 716. [CrossRef]
45. Jaber, V.; Zhao, Y.; Lukiw, W.J. Alterations in micro RNA-messenger RNA (miRNA-mRNA) coupled signaling networks in sporadic Alzheimer's disease (AD) hippocampal CA1. *J. Alzheimers Dis. Parkinsonism* **2017**, *7*, 312. [CrossRef]
46. Mai, H.; Fan, W.; Wang, Y.; Cai, Y.; Li, X.; Chen, F.; Chen, X.; Yang, J.; Tang, P.; Chen, H.; et al. Intranasal Administration of miR-146a Agomir Rescued the Pathological Process and Cognitive Impairment in an AD Mouse Model. *Mol. Ther. Nucleic Acids* **2019**, *18*, 681–695. [CrossRef] [PubMed]
47. Mujica, M.L.; Gallay, P.A.; Perrachione, F.; Montemerlo, A.E.; Tamborelli, L.A.; Vaschetti, V.; Reartes, D.; Bollo, S.; Rodríguez, M.C.; Dalmasso, P.D.; et al. New trends in the development of electrochemical biosensors for the quantification of microRNAs. *J. Pharm. Biomed. Anal.* **2020**, *189*, 113478. [CrossRef] [PubMed]
48. Alexandrov, P.N.; Dua, P.; Hill, J.M.; Bhattacharjee, S.; Zhao, Y.; Lukiw, W.J. microRNA (miRNA) speciation in Alzheimer's disease (AD) cerebrospinal fluid (CSF) and extracellular fluid (ECF). *Int. J. Biochem. Mol. Biol.* **2012**, *3*, 365–373. [PubMed]
49. Slota, J.A.; Booth, S.A. MicroRNAs in neuroinflammation: Implications in disease pathogenesis, biomarker discovery and therapeutic applications. *Noncoding RNA* **2019**, *5*, 35. [CrossRef]
50. Zhao, Y.; Bhattacharjee, S.; Jones, B.M.; Hill, J.; Dua, P.; Lukiw, W.J. Regulation of neurotropic signaling by the inducible, NF-kB-sensitive miRNA-125b in Alzheimer's disease (AD) and in primary human neuronal-glial (HNG) cells. *Mol. Neurobiol.* **2014**, *50*, 97–106. [CrossRef]
51. Jaber, V.R.; Zhao, Y.; Sharfman, N.M.; Li, W.; Lukiw, W.J. Addressing Alzheimer's Disease (AD) Neuropathology Using Anti-microRNA (AM) Strategies. *Mol. Neurobiol.* **2019**, *56*, 8101–8108. [CrossRef]
52. Kaipainen, A.; Jääskeläinen, O.; Liu, Y.; Haapalinna, F.; Nykänen, N.; Vanninen, R.; Koivisto, A.M.; Julkunen, V.; Remes, A.M.; Herukka, S.K. Cerebrospinal Fluid and MRI Biomarkers in Neurodegenerative Diseases: A Retrospective Memory Clinic-Based Study. *J. Alzheimers Dis.* **2020**, *75*, 751–765. [CrossRef]
53. Kamagata, K.; Andica, C.; Hatano, T.; Ogawa, T.; Takeshige-Amano, H.; Ogaki, K.; Akashi, T.; Hagiwara, A.; Fujita, S.; Aoki, S.; et al. Advanced diffusion magnetic resonance imaging in patients with Alzheimer's and Parkinson's diseases. *Neural Regen. Res.* **2020**, *15*, 1590–1600. [CrossRef]
54. Lo Buono, V.; Palmeri, R.; Corallo, F.; Allone, C.; Pria, D.; Bramanti, P.; Marino, S. Diffusion tensor imaging of white matter degeneration in early stage of Alzheimer's disease: A review. *Int. J. Neurosci.* **2020**, *130*, 243–250. [CrossRef]
55. Lombardi, G.; Crescioli, G.; Cavedo, E.; Lucenteforte, E.; Casazza, G.; Bellatorre, A.; Lista, C.; Costantino, G.; Frisoni, G.; Virgili, G.; et al. Structural magnetic resonance imaging for the early diagnosis of dementia due to Alzheimer's disease in people with mild cognitive impairment. *Cochrane Database Syst. Rev.* **2020**, *3*. [CrossRef]
56. Blennow, K.; Zetterberg, H. Biomarkers for Alzheimer's disease: Current status and prospects for the future. *J. Intern. Med.* **2018**, *284*, 643–663. [CrossRef]

57. Donatelli, G.; Ceravolo, R.; Frosini, D.; Tosetti, M.; Bonuccelli, U.; Cosottini, M. Present and future of ultra-high field MRI in neurodegenerative disorders. *Curr. Neurol. Neurosci. Rep.* **2018**, *18*, 31. [CrossRef] [PubMed]
58. Sherva, R.; Tripodis, Y.; Bennett, D.A.; Chibnik, L.B.; Crane, P.K.; de Jager, P.L.; Farrer, L.A.; Saykin, A.J.; Shulman, J.M.; Naj, A.; et al. Genome-wide association study of the rate of cognitive decline in Alzheimer's disease. *Alzheimers Dement.* **2014**, *10*, 45–52. [CrossRef] [PubMed]
59. Dong, A.; Toledo, J.B.; Honnorat, N.; Doshi, J.; Varol, E.; Sotiras, A.; Wolk, D.; Trojanowski, J.Q.; Davatzikos, C. Alzheimer's Disease Neuroimaging Initiative. Heterogeneity of neuroanatomical patterns in prodromal Alzheimer's disease: Links to cognition, progression and biomarkers. *Brain* **2017**, *140*, 735–747. [CrossRef] [PubMed]
60. Gibney, B.; Redmond, C.E.; Byrne, D.; Mathur, S.; Murray, N. A review of the applications of dual-energy CT in acute neuroimaging. *Can. Assoc. Radiol. J.* **2020**, *71*, 253–265. [CrossRef] [PubMed]
61. Koychev, I.; Hofer, M.; Friedman, N.C. Correlation of Alzheimer's disease neuropathologic staging with amyloid and tau scintigraphic imaging biomarkers. *J. Nucl. Med.* **2020**. [CrossRef] [PubMed]
62. Tetreault, A.M.; Phan, T.; Orlando, D.; Lyu, I.; Kang, H.; Landman, B.; Darby, R. Network localization of clinical, cognitive, and neuropsychiatric symptoms in Alzheimer's disease. *Brain* **2020**, *143*, 1249–1260. [CrossRef]
63. Emrani, S.; Lamar, M.; Price, C.C.; Wasserman, V.; Matusz, E.; Au, R.; Swenson, R.; Nagele, R.; Heilman, K.M.; Libon, D.J. Alzheimer's/vascular spectrum dementia: Classification in addition to diagnosis. *J. Alzheimers Dis.* **2020**, *73*, 63–71. [CrossRef] [PubMed]
64. Habes, M.; Grothe, M.J.; Tunc, B.; McMillan, C.; Wolk, D.A.; Davatzikos, C. Disentangling heterogeneity in Alzheimer's disease and related dementias using data-driven methods. *Biol. Psychiatry* **2020**, *88*, 70–72. [CrossRef]
65. Hampel, H.; Goetzl, E.J.; Kapogiannis, D.; Lista, S.; Vergallo, A. Biomarker-Drug and Liquid Biopsy Co-development for Disease Staging and Targeted Therapy: Cornerstones for Alzheimer's Precision Medicine and Pharmacology. *Front. Pharmacol.* **2019**, *10*, 310. [CrossRef]
66. Lewczuk, P.; Łukaszewicz-Zając, M.; Mroczko, P.; Kornhuber, J. Clinical significance of fluid biomarkers in Alzheimer's disease. *Pharmacol. Rep.* **2020**. [CrossRef] [PubMed]
67. Pulliam, L.; Sun, B.; Mustapic, M.; Chawla, S.; Kapogiannis, D. Plasma neuronal exosomes serve as biomarkers of cognitive impairment in HIV infection and Alzheimer's disease. *J. Neurovirol.* **2019**, *25*, 702–709. [CrossRef] [PubMed]
68. Hampel, H.; Vergallo, A.; Perry, G.; Lista, S.; Alzheimer Precision Medicine Initiative (APMI). The Alzheimer precision medicine initiative. *J. Alzheimers Dis.* **2019**, *68*, 1–24. [CrossRef] [PubMed]
69. Guerreiro, R.J.; Gustafson, D.R.; Hardy, J. The genetic architecture of Alzheimer's disease: Beyond APP, PSENs and APOE. *Neurobiol. Aging.* **2012**, *33*, 437–456. [CrossRef]
70. Cole, M.A.; Seabrook, G.R. On the horizon-the value and promise of the global pipeline of Alzheimer's disease therapeutics. *Alzheimers Dement. (N. Y.)* **2020**, *6*, e12009. [CrossRef]
71. Jellinger, K.A. Neuropathological assessment of the Alzheimer spectrum. *J. Neural. Transm.* **2020**, *127*, 1229–1256. [CrossRef]

6

Use of Biomarkers in Ongoing Research Protocols on Alzheimer's Disease

Marco Canevelli [1,2,*], Giulia Remoli [1], Ilaria Bacigalupo [2], Martina Valletta [1], Marco Toccaceli Blasi [1], Francesco Sciancalepore [1], Giuseppe Bruno [1], Matteo Cesari [3,4] and Nicola Vanacore [2]

1 Department of Human Neuroscience, Sapienza University, 00185 Rome, Italy; remoligiulia92@gmail.com (G.R.); m.valletta@live.it (M.V.); toccaceliblasi.1529394@studenti.uniroma1.it (M.T.B.); sciancalepore.1679543@studenti.uniroma1.it (F.S.); giuseppe.bruno@uniroma1.it (G.B.)
2 National Center for Disease Prevention and Health Promotion, Italian National Institute of Health, 00161 Rome, Italy; ilaria.bacigalupo@iss.it (I.B.); nicola.vanacore@iss.it (N.V.)
3 Department of Clinical Sciences and Community Health, University of Milan, 20122 Milan, Italy; macesari@gmail.com
4 Geriatric Unit, Fondazione IRCCS Ca' Granda Ospedale Maggiore Policlinico, 20122 Milan, Italy
* Correspondence: marco.canevelli@gmail.com

Abstract: The present study aimed to describe and discuss the state of the art of biomarker use in ongoing Alzheimer's disease (AD) research. A review of 222 ongoing phase 1, 2, 3, and 4 protocols registered in the clinicaltrials.gov database was performed. All the trials (i) enrolling subjects with clinical disturbances and/or preclinical diagnoses falling within the AD continuum; and (ii) testing the efficacy and/or safety/tolerability of a therapeutic intervention, were analyzed. The use of biomarkers of amyloid deposition, tau pathology, and neurodegeneration among the eligibility criteria and/or study outcomes was assessed. Overall, 58.2% of ongoing interventional studies on AD adopt candidate biomarkers. They are mostly adopted by studies at the preliminary stages of the drug development process to explore the safety profile of novel therapies, and to provide evidence of target engagement and disease-modifying properties. The biologically supported selection of participants is mostly based on biomarkers of amyloid deposition, whereas the use of biomarkers as study outcomes mostly relies on markers of neurodegeneration. Biomarkers play an important role in the design and conduction of research protocols targeting AD. Nevertheless, their clinical validity, utility, and cost-effectiveness in the "real world" remain to be clarified.

Keywords: Alzheimer's disease; biomarkers; drug development; clinical trials; diagnostic research

1. Introduction

In the last few decades, the notion of Alzheimer's disease (AD) has substantially changed. The enhanced understanding of the underlying neuropathophysiological mechanisms has supported a gradual shift from a clinical-pathological conception of AD [1] to a more biology-oriented framework [2,3].

The progressive evolution of the AD construct has been mainly sustained by the identification of key biomarkers of the AD neuropathological process [4]. According to the latest research definition, AD can be diagnosed in vivo, independently of cognitive manifestations, by the means of biomarkers reflecting β-amyloid deposition, tau pathology, and neurodegeneration [3]. Although their use is currently recommended only for research purposes [3,5], biomarkers are increasingly used in specialist clinical settings [6,7]. Nevertheless, some concerns and methodological shortcomings still affect the use of candidate AD biomarkers in routine clinical care. First, their clinical validity and utility have not yet been fully proven, and inconclusive evidence exists about their analytical validity [8]. Moreover, the lifetime risk of dementia among individuals with positive AD biomarkers varies considerably. In this regard, it is estimated that most persons affected by preclinical AD based on abnormal biomarker status will not develop dementia in their lifetimes [9]. Furthermore, they are either expensive, invasive, or both.

Biomarkers often play an important role in the design and conduction of research protocols targeting AD [10]. They may improve the selection of participants and render more biologically homogeneous the sampled populations. Moreover, their use may help demonstrating target engagement by tested intervention, providing evidence on disease modification, informing analytic stratification, and monitoring adverse effects [10]. At the same time, the sustainability of biomarker's translation into care models and the generalizability (i.e., transferability) of interventions to the "real world" should always be taken into account [11].

In the present study, we describe and discuss the state of the art of biomarker use in AD research by reviewing the ongoing protocols registered in the clinicaltrials.gov database, updating and extending previous analyses on the topic [12]. In particular, we focus on the adoption of candidate biomarkers of amyloid deposition, tau pathology, and neurodegeneration as (i) eligibility criteria; and (ii) study outcomes. This analysis may inform how AD biomarkers are currently adopted in the drug development process, shedding a light on potential methodological, clinical, and ethical issues. Moreover, this approach may provide useful insights into a public health perspective considering that AD biomarkers and diagnostic procedures tested in research protocols will likely be increasingly translated in the daily practice to support clinical activities (e.g., risk prediction [13]) and regulatory decisions (e.g., drug accessibility and reimbursability [14]).

2. Materials and Methods

2.1. Data Source and Search Strategy

Clinicaltrials.gov was used as the reference source for the present study. Clinicaltrials.gov is an online database provided by the U.S. National Library of Medicine, which collects information from clinical studies that are conducted worldwide on a wide range of diseases and conditions.

The database was explored on 10 May 2020, by using the following terms and fields in the advanced search function: "Alzheimer" [CONDITION OR DISEASE] AND "interventional studies (clinical trials)" [STUDY TYPE] AND ("not yet recruiting" OR "recruiting" OR "enrolling by invitation" OR "active, not recruiting") [STATUS: RECRUITMENT] AND ("phase 1" OR "phase 2" OR "phase 3" OR "phase 4") [PHASE]. No restriction on age, sex, date, and location was applied.

Two authors (M.V. and G.R.) independently screened the resulting records and assessed their adherence to the following inclusion criteria:

i) Enrolling subjects with clinical disturbances and/or preclinical diagnoses falling within the AD continuum (i.e., preclinical AD, subjective cognitive decline, mild cognitive impairment, prodromal AD, and AD dementia) [3];
ii) Testing the efficacy and/or safety/tolerability of a therapeutic (both pharmacological and non-pharmacological) intervention.

Thus, trials enrolling participants with non-AD dementias or healthy volunteers, and primarily aiming at investigating diagnostic procedures (e.g., a novel neuroimaging technique) were excluded.

The flow chart presented in Figure 1 shows the process of protocols selection.

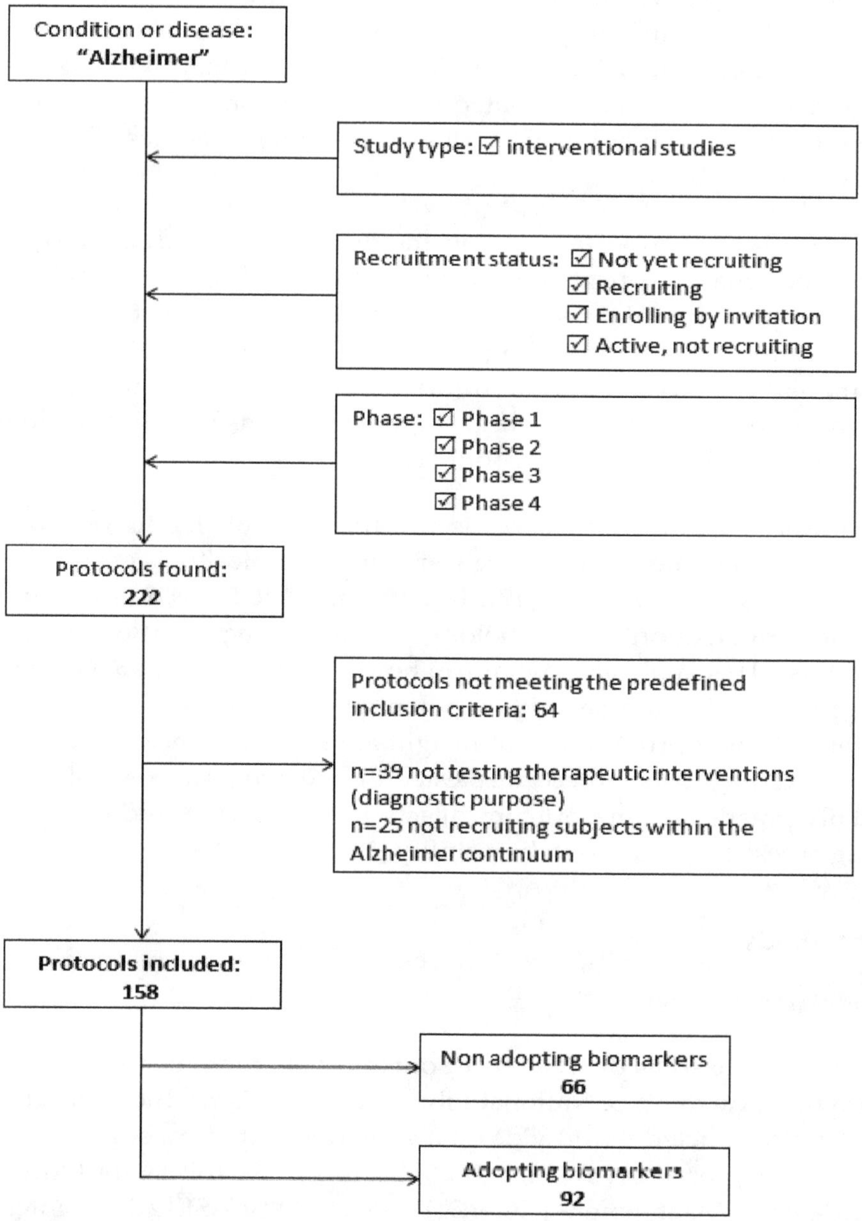

Figure 1. Flow-chart of protocols' selection.

2.2. Data Extraction

Two reviewers (M.V. and G.R.) independently extracted the following data from the selected protocols: NCT number; phase; status; study design; expected end date; sponsor; target condition; intervention; mechanism of action; primary and secondary outcome measure (s); planned number of participants. The use of the following AD biomarkers among the eligibility criteria and/or study outcomes was also assessed according to the AT (N) biomarker grouping [3]:

- A, amyloid deposition: (i) low cerebrospinal fluid (CSF) Aβ42 or Aβ42/Aβ40 ratio; and (ii) positive amyloid positron emission tomography (PET) scan;
- T, tau pathology: (i) elevated CSF phospho-tau (*p*-tau); and (ii) positive tau PET scan;
- N, neurodegeneration: (i) atrophy on anatomic magnetic resonance imaging (MRI); (ii) elevated CSF total tau (*t*-tau); and (iii) fluorodeoxyglucose (FDG) PET hypometabolism.

Disagreements in the selection process and/or extraction of data were solved by consensus or by involving two additional reviewers (M.C. and M.T.B.).

2.3. Data Analysis

Data were provided for two categories of protocols: (i) those using biomarkers in the selection of participants; and (ii) those using biomarkers as study outcomes. These categories were partially overlapping because some studies adopted biomarkers both as eligibility criteria and endpoints. Percentages and median values were calculated to summarize the abstracted categorical and continuous variables. Chi-square and median tests were used to compare the methodological characteristics of protocols adopting versus non-adopting biomarkers to ascertain eligibility and/or as endpoints. Statistical significance was set at $p < 0.05$.

3. Results

3.1. Search Results

A total of 222 protocols of phase 1, 2, 3, and 4 interventional studies were retrieved by the structured search on clinicaltrials.gov. Sixty-four of them were subsequently excluded because they did not fulfill the predefined set of inclusion criteria. Specifically, 39 studies were not testing therapeutic interventions, but were evaluated novel diagnostic procedures. Moreover, 25 trials were recruiting participants with clinical conditions not falling within the AD continuum (e.g., healthy volunteers, patients with other neurodegenerative dementias). Thus, 158 protocols were ultimately included in the analysis, as shown in Figure 1. A high agreement (>90%) was reported by the two reviewers involved in the selection process.

3.2. Characteristics of Protocols Adopting Biomarkers

Overall, 92 out of the 158 identified interventional studies (58.2%) adopted candidate AD biomarkers (Table 1). Compared with protocols not using biomarkers (n = 66), these studies were more frequently in the earlier phases of drug development (i.e., phase 1 and 2), more commonly aimed at evaluating the safety/tolerability of the tested interventions or their impact on AD underlying pathophysiological mechanisms (e.g., amyloid deposition, tau pathology, neuroinflammation), and almost exclusively focused on the assessment of pharmacological therapies (Table 1). On the contrary, studies not adopting biomarkers mostly adopted cognitive, functional, and neuropsychiatric measures as primary outcomes and were more commonly finalized at testing non-pharmacological interventions.

A total of 27,566 participants will tentatively be enrolled in the 92 protocols using biomarkers, with estimated sample sizes ranging between 12 and 2400 (median 120) subjects. These protocols are mostly conducted in the U.S. and funded by the biopharma industry. Their reported starting dates vary from November 2010 to January 2021, with completion dates indicated as ranging between December 2019 and August 2026. In the majority of studies, patients with overt AD dementia were indicated as eligible for participation, whereas nearly 20% of protocols restricted participation to subjects with preclinical or prodromal AD. Measures of clinical improvement were indicated as primary outcomes by 41.3% of studies with biomarkers.

Concerning how biomarkers are planned to be used, 62 studies adopt biomarkers to ascertain the eligibility of participants, 66 as study outcomes, whereas 36 both as inclusion criteria and endpoints.

The main characteristics of the ongoing protocols on AD using biomarkers are resumed in the Supplementary Material.

Table 1. Characteristics of the included protocols according to the adoption of biomarkers.

	Adopting Biomarkers (n = 92)	**Non Adopting Biomarkers (n = 66)**	p
Participants per study (n)	120 (43–382)	133 (43–267)	0.77
Phases			<0.01
Phase 1 and Phase 1–2	22 (23.9)	14 (21.2)	
Phase 2 and Phase 2–3	52 (56.5)	24 (36.4)	
Phase 3	15 (16.3)	18 (27.3)	
Phase 4	3 (3.3)	10 (15.2)	
Condition			0.21
Enrolling participants with AD dementia	74 (80.4)	58 (87.9)	
Not enrolling participants with AD dementia	18 (19.6)	8 (12.1)	
Main sponsor			0.12
Industry	56 (60.9)	32 (48.5)	
Other	36 (39.1)	34 (51.5)	
Primary outcome			<0.001
Safety	33 (35.9)	17 (25.8)	
Clinical improvement	38 (41.3)	47 (71.2)	
AD biological change	21 (14.6)	2 (3.0)	
Intervention			0.04
Pharmacological	87 (94.6)	56 (84.8)	
Non-pharmacological	5 (5.4)	10 (15.2)	

AD: Alzheimer's disease; MCI: Mild cognitive impairment; SCD: Subjective cognitive decline. Data are shown as median (IQR) or n (%).

3.3. *Use of Biomarkers in the Selection of Participants*

A total of 62 phase 1 (n = 7), phase 1–2 (n = 11), phase 2 (n = 26), phase 2–3 (n = 3), phase 3 (n = 14), and phase 4 (n = 1) studies are currently using AD biomarkers in the selection of participants. Twenty-one studies are testing anti-amyloid therapies, 7 anti-tau compounds, and 34 novel treatments with other mechanisms of action.

The biomarker-based criteria that is most commonly adopted to determine the eligibility of participants in the selected protocols are a positive amyloid PET scan (72.6% of the protocols) and a low CSF Aβ42 or Aβ42/Aβ40 ratio (48.4% of the protocols) (Figure 2). These two criteria are interchangeably used in 21 studies (33.9%). No study requires the documentation of amyloid positivity at both the CSF and PET assessment. CSF t-tau and p-tau levels, tau-PET, volumetric MRI, and FDG PET are instead less commonly used. The biologically supported selection of participants is mostly based on biomarkers of amyloid deposition (87.1% of the cases) rather than on those reflective of neurodegeneration (21.0%) or tau pathology (9.7%). Few studies are using combinations of biomarkers, often simultaneously measuring those indicative of amyloid deposition and neuronal injury (11.3% of the protocols) (Figure 2). No statistically significant difference was found when comparing the biomarkers adopted by phase 1 and 2 studies versus phase 3 and 4 studies (data not shown).

Only 6 out of the 36 protocols adopting CSF measurements in the ascertainment of participants' eligibility indicated the considered cut-points (Table 2). The majority of protocols performing amyloid PET in the screening phase does not provide sufficient information about the adopted radiotracer (e.g., florbetapir, florbetaben).

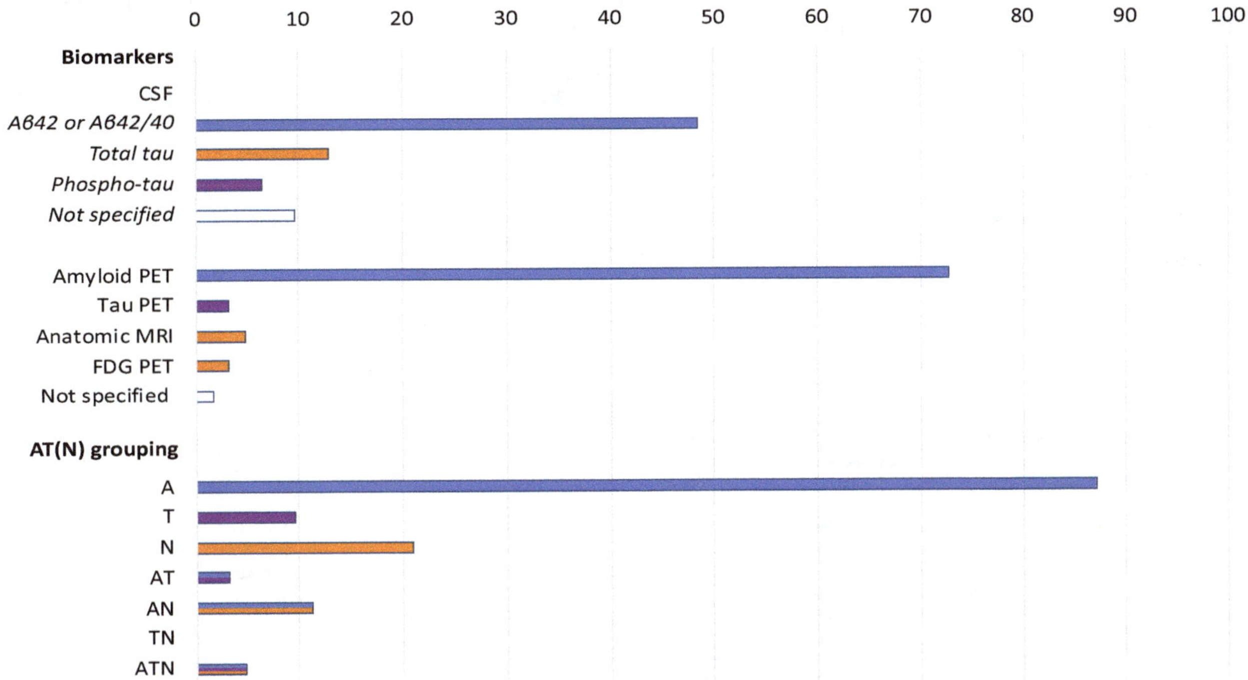

Figure 2. Biomarkers adopted to ascertain eligibility in the selected protocols ($n = 62$) according to the AT (N) grouping. Data are shown as %. A: aggregated Aβ or associated pathologic state; T: aggregated tau (neurofibrillary tangles) or associated pathologic state; N: neurodegeneration or neuronal injury. Colors refer to AT (N) biomarker grouping: blue: A; purple: T; orange: N.

Table 2. CSF cut-offs adopted in the six protocols with available information.

	CSF Cut-Offs
NCT02547818	Aβ42 ≥ 180 pg/mL and ≤ 690 pg/mL
NCT02947893	Aβ42 < 600 ng/mL
NCT03061474	Aβ42 ≤ 600 pg/mL or *t*-tau/Aβ42 ratio ≥ 0.39
NCT03069014	Aβ42 < 550 ng/L or Aβ40/42 ratio < 0.89
NCT04079803	*t*-tau/Aβ42 ratio ≥ 0.28
NCT04191486	Aβ ≤ 1000 pg/mL and *p*-tau 181 ≥ 19 pg/mL

Values and measurement units are reported as specified in the protocols.

3.4. Use of Biomarkers as Study Outcomes

Overall, 66 phase 1 ($n = 8$), phase 1–2 ($n = 9$), phase 2 ($n = 31$), phase 2–3 ($n = 7$), phase 3 ($n = 9$), and phase 4 ($n = 2$) studies are using AD biomarkers as study outcomes. Eighteen of them are testing anti-amyloid therapies, 3 anti-tau molecules, and 45 novel compounds with different biological properties. Eight protocols indicate biomarkers as primary outcomes, 46 as secondary outcomes, whereas 12 both as primary and secondary outcomes.

Changes of MRI or FDG PET findings are the most commonly adopted biomarker-based primary endpoints, being selected by 5 out of the 20 studies using biomarkers as primary outcome measures (Figure 3). Among protocols using biomarkers as secondary outcomes, the most frequently adopted measures are brain MRI (56.9% of the studies), CSF *t*-tau (36.2%), Aβ42 or Aβ42/Aβ40 (34.5%), *p*-tau (32.8%), and amyloid PET (31.0%). The use of biomarkers as study outcomes mostly relies on markers of neurodegeneration (48.1% of the cases) rather than on those of amyloid (21.6%) and tau (21.6%) pathology (Figure 3). In 21 studies, an ATN combination of biomarkers is adopted. No statistically significant difference was observed when comparing the biomarkers used as outcomes by phase 1 and 2 studies versus phase 3 and 4 studies (data not shown).

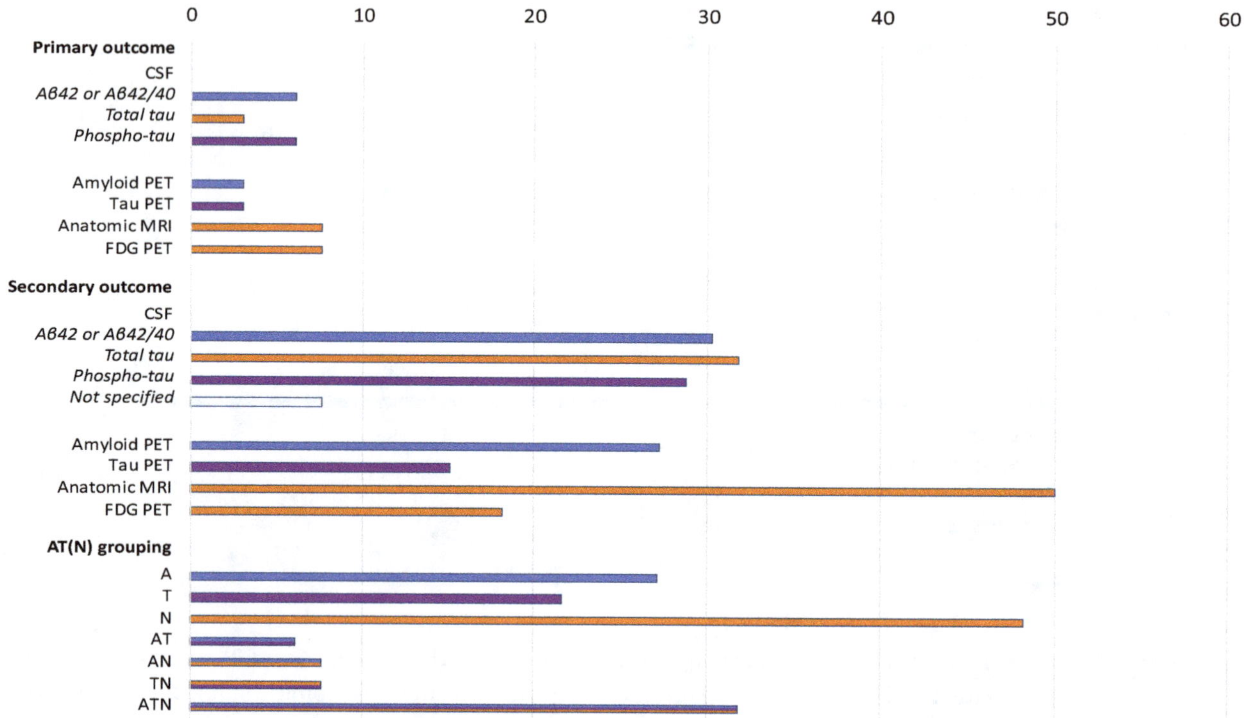

Figure 3. Biomarkers adopted as primary or secondary outcomes in the selected protocols (n = 66) according to the AT (N) grouping. Data are shown as %. A: aggregated Aβ or associated pathologic state; T: aggregated tau (neurofibrillary tangles) or associated pathologic state; N: neurodegeneration or neuronal injury. Colors refer to AT (N) biomarker grouping blue: A; purple: T; orange: N.

For the studies with biomarkers as primary outcomes, information on the sample size calculation has never been provided.

3.5. *Use of Biomarkers Both as Eligibility Criteria and Study Outcomes*

A total of 36 phase 1 (n = 5), phase 1–2 (n = 8), phase 2 (n = 13), phase 2–3 (n = 2), and phase 3 (n = 8) studies are using AD biomarkers both in the selection of participants and as study outcomes. These studies mostly include biomarkers of amyloid deposition among the eligibility criteria (91.7% of studies) and biomarkers of amyloid pathology (75.0%) and/or neuronal injury (75.0%) as endpoints.

4. Conclusions

In the present study, we provided a snapshot of the current use of candidate biomarkers in AD research protocols based on the data registered on the clinicaltrials.gov database. Overall, more than half of ongoing interventional studies targeting the AD continuum are adopting measures of amyloid deposition and/or tau pathology and/or neuronal injury. Biomarkers are used both for the selection of participants and to ascertain the efficacy of the tested interventions. They are mostly adopted by studies at the preliminary stages of the drug development process to explore the safety profile of novel therapies, and to provide evidence of target engagement (e.g., receptor occupancy) and disease-modifying properties. On the contrary, their use in trials primarily looking at improving the clinical manifestations of the disease is still limited. Indeed, only nearly 40% of studies with biomarkers adopted cognitive, functional, neuropsychiatric, and other clinical measures as their primary outcomes.

Based on our findings, a relevant number of clinical trials are incorporating measures of A to refine the clinical diagnosis of AD in participating subjects with dementia. It is well-established that a sizeable proportion of individuals clinically diagnosed with AD dementia have amyloid biomarkers incompatible with the diagnosis [15]. Patients with negative amyloid status tend to exhibit a slower clinical progression over time as compared with patients with amyloid positivity at the CSF and/or PET [15]. Introducing these procedures as enrichment tools can, therefore, allow to homogenize study samples, reduce the heterogeneity in clinical outcomes, and increase the probability of detecting drug-placebo differences. The same considerations can be extended to participants with mild cognitive impairment (MCI) in whom the demonstration of underlying amyloid pathology reduces the chance of observing alternative clinical trajectories (e.g., reversion to normal cognition) that may bias the study findings and their interpretation [16].

Different reflections may instead be applied to the preclinical stages of AD. In fact, among cognitively intact individuals, the detection of isolated amyloid positivity (or "Alzheimer's pathological change" [3]) is associated with a more considerable heterogeneity of clinical outcomes, thus complicating the assessment of clinical endpoints. Moreover, most of the subjects testing positive for A biomarkers will likely not exhibit a significant cognitive and functional worsening over time [9,17,18]. For instance, it has been calculated that the lifetime risks of developing AD dementia of a 60-year-old man and a 60-year-old woman with amyloidosis are only 23% and 31%, respectively [9]. Therefore, there is the risk of including in research protocols a disproportionate number of subjects who will never develop the target condition, thus only exposing them to the risk of serious adverse events with an unfavorable harm/benefit balance. For these reasons, it is fundamental to develop and implement appropriate and ethical strategies of risk disclosure to avoid the misinterpretation of testing results and the generation of adverse psychological reactions [19]. It is noteworthy that only a few studies combined biomarkers of A and T in the selection of participants. Including measures of tau pathology is instead required to determine if someone who is in the Alzheimer's disease continuum has indeed AD [3], consequently making more uniform the study populations and risk profiles of participants in clinical trials.

Other important considerations are raised concerning the use of biomarkers as screening tools in clinical trials [20]. In particular, the "real world" transferability of interventions emerging as effective in restricted samples of asymptomatic individuals with positive biomarkers will hardly be sustainable for our healthcare systems. Pathological AD markers are very common (i.e., 46%) in representative samples of older people [21], and it has been estimated that about 46.7 million Americans had preclinical AD in 2017 [22]. So, how can we translate these procedures on such a large scale to identify candidates for future disease-modifying treatments? Other controversies such as the standardization of CSF cut-points, the interchangeability of PET radiotracers and CSF assays, and the agreement between amyloid testing procedures remain to be addressed.

Candidate AD biomarkers are also frequently used as study outcomes. Specifically, measures of neurodegeneration are often adopted as downstream biomarkers to provide objective evidence that a drug ameliorates neurodegeneration. Indeed, the attenuation of the neurodegenerative process may be demonstrated (or at least suggested) by changes in the rates of glucose metabolism in cortical neurons (FDG PET), brain atrophy (volumetric MRI), and neuronal injury (CSF *t*-tau) [23]. N biomarkers may, therefore, support disease modification if a drug–placebo difference is detected and coupled with a similar clinical benefit [10,24,25]. It is noteworthy that, to date, no AD biomarker has yet qualified as a surrogate endpoint [26], which is a measurement that substitutes for clinical endpoints and is expected to predict clinical benefit [25]. Different to other areas of clinical neuroscience, such as multiple sclerosis, no AD biomarker has been consistently associated with the clinical trajectory of the disease, especially in its preclinical and prodromal stages [25]. Markers of amyloid and tau pathology as outcome measures are instead mostly useful to demonstrate drug engagement. Especially in the early phases of drug development, longitudinal CSF and PET measures of amyloid and tau pathology may confirm that a given compound affects the target brain protein [10]. For instance, several anti-Aβ monoclonal antibodies have shown a dose and time-dependent plaque reduction at the amyloid imaging, reflecting target engagement [27].

All these reflections on the use of biomarkers in AD research reinforce the need pursue their thorough clinical validation, as various methodological issues still limit their translation in the daily practice [8]. In particular, there is a lack of studies analyzing the distribution of biomarkers in healthy subjects and their interindividual variability according to major clinical and biological characteristics (e.g., age, sex, frailty) [28]. This information would be of great relevance in the promise of personalized medicine approaches. Moreover, no candidate AD biomarker has yet passed all the phases on which the architecture of diagnostic research is based [29].

The present study has some limitations to be mentioned and discussed. Our analysis cannot constitute an exhaustive overview on the topic because there are other registries for clinical trials on AD ongoing worldwide besides clinicaltrials.gov. Only a limited amount of information is available in the registered protocols, making it challenging to achieve an unbiased analysis of the methodological aspects of the studies. For example, in most of the selected protocols, brain MRI was simply mentioned among the participant selection procedures to exclude non-AD diagnoses. However, we cannot determine whether, in some cases, volumetric sequences were performed. This may have led to an underestimation of results concerning the use of MRI as a biomarker of neurodegeneration. Moreover, only the biomarkers incorporated in the AT (N) framework were considered. There is emerging evidence that other measures may represent promising biomarkers to be used in clinical trials [10,25].

In conclusion, biomarkers are largely used in ongoing clinical trials targeting the AD continuum. Their adoption may relevantly improve the selection of participants and the assessment of the efficacy and safety/tolerability of novel treatments. Nevertheless, their use in drug development must be accompanied by a demonstration of their clinical validity, utility, and cost-effectiveness in the "real world". Otherwise, there is a risk of an experimenting model of care and access to treatments that are unsustainable for our healthcare systems.

Author Contributions: M.C. (Marco Canevelli): Conception and design of the study, writing of the manuscript. G.R.: Data collection, drafting of the manuscript. I.B.: Data collection, drafting of the manuscript. M.V.: Data collection, drafting of the manuscript. M.T.B.: Data collection, drafting of the manuscript. F.S.: Data collection, drafting of the manuscript. G.B.: revising the manuscript critically for important intellectual content. M.C. (Matteo Cesari): Revising the manuscript critically for important intellectual content. N.V.: Conception of the study, writing of the manuscript. All authors have read and agreed to the published version of the manuscript.

Acknowledgments: Marco Canevelli is supported by a research grant of the Italian Ministry of Health (GR-2016-02364975) for the project "Dementia in immigrants and ethnic minorities living in Italy: clinical-epidemiological aspects and public health perspectives" (ImmiDem). Matteo Cesari has received honoraria for presentations at scientific meetings and/or research funding from Nestlé and Pfizer. He is involved in the coordination of an Innovative Medicines Initiative-funded project (including partners from the European Federation Pharmaceutical Industries and Associates [Sanofi, Novartis, Servier, GSK, Lilly]).

References

1. McKhann, G.; Drachman, D.; Folstein, M.; Katzman, R.; Price, D.; Stadlan, E.M. Clinical diagnosis of Alzheimer's disease: Report of the NINCDS-ADRDA Work Group under the auspices of Department of Health and Human Services Task Force on Alzheimer's Disease. *Neurology* **1984**, *34*, 939–944. [CrossRef] [PubMed]
2. Jack, C.R.; Albert, M.S.; Knopman, D.S.; McKhann, G.M.; Sperling, R.A.; Carrillo, M.C.; Thies, B.; Phelps, C.H. Introduction to the recommendations from the National Institute on Aging-Alzheimer's Association workgroups on diagnostic guidelines for Alzheimer's disease. *Alzheimers Dement.* **2011**, *7*, 257–262. [CrossRef] [PubMed]
3. Jack, C.R.; Bennett, D.A.; Blennow, K.; Carrillo, M.C.; Dunn, B.; Haeberlein, S.B.; Holtzman, D.M.; Jagust, W.; Jessen, F.; Karlawish, J.; et al. NIA-AA Research Framework: Toward a biological definition of Alzheimer's disease. *Alzheimers Dement.* **2018**, *14*, 535–562. [CrossRef] [PubMed]

4. Jack, C.R.; Bennett, D.A.; Blennow, K.; Carrillo, M.C.; Feldman, H.H.; Frisoni, G.B.; Hampel, H.; Jagust, W.J.; Johnson, K.A.; Knopman, D.S.; et al. A/T/N: An unbiased descriptive classification scheme for Alzheimer disease biomarkers. *Neurology* **2016**, *87*, 539–547. [CrossRef] [PubMed]
5. McKhann, G.M.; Knopman, D.S.; Chertkow, H.; Hyman, B.T.; Jack, C.R.; Kawas, C.H.; Klunk, W.E.; Koroshetz, W.J.; Manly, J.J.; Mayeux, R.; et al. The diagnosis of dementia due to Alzheimer's disease: Recommendations from the National Institute on Aging-Alzheimer's Association workgroups on diagnostic guidelines for Alzheimer's disease. *Alzheimers Dement.* **2011**, *7*, 263–269. [CrossRef]
6. Frisoni, G.B.; Boccardi, M.; Barkhof, F.; Blennow, K.; Cappa, S.; Chiotis, K.; Démonet, J.-F.; Garibotto, V.; Giannakopoulos, P.; Gietl, A.; et al. Strategic roadmap for an early diagnosis of Alzheimer's disease based on biomarkers. *Lancet Neurol.* **2017**, *16*, 661–676. [CrossRef]
7. Sancesario, G.M.; Toniolo, S.; Chiasserini, D.; Di Santo, S.G.; Zegeer, J.; Bernardi, G.; Musicco, M.; Caltagirone, C.; Parnetti, L.; Bernardini, S. The Clinical Use of Cerebrospinal Fluid Biomarkers for Alzheimer's Disease Diagnosis: The Italian Selfie. *J. Alzheimers Dis.* **2017**, *55*, 1659–1666. [CrossRef]
8. Canevelli, M.; Bacigalupo, I.; Gervasi, G.; Lacorte, E.; Massari, M.; Mayer, F.; Vanacore, N.; Cesari, M. Methodological Issues in the Clinical Validation of Biomarkers for Alzheimer's Disease: The Paradigmatic Example of CSF. *Front. Aging Neurosci.* **2019**, *11*. [CrossRef]
9. Brookmeyer, R.; Abdalla, N. Estimation of lifetime risks of Alzheimer's disease dementia using biomarkers for preclinical disease. *Alzheimers Dement.* **2018**, *14*, 981–988. [CrossRef]
10. Cummings, J. The Role of Biomarkers in Alzheimer's Disease Drug Development. *Adv. Exp. Med. Biol.* **2019**, *1118*, 29–61. [CrossRef]
11. Rothwell, P.M. External validity of randomised controlled trials: "To whom do the results of this trial apply?". *Lancet* **2005**, *365*, 82–93. [CrossRef]
12. Cummings, J.; Lee, G.; Ritter, A.; Sabbagh, M.; Zhong, K. Alzheimer's disease drug development pipeline: 2019. *Alzheimers Dement.* **2019**, *5*, 272–293. [CrossRef] [PubMed]
13. Van Maurik, I.S.; Slot, R.E.R.; Verfaillie, S.C.J.; Zwan, M.D.; Bouwman, F.H.; Prins, N.D.; Teunissen, C.E.; Scheltens, P.; Barkhof, F.; Wattjes, M.P.; et al. Personalized risk for clinical progression in cognitively normal subjects-the ABIDE project. *Alzheimers Res. Ther.* **2019**, *11*, 33. [CrossRef]
14. Rossini, P.M.; Cappa, S.F.; Lattanzio, F.; Perani, D.; Spadin, P.; Tagliavini, F.; Vanacore, N. The Italian INTERCEPTOR Project: From the Early Identification of Patients Eligible for Prescription of Antidementia Drugs to a Nationwide Organizational Model for Early Alzheimer's Disease Diagnosis. *J. Alzheimers Dis.* **2019**, *72*, 373–388. [CrossRef] [PubMed]
15. Landau, S.M.; Horng, A.; Fero, A.; Jagust, W.J. Alzheimer's Disease Neuroimaging Initiative Amyloid negativity in patients with clinically diagnosed Alzheimer disease and MCI. *Neurology* **2016**, *86*, 1377–1385. [CrossRef] [PubMed]
16. Canevelli, M.; Grande, G.; Lacorte, E.; Quarchioni, E.; Cesari, M.; Mariani, C.; Bruno, G.; Vanacore, N. Spontaneous Reversion of Mild Cognitive Impairment to Normal Cognition: A Systematic Review of Literature and Meta-Analysis. *J. Am. Med. Dir. Assoc.* **2016**, *17*, 943–948. [CrossRef]
17. Rosenberg, A.; Solomon, A.; Jelic, V.; Hagman, G.; Bogdanovic, N.; Kivipelto, M. Progression to dementia in memory clinic patients with mild cognitive impairment and normal β-amyloid. *Alzheimers Res. Ther.* **2019**, *11*, 99. [CrossRef]
18. Jansen, W.J.; Ossenkoppele, R.; Knol, D.L.; Tijms, B.M.; Scheltens, P.; Verhey, F.R.J.; Visser, P.J.; Amyloid Biomarker Study Group; Aalten, P.; Aarsland, D.; et al. Prevalence of cerebral amyloid pathology in persons without dementia: A meta-analysis. *JAMA* **2015**, *313*, 1924–1938. [CrossRef]
19. Roberts, J.S.; Dunn, L.B.; Rabinovici, G.D. Amyloid imaging, risk disclosure and Alzheimer's disease: Ethical and practical issues. *Neurodegener. Dis. Manag.* **2013**, *3*, 219–229. [CrossRef]
20. Mattsson, N.; Carrillo, M.C.; Dean, R.A.; Devous, M.D.; Nikolcheva, T.; Pesini, P.; Salter, H.; Potter, W.Z.; Sperling, R.S.; Bateman, R.J.; et al. Revolutionizing Alzheimer's disease and clinical trials through biomarkers. *Alzheimer's Dement. Diagn. Assess. Dis. Monit.* **2015**, *1*, 412–419. [CrossRef]
21. Kern, S.; Zetterberg, H.; Kern, J.; Zettergren, A.; Waern, M.; Höglund, K.; Andreasson, U.; Wetterberg, H.; Börjesson-Hanson, A.; Blennow, K.; et al. Prevalence of preclinical Alzheimer disease. *Neurology* **2018**, *90*, e1682–e1691. [CrossRef] [PubMed]
22. Brookmeyer, R.; Abdalla, N.; Kawas, C.H.; Corrada, M.M. Forecasting the prevalence of preclinical and clinical Alzheimer's disease in the United States. *Alzheimers Dement.* **2018**, *14*, 121–129. [CrossRef] [PubMed]

23. Blennow, K.; Hampel, H.; Zetterberg, H. Biomarkers in amyloid-β immunotherapy trials in Alzheimer's disease. *Neuropsychopharmacology* **2014**, *39*, 189–201. [CrossRef]
24. Cummings, J. Disease modification and Neuroprotection in neurodegenerative disorders. *Transl. Neurodegener.* **2017**, *6*, 25. [CrossRef] [PubMed]
25. Vellas, B.; Andrieu, S.; Sampaio, C.; Wilcock, G. Disease-modifying trials in Alzheimer's disease: A European task force consensus. *Lancet Neurol.* **2007**, *6*, 56–62. [CrossRef]
26. Barcikowska, M. European Medicines Agency Guideline on the clinical investigation of medicines for the treatment of Alzheimer's disease. *Lek. POZ* **2018**, *4*, 370–374.
27. Cummings, J.; Feldman, H.H.; Scheltens, P. The "rights" of precision drug development for Alzheimer's disease. *Alzheimer's Res. Ther.* **2019**, *11*, 76. [CrossRef]
28. Wallace, L.M.K.; Theou, O.; Godin, J.; Andrew, M.K.; Bennett, D.A.; Rockwood, K. Investigation of frailty as a moderator of the relationship between neuropathology and dementia in Alzheimer's disease: A cross-sectional analysis of data from the Rush Memory and Aging Project. *Lancet Neurol.* **2019**, *18*, 177–184. [CrossRef]
29. Sackett, D.L.; Haynes, R.B. The architecture of diagnostic research. *BMJ* **2002**, *324*, 539–541. [CrossRef]

7

Preventive Effects of Dairy Products on Dementia and the Underlying Mechanisms

Yasuhisa Ano [1,*] and Hiroyuki Nakayama [2]

1 Research Laboratories for Health Science & Food Technologies, Kirin Company Ltd., 1-13-5 Fukuura Kanazawa-ku, Yokohama-shi, Kanagawa 236-0004, Japan
2 Laboratory of Veterinary Pathology, Graduate School of Agricultural and Life Sciences, the University of Tokyo, 1-1-1 Yayoi, Bunkyo-ku, Tokyo 113-8657, Japan; anakaya@mail.ecc.u-tokyo.ac.jp
* Correspondence: Yasuhisa_Ano@kirin.co.jp

Abstract: Alongside the rapid population aging occurring worldwide, the prevention of age-related memory decline and dementia has become a high priority. Dairy products have many physiological effects owing to their contents of lactic acid bacteria and the fatty acids and peptides generated during their fermentation. In particular, several recent studies have elucidated the effects of fermented dairy products on cognitive function. Epidemiological and clinical evidence has indicated that fermented dairy products have preventive effects against dementia, including Alzheimer's disease. Recent preclinical studies have identified individual molecules generated during fermentation that are responsible for those preventive effects. Oleamide and dehydroergosterol have been identified as the agents responsible for reducing microglial inflammatory responses and neurotoxicity. In this review, the protective effects of fermented dairy products and their components on cognitive function, the mechanisms underlying those effects, and the prospects for their future clinical development will be discussed.

Keywords: amyloid β; Alzheimer's disease; cognitive function; dairy products; dementia; inflammation; microglia

1. Introduction

With the rapid aging of the population worldwide, cognitive decline and dementia are becoming increasing burdens not only on patients and their families, but also on national healthcare systems. Dementia is a general term for memory loss and other mental abilities severe enough to interfere with daily life. It is caused by physical changes in the brain. The most common type of dementia is Alzheimer's disease, which comprises 50–70% of dementia cases. Alzheimer's disease is histopathologically characterized by the presence of amyloid beta (Aβ) plaques and intracellular neurofibrillary tangles (NFTs) consisting of hyperphosphorylated tau. Both Aβ senile plaques and NFTs are formed of insoluble, densely-packed protein filaments. The accumulation of Aβ plaques and NFTs correlates with the symptoms of Alzheimer's disease and results in neuronal damage and death [1–4]. Other common types of dementia include vascular dementia [5], Lewy body dementia [6], and front temporal dementia [7]. Numerous reports have demonstrated that the formation of Aβ plaques is followed by inflammation in the brain, which is closely associated with NFTs and accelerates the development and progression of Alzheimer's disease [3,4,8,9]. The mechanisms that regulate Aβ plaques, NFTs, and inflammation are important targets for the therapy and prevention of Alzheimer's disease. However, owing to the lack of a disease-modifying therapy for dementia, preventive approaches such as diet, exercise, and active learning are being explored. In addition, high blood pressure, smoking, diabetes, and obesity are risk factors for dementia [10]. A recent study suggested that stress is also a risk factor for Alzheimer's disease [11]. Therefore, it is important to reduce these risk factors through adopting appropriate lifestyle habits.

There is now substantial evidence that dietary factors can modify the risk of dementia. Based on the results of several epidemiological investigations, the Mediterranean diet has been receiving increasing attention as a nutritional approach for lowering the risks of dementia [12–14]. In addition, specific dietary components including docosahexaenoic acid (DHA) from fish oil [15–18], resveratrol from red grapes [19–21], and curcumin from turmeric [22–24] have been evaluated for their potential protective effects against dementia or cognitive decline in several clinical trials. Recent epidemiological and clinical studies have indicated that fermented dairy products and their components, including lactic acid bacteria as well as peptides and fatty acids generated during fermentation, may also protect against dementia or cognitive decline. In this review, the recent studies investigating the effects of the intake of fermented dairy products on the risks of dementia and the underlying mechanisms demonstrated by recent studies will be discussed.

2. Epidemiological Studies on the Relationship between Fermented Dairy Product Consumption and Cognitive Function

Recent epidemiological studies have suggested that the consumption of dairy products, including yogurt and low-fat cheese, may reduce the risk of cognitive decline in the elderly and contribute to the prevention of Alzheimer's disease. Camfield et al. [25] suggested in their review that specific components of dairy products including bioactive peptides, colostrinin, proline-rich polypeptides, α-lactalbumin, vitamin B12, calcium, and probiotics might promote healthy brain function during aging. They also suggested that low-fat dairy products, when consumed regularly as part of a balanced diet, may have several beneficial outcomes for neurocognitive health during aging. However, the underlying mechanisms that benefit cognitive function have not been elucidated.

Crichton et al. [26,27] revealed that individuals who consumed low-fat dairy products, including yogurt and cheese, once a week had a higher cognitive function than those who did not. Previous reports had suggested that low-fat dairy products might lower the risks of obesity [28–30], type 2 diabetes [31,32], and cardiovascular diseases, which are all linked with the risks of cognitive decline and dementia [33–35]. They evaluated pre-existing data from 1183 participants and examined associations between dairy intake and self-reported cognitive and memory functions, self-esteem, stress, anxiety, mood, and psychological well-being. Dairy intake was calculated using a self-completed, quantified food frequency questionnaire (FFQ) and detailed information regarding the intakes of milk, cheese, ice cream, cream, yogurt, and dairy desserts as well as the fat content of each item was analyzed from the FFQ. The results revealed that the intakes of dairy and macronutrients were significantly associated with psychological health measures. In men, a higher protein intake was associated with lower perceived stress scores. Analyses of individual dairy foods found that the consumption of low-fat yogurt was positively associated with memory performance (quality of recall) in men. In women, the consumption of low-fat cheese was positively associated with social functioning and negatively associated with perceived stress levels. The intake of cheese was reported to be associated with decreased cognitive impairment in a population of late middle-aged to elderly people [36]. These results suggested that low-fat yogurt and cheese are beneficial for cognitive functions.

Ozawa et al. [37] surveyed more than 1000 Japanese subjects who were living in a local community, aged 60–79 years, and free from dementia to investigate any potential association between their diet and their risks of dementia. Their dietary patterns were surveyed using a 70-item semi-quantitative FFQ, and their average daily nutritional intakes were calculated from the weekly frequency and portion size of various foods. Their health status was monitored by several methods including a neuropsychological test. Dietary patterns associated with the risk of dementia were assessed using a reduced rank regression analysis [38]. This analysis extracted seven dietary patterns that explained 87.1% of the total variation in the intakes of the following seven nutrients, which were selected as responsible variables: saturated fatty acid, monounsaturated fatty acid, polyunsaturated fatty acid, vitamin C, potassium, calcium, and magnesium. Seven dietary factors were associated with a preventive effect against the risks of dementia that was greater than 20% in magnitude. These protective factors were soybeans and soybean products, green vegetables, other vegetables, algae, and milk and dairy products. In contrast, a high intake of rice was associated with an increase in the risks of dementia greater than 20% in magnitude. Thus, a dietary pattern characterized by high intakes of soybeans and soybean products, vegetables, algae, and milk or dairy products together with a low intake of rice was associated with a reduced risk of dementia. These results support the contention that a high intake of milk and dairy products helps to prevent cognitive decline.

The subsequent research of Ozawa et al. [39] focused on the effects of milk and dairy intake on the development of all-cause dementia and its subtypes in an elderly Japanese population. During 17 years of follow-up on individuals aged 60 years or older who did not initially have dementia (N = 1081), 303 subjects developed all-cause dementia. The age- and sex-adjusted incidences of all-cause dementia, Alzheimer's disease, and vascular dementia all showed a significant inverse correlation with the intake of milk and dairy products. After adjusting for potential confounders, the linear inverse relationship between the intake of milk and dairy products and the development of Alzheimer's disease remained significant, whereas the relationships with all-cause dementia and vascular dementia were not significant. The investigation showed that a greater intake of milk and dairy products was associated with a reduced risk of dementia, especially Alzheimer's disease, in the general Japanese population.

3. Clinical Trials for the Improvement of Cognitive Function by Dairy Products

In a clinical trial, Ogata et al. [40] found that the intake of dairy products was strongly associated with better short-term memory. The association was significant both with and without adjustment for genetic and family environment factors using a sample of twin pairs. Short-term memory was evaluated using the "logical memory I" (LM-I) scores from the Japanese version of the revised Wechsler memory scale. Participants were asked to listen to two short stories and immediately recall the details. The final analysis was performed using data from 78 men and 278 women. All individual-level analyses using generalized estimating equations showed that dairy product intake was significantly associated with the LM-I scores in men. In addition, a within-pair analysis using within-monozygotic and within–dizygotic pair-difference scores showed a significant association between the intake of dairy products and LM-I scores in men. Furthermore, a within-pair analysis using within-monozygotic pair-difference scores indicated a significant association between the intake of dairy products and LM-I scores in men. Among men, a high intake of dairy products was significantly associated with better short-term memory after adjustment for possible covariates. The authors concluded that the intake of dairy products may prevent cognitive decline regardless of genetic and family environment factors in men.

Markus et al. [41,42] demonstrated that the intakes of α-lactalbumin-rich whey protein isolate improved cognitive performance in stress-vulnerable subjects. They evaluated the effects of the intake of tryptophan-rich whey protein on the ratio of plasma tryptophan to the sum of the other large neutral amino acids (Trp-LNAA ratio) and cognitive performance in high stress-vulnerable subjects. Their double-blind, placebo-controlled, crossover study included 29 high stress-vulnerable subjects and 29 low stress-vulnerable subjects. A significantly greater increase in the plasma Trp-LNAA ratio was observed after the consumption of the α-lactalbumin-rich diet than after the consumption of the control diet. Cognitive performance was evaluated using a computerized Sternberg memory scanning task, and the subjects' reaction time and amount of errors across the different subtasks were measured. The mean reaction time showed a significant difference between the high and low stress-vulnerable subjects. Furthermore, the reaction time of the high-stress-vulnerable subjects was significantly lower after consuming the α-lactalbumin diet (758 $\pm$ 137 ms) than it was after consuming the control diet (800 $\pm$ 173 ms). An increase in the plasma Trp-LNAA ratio is considered to be an indirect indicator of increased brain serotonin function, which results in the improvement of cognitive performance.

The authors suggested that the intake of an α-lactalbumin-rich diet increases the level of tryptophan and serotonin in the brain and improves cognitive performance in stress-vulnerable subjects.

4. Preventive Effects of Dairy Products Fermented with *Penicillium candidum* against the Pathology of Alzheimer's Disease

Recent epidemiological and clinical studies have suggested that a high intake of dairy products may have preventive effects against cognitive decline and Alzheimer's disease. Following this finding, it is important to elucidate the mechanism and responsible molecular components. Using transgenic model mice, Ano et al. [43] demonstrated that the intake of Camembert cheese, which is a fermented dairy product, displayed preventive effects against Alzheimer's disease. In the experiment, 5xFAD mice were used as an Alzheimer's disease model. These mice overexpress mutant human amyloid precursor protein with the Swedish (K670N, M671L), Florida (I716V), and London (V717I) familial Alzheimer's disease mutations along with human presenilin 1 harboring two familial Alzheimer's disease mutations, namely M146L and L286V. The 5xFAD mice display Aβ depositions, plaques, and severe inflammation in the brain in addition to impaired cognitive function. 5xFAD mice aged 3–6 months were given food with or without an extract from Camembert cheese. The brain tissues of mice fed with the Camembert cheese extract showed reduced levels of inflammatory cytokines including tumor necrosis factor α (TNF-α) and macrophage inflammatory protein 1α. The amounts of $A\beta_{1\text{-}42}$ quantified by enzyme-linked immunosorbent assay (ELISA) and detected immunohistochemically were reduced in the group fed with the Camembert cheese extract. The abundances of the brain-derived and glial-derived neurotropic factors increased. These results showed that certain components of Camembert cheese contribute to the suppression of the inflammation and reduction of Aβ in the brain. In subsequent studies of the same research group, the responsible agents in Camembert cheese that contribute to the prevention of Alzheimer's disease pathology, especially inflammation in the brain, were explored.

5. Neuronal Inflammation Accelerates the Pathology of Alzheimer's Disease

Several reports have demonstrated that inflammation in the brain following the formation of Aβ plaques and NFTs is closely associated with the development and progression of Alzheimer's disease [3,8,9]. Inflammation in the brain is mainly regulated by microglia, which remove apoptotic cells and waste products such as Aβ through phagocytosis and also contribute to the host defense against virus infection in the central nervous system [44,45]. Microglia play an important role in clearing Aβ to regulate the pathology of Alzheimer's disease [46]. Recent studies revealed the crucial roles of microglia in maintaining the brain environment and cognitive function. However, in the brain tissues of patients with Alzheimer's disease, microglia infiltrate around the Aβ plaques, become excessively activated, and chronically produce inflammatory mediators such as TNF-α, macrophage inflammatory protein 1α, reactive oxygen species, and nitric oxide. These inflammatory mediators are toxic to neurons and cause neuronal cell death subsequent to Aβ deposition [47]. Under normal physiological conditions, microglia are important for the maintenance of brain environment; however, under pathological conditions, microglia can become excessively activated and negatively contribute to the brain environment.

Numerous reports have suggested that controlling the activities of microglia may contribute to the prevention and cure of Alzheimer's disease and cognitive decline. Epidemiological studies have suggested that the prolonged use of nonsteroidal anti-inflammatory drugs, including a common medication, ibuprofen, significantly reduces the risk of developing Alzheimer's disease [48–51]. Consistent with those results, a long-term ibuprofen treatment was found to significantly suppress microglial inflammation and the development of Aβ plaques in a transgenic mouse model of Alzheimer's disease [52,53].

Before Ano et al. evaluated the effects of a Camembert cheese extract using 5xFAD transgenic Alzheimer's model mice, they assessed the effects of various fermented dairy products on microglia [43]. Their results indicated that dairy products fermented with the fungi *Penicillium candidum* and *Penicillium roqueforti* suppressed the inflammatory responses of primary microglia. Their findings suggested that *Penicillium* fermentation is essential for the anti-inflammatory activity, although other dairy products that were unfermented or fermented did not suppress the microglial inflammatory responses. The intake of Camembert cheese extract reduced inflammatory responses and Aβ production in the hippocampus of 5xFAD transgenic mice, while it increased the production of the brain-derived and glial-derived neurotropic factors. Various fatty acids and peptides were also generated during the fermentation of dairy products with the *Penicillium* fungi. Ano et al., in addition, investigated the molecular components of Camembert cheese that are responsible for preventing the development of Alzheimer's disease pathology.

6. Effects of Oleamide and Dehydroergosterol Generated during the Fermentation of Dairy Products with *Penicillium* Fungi on Brain Inflammation

Ano et al. [43,54] identified oleamide and dehydroergosterol as two components of Camembert cheese that were responsible for suppressing microglial inflammation. Oleamide is an amide of oleic acid [55,56] (Figure 1) that forms naturally in the body of animals and might be synthesized during the fermentation of dairy products by *Penicillium* fungi [57]. Oleamide accumulates in the cerebrospinal fluid during sleep deprivation and induces sleep in animals; thus, it has potential applications in the treatment of mood and sleep disorders [58,59]. Oleamide not only suppresses the production of inflammatory cytokines and chemokines but also increases the microglial phagocytosis of Aβ. In addition, it induces the differentiation of microglia into the anti-inflammatory M2 type. A recent study using murine macrophages showed that oleamide suppressed the induction of iNOS and COX-2 by lipopolysaccharides (LPS) via preventing the nuclear translocation of NF-κβ by suppressing the phosphorylation of Iκβ-α [60]. Oleamide is also known as an endogenous substance that binds to cannabinoid receptor 2 (CB2), which is mainly expressed on the surface of immune cells (monocytes, macrophages, and B cells). CB2 is also expressed on microglia and contributes to the inhibition of microglia-mediated neurotoxicity by reducing the production of pro-inflammatory molecules [61]. In addition, CB2 activity facilitates the transformation of microglial cells from the M1 to M2 phenotype, which is suggested to favor phagocytosis and reparative mechanisms [62]. Several studies have proposed a direct role for CB2 in the modulation of Aβ peptide levels in the brain. Most of those studies have suggested that CB2 participates in Aβ clearance rather than in Aβ production and aggregation. In the case of amyloid precursor protein/presenilin 1 mice lacking CB2, the increased Aβ deposition observed may be related to a reduced phagocytotic activity of microglia in their brains [63], considering the role of CB2 activity in promoting microglial-induced Aβ phagocytosis [64,65]. These reports support the contention that oleamide, which is an agonist of CB2, suppresses the microglial inflammation and enhances the phagocytosis of Aβ, resulting in a preventive action against Alzheimer's disease. CB2 has been receiving increasing attention as a therapeutic target for Alzheimer's disease [66–68]. Ano et al. discovered that the concentration of oleamide in dairy products depends on the type of dairy product and the fermentation process used. Therefore, the dietary intake of oleamide can be increased via supplementation or the consumption of specific dairy products.

Dehydroergosterol was also discovered as a component of Camembert cheese that suppressed microglial inflammation. Dehydroergosterol is an analogue of ergosterol, which is a sterol found in the cell membrane of fungi [69,70] (Figure 1). Dehydroergosterol is generated by fungi during fermentation. Dehydroergosterol suppresses the LPS-induced inflammatory response (including TNF-α production) of primary microglia in a concentration-dependent manner, whereas ergosterol does not display this activity. Microglia treated with dehydroergosterol were observed to differentiate into the anti-inflammatory M2 phenotype. The number of apoptotic neurons detected by staining for caspase 3/7 decreased after co-culturing the cells with a microglial culture supernatant treated with dehydroergosterol and LPS as compared with an LPS-only control. These results suggested that dehydroergosterol suppresses the inflammatory responses of microglia and exerts a neuroprotective effect via promoting synaptic extension and neuronal survival [71]. The amount of dehydroergosterol produced during fermentation varies among different *Penicillium* strains, so it might be possible to increase the amount of dehydroergosterol in dairy products by optimizing the fermentation processes.

The mechanisms by which oleamide and dehydroergosterol regulate inflammation in the brain have been receiving increasing attention, because neural inflammation is involved not only in dementia but also in other neuronal disorders [72,73] including depression [74,75], anxiety disorder [76], and chronic fatigue [77]. A recent study demonstrated that the intakes of oleamide shows antidepressant-like effects in mice subjected to the forced swimming test via the activation of cannabinoid receptors [78]. In another demonstration, oleamide improved schizophrenia-like symptoms in mice treated with an NMDA receptor antagonist, MK-801 [79]. The balance of microglial differentiation between M1 pro-inflammatory type and M2 anti-inflammatory type is important to maintain homeostasis in the central nervous system. Oleamide has the potential to have preventive effects against the development of several brain disorders. Daily habits including nutrition, sleep, and exercise are closely related to the maintenance of the microglial balance and the prevention of neuronal disorders. Future studies will further elucidate the effects of active ingredients of fermented dairy products against depression and other brain diseases.

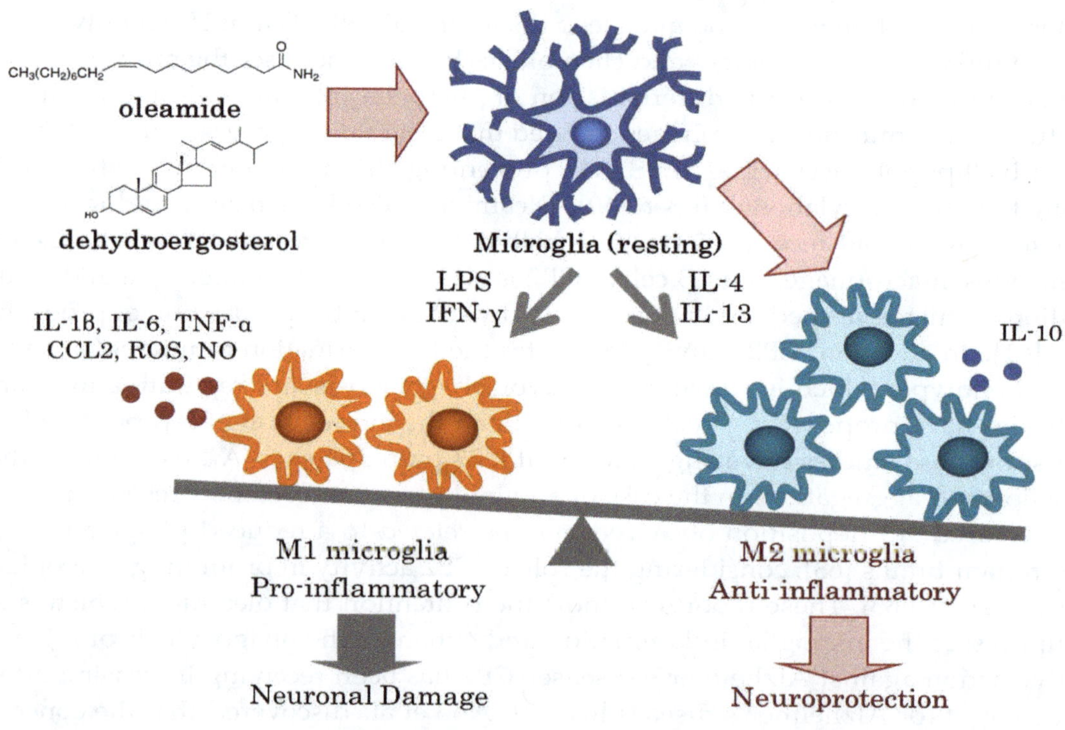

Figure 1. Modulation of microglial activation by dairy products.

7. Conclusions

This review introduced recent advances regarding the protective effects of dairy product intake against dementia and cognitive decline. The reports regarding these issues will help with the development of new approaches for the prevention of dementia. Oleamide and dehydroergosterol were discussed in this review as responsible agents for these protective effects of dairy products (Figure 1). However, the functions of the other various fatty acids and peptides generated during fermentation have not yet been elucidated. Future studies are expected to elucidate the mechanisms underlying the physiological benefits of dairy products in more detail. Based on the current evidence, the regular intake of dairy products and their molecular or microbial components seems to have the potential to contribute to the prevention of dementia and cognitive decline.

Oleamide and dehydroergosterol identified from Camembert cheese induce microglia into the M2 anti-inflammatory phenotype, leading to neuroprotection. The mechanisms that regulate microglial activation and inflammation in Alzheimer's disease are important targets for disease prevention. The regulation of microglia via daily lifestyle habits has been receiving increasing attention. The intake of neuroprotective and anti-inflammatory compounds including oleamide and dehydroergosterol in meals is safe and easy, so nutritional approaches are promising for the prevention of neurodegenerative disorders.

Abbreviations

Aβ	Amyloid β
CB2	Cannabinoid receptor 2
FAD	Familial Alzheimer's disease
FFQ	Food frequency questionnaire
LM-I	Logical memory I
LPS	Lipopolysaccharides
NFT	Neurofibrillary tangle
TNF-α	Tumor necrosis factor α

References

1. Bloom, G.S. Amyloid-β and tau: The trigger and bullet in Alzheimer disease pathogenesis. *JAMA Neurol.* **2014**, *71*, 505–508. [CrossRef] [PubMed]
2. Polanco, J.C.; Li, C.; Bodea, L.G.; Martinez-Marmol, R.; Meunier, F.A.; Gotz, J. Amyloid-β and tau complexity—Towards improved biomarkers and targeted therapies. *Nat. Rev. Neurol.* **2018**, *14*, 22–39. [CrossRef] [PubMed]
3. Takashima, A. Amyloid-β, tau, and dementia. *J. Alzheimer Dis. JAD* **2009**, *17*, 729–736. [CrossRef] [PubMed
4. Congdon, E.E.; Sigurdsson, E.M. Tau-targeting therapies for Alzheimer disease. *Nat. Rev. Neurol.* **2018** [CrossRef] [PubMed]]
5. Kalaria, R.N. The pathology and pathophysiology of vascular dementia. *Neuropharmacology* **2018**, *134 Pt B*· 226–239. [CrossRef] [PubMed]
6. Mueller, C.; Ballard, C.; Corbett, A.; Aarsland, D. The prognosis of dementia with Lewy bodies. *Lancet Neurol* **2017**, *16*, 390–398. [CrossRef]
7. Silveri, M.C. Frontotemporal dementia to Alzheimer's disease. *Dialogues Clin. Neurosci.* **2007**, *9*, 153–160. [PubMed]
8. Heppner, F.L.; Ransohoff, R.M.; Becher, B. Immune attack: The role of inflammation in Alzheimer disease. *Nat. Rev. Neurosci.* **2015**, *16*, 358–372. [CrossRef] [PubMed]
9. Ransohoff, R.M. Specks of insight into Alzheimer's disease. *Nature* **2017**, *552*, 342–343. [CrossRef] [PubMed
10. Livingston, G.; Sommerlad, A.; Orgeta, V.; Costafreda, S.G.; Huntley, J.; Ames, D.; Ballard, C.; Banerjee, S.; Burns, A.; Cohen-Mansfield, J.; et al. Dementia prevention, intervention, and care. *Lancet* **2017**, *390* 2673–2734. [CrossRef]
11. Caruso, A.; Nicoletti, F.; Mango, D.; Saidi, A.; Orlando, R.; Scaccianoce, S. Stress as risk factor for Alzheimer's disease. *Pharmacol. Res.* **2018**, *132*, 130–134. [CrossRef] [PubMed]
12. Petersson, S.D.; Philippou, E. Mediterranean Diet, Cognitive Function, and Dementia: A Systematic Review of the Evidence. *Adv. Nutr.* **2016**, *7*, 889–904. [CrossRef] [PubMed]
13. Singh, B.; Parsaik, A.K.; Mielke, M.M.; Erwin, P.J.; Knopman, D.S.; Petersen, R.C.; Roberts, R.O. Association of mediterranean diet with mild cognitive impairment and Alzheimer's disease: A systematic review and meta-analysis. *J. Alzheimer Dis. JAD* **2014**, *39*, 271–282. [CrossRef] [PubMed]
14. Lourida, I.; Soni, M.; Thompson-Coon, J.; Purandare, N.; Lang, I.A.; Ukoumunne, O.C.; Llewellyn, D.J. Mediterranean diet, cognitive function, and dementia: A systematic review. *Epidemiology* **2013**, *24*, 479–489. [CrossRef] [PubMed]

15. Freitas, H.R.; Ferreira, G.D.C.; Trevenzoli, I.H.; Oliveira, K.J.; de Melo Reis, R.A. Fatty Acids, Antioxidants and Physical Activity in Brain Aging. *Nutrients* **2017**, *9*. [CrossRef] [PubMed]
16. Heras-Sandoval, D.; Pedraza-Chaverri, J.; Perez-Rojas, J.M. Role of docosahexaenoic acid in the modulation of glial cells in Alzheimer's disease. *J. Neuroinflamm.* **2016**, *13*, 61. [CrossRef] [PubMed]
17. Dyall, S.C. Long-chain omega-3 fatty acids and the brain: A review of the independent and shared effects of EPA, DPA and DHA. *Front. Aging Neurosci.* **2015**, *7*, 52. [CrossRef] [PubMed]
18. Crupi, R.; Marino, A.; Cuzzocrea, S. n-3 fatty acids: Role in neurogenesis and neuroplasticity. *Curr. Med. Chem.* **2013**, *20*, 2953–2963. [CrossRef] [PubMed]
19. Sawda, C.; Moussa, C.; Turner, R.S. Resveratrol for Alzheimer's disease. *Ann. N. Y. Acad. Sci.* **2017**, *1403*, 142–149. [CrossRef] [PubMed]
20. Bastianetto, S.; Menard, C.; Quirion, R. Neuroprotective action of resveratrol. *Biochim. Biophys. Acta* **2015**, *1852*, 1195–1201. [CrossRef] [PubMed]
21. Turner, R.S.; Thomas, R.G.; Craft, S.; van Dyck, C.H.; Mintzer, J.; Reynolds, B.A.; Brewer, J.B.; Rissman, R.A.; Raman, R.; Aisen, P.S. A randomized, double-blind, placebo-controlled trial of resveratrol for Alzheimer disease. *Neurology* **2015**, *85*, 1383–1391. [CrossRef] [PubMed]
22. Goozee, K.G.; Shah, T.M.; Sohrabi, H.R.; Rainey-Smith, S.R.; Brown, B.; Verdile, G.; Martins, R.N. Examining the potential clinical value of curcumin in the prevention and diagnosis of Alzheimer's disease. *Br. J. Nutr.* **2016**, *115*, 449–465. [CrossRef] [PubMed]
23. Hemachandra Reddy, P.; Manczak, M.; Yin, X.; Grady, M.C.; Mitchell, A.; Tonk, S.; Kuruva, C.S.; Bhatti, J.S.; Kandimalla, R.; Vijayan, M.; et al. Protective Effects of Indian Spice Curcumin Against Amyloid-β in Alzheimer's Disease. *J. Alzheimer Dis. JAD* **2018**, *61*, 843–866. [CrossRef] [PubMed]
24. Botchway, B.O.A.; Moore, M.K.; Akinleye, F.O.; Iyer, I.C.; Fang, M. Nutrition: Review on the Possible Treatment for Alzheimer's Disease. *J. Alzheimer Dis. JAD* **2018**, *61*, 867–883. [CrossRef] [PubMed]
25. Camfield, D.A.; Owen, L.; Scholey, A.B.; Pipingas, A.; Stough, C. Dairy constituents and neurocognitive health in ageing. *Br. J. Nutr.* **2011**, *106*, 159–174. [CrossRef] [PubMed]
26. Crichton, G.E.; Murphy, K.J.; Bryan, J. Dairy intake and cognitive health in middle-aged South Australians. *Asia Pac. J. Clin. Nutr.* **2010**, *19*, 161–171. [PubMed]
27. Crichton, G.E.; Bryan, J.; Murphy, K.J.; Buckley, J. Review of dairy consumption and cognitive performance in adults: Findings and methodological issues. *Dement. Geriatr. Cogn. Disord.* **2010**, *30*, 352–361. [CrossRef] [PubMed]
28. Major, G.C.; Chaput, J.P.; Ledoux, M.; St-Pierre, S.; Anderson, G.H.; Zemel, M.B.; Tremblay, A. Recent developments in calcium-related obesity research. *Obes. Rev.* **2008**, *9*, 428–445. [CrossRef] [PubMed]
29. Zemel, M.B. Role of calcium and dairy products in energy partitioning and weight management. *Am. J. Clin. Nutr.* **2004**, *79*, 907S–912S. [CrossRef] [PubMed]
30. Azadbakht, L.; Mirmiran, P.; Esmaillzadeh, A.; Azizi, T.; Azizi, F. Beneficial effects of a Dietary Approaches to Stop Hypertension eating plan on features of the metabolic syndrome. *Diabetes Care* **2005**, *28*, 2823–2831. [CrossRef] [PubMed]
31. Choi, H.K.; Willett, W.C.; Stampfer, M.J.; Rimm, E.; Hu, F.B. Dairy consumption and risk of type 2 diabetes mellitus in men: A prospective study. *Arch. Intern. Med.* **2005**, *165*, 997–1003. [CrossRef] [PubMed]
32. Liu, S.; Choi, H.K.; Ford, E.; Song, Y.; Klevak, A.; Buring, J.E.; Manson, J.E. A prospective study of dairy intake and the risk of type 2 diabetes in women. *Diabetes Care* **2006**, *29*, 1579–1584. [CrossRef] [PubMed]
33. Dik, M.G.; Jonker, C.; Comijs, H.C.; Deeg, D.J.; Kok, A.; Yaffe, K.; Penninx, B.W. Contribution of metabolic syndrome components to cognition in older individuals. *Diabetes Care* **2007**, *30*, 2655–2660. [CrossRef] [PubMed]
34. Crichton, G.E.; Elias, M.F.; Buckley, J.D.; Murphy, K.J.; Bryan, J.; Frisardi, V. Metabolic syndrome, cognitive performance, and dementia. *J. Alzheimer Dis. JAD* **2012**, *30* (Suppl. 2), S77–S87. [CrossRef] [PubMed]
35. Raffaitin, C.; Gin, H.; Empana, J.P.; Helmer, C.; Berr, C.; Tzourio, C.; Portet, F.; Dartigues, J.F.; Alperovitch, A.; Barberger-Gateau, P. Metabolic syndrome and risk for incident Alzheimer's disease or vascular dementia: The Three-City Study. *Diabetes Care* **2009**, *32*, 169–174. [CrossRef] [PubMed]
36. Rahman, A.; Sawyer Baker, P.; Allman, R.M.; Zamrini, E. Dietary factors and cognitive impairment in community-dwelling elderly. *J. Nutr. Health Aging* **2007**, *11*, 49–54. [PubMed]

37. Ozawa, M.; Ninomiya, T.; Ohara, T.; Doi, Y.; Uchida, K.; Shirota, T.; Yonemoto, K.; Kitazono, T.; Kiyohara, Y. Dietary patterns and risk of dementia in an elderly Japanese population: The Hisayama Study. *Am. J. Clin. Nutr.* **2013**, *97*, 1076–1082. [CrossRef] [PubMed]
38. Hoffmann, K.; Schulze, M.B.; Schienkiewitz, A.; Nothlings, U.; Boeing, H. Application of a new statistical method to derive dietary patterns in nutritional epidemiology. *Am. J. Epidemiol.* **2004**, *159*, 935–944. [CrossRef] [PubMed]
39. Ozawa, M.; Ohara, T.; Ninomiya, T.; Hata, J.; Yoshida, D.; Mukai, N.; Nagata, M.; Uchida, K.; Shirota, T.; Kitazono, T.; et al. Milk and dairy consumption and risk of dementia in an elderly Japanese population: The Hisayama Study. *J. Am. Geriatr. Soc.* **2014**, *62*, 1224–1230. [CrossRef] [PubMed]
40. Ogata, S.; Tanaka, H.; Omura, K.; Honda, C.; Osaka Twin Research, G.; Hayakawa, K. Association between intake of dairy products and short-term memory with and without adjustment for genetic and family environmental factors: A twin study. *Clin. Nutr.* **2016**, *35*, 507–513. [CrossRef] [PubMed]
41. Markus, C.R.; Olivier, B.; Panhuysen, G.E.; Van Der Gugten, J.; Alles, M.S.; Tuiten, A.; Westenberg, H.G.; Fekkes, D.; Koppeschaar, H.F.; de Haan, E.E. The bovine protein alpha-lactalbumin increases the plasma ratio of tryptophan to the other large neutral amino acids, and in vulnerable subjects raises brain serotonin activity, reduces cortisol concentration, and improves mood under stress. *Am. J. Clin. Nutr.* **2000**, *71*, 1536–1544. [CrossRef] [PubMed]
42. Markus, C.R.; Olivier, B.; de Haan, E.H. Whey protein rich in alpha-lactalbumin increases the ratio of plasma tryptophan to the sum of the other large neutral amino acids and improves cognitive performance in stress-vulnerable subjects. *Am. J. Clin. Nutr.* **2002**, *75*, 1051–1056. [CrossRef] [PubMed]
43. Ano, Y.; Ozawa, M.; Kutsukake, T.; Sugiyama, S.; Uchida, K.; Yoshida, A.; Nakayama, H. Preventive effects of a fermented dairy product against Alzheimer's disease and identification of a novel oleamide with enhanced microglial phagocytosis and anti-inflammatory activity. *PLoS ONE* **2015**, *10*, e0118512. [CrossRef] [PubMed]
44. Sarlus, H.; Heneka, M.T. Microglia in Alzheimer's disease. *J. Clin. Investig.* **2017**, *127*, 3240–3249. [CrossRef] [PubMed]
45. Visan, I. Alzheimer's disease microglia. *Nat. Immunol.* **2017**, *18*, 876. [CrossRef] [PubMed]
46. Lee, C.Y.; Landreth, G.E. The role of microglia in amyloid clearance from the AD brain. *J. Neural Transm.* **2010**, *117*, 949–960. [CrossRef] [PubMed]
47. Hansen, D.V.; Hanson, J.E.; Sheng, M. Microglia in Alzheimer's disease. *J. Cell Biol.* **2018**, *217*. [CrossRef] [PubMed]
48. Stewart, W.F.; Kawas, C.; Corrada, M.; Metter, E.J. Risk of Alzheimer's disease and duration of NSAID use. *Neurology* **1997**, *48*, 626–632. [CrossRef] [PubMed]
49. Wang, J.; Tan, L.; Wang, H.F.; Tan, C.C.; Meng, X.F.; Wang, C.; Tang, S.W.; Yu, J.T. Anti-inflammatory drugs and risk of Alzheimer's disease: An updated systematic review and meta-analysis. *J. Alzheimer Dis. JAD* **2015**, *44*, 385–396. [CrossRef] [PubMed]
50. Imbimbo, B.P.; Solfrizzi, V.; Panza, F. Are NSAIDs useful to treat Alzheimer's disease or mild cognitive impairment? *Front. Aging Neurosci.* **2010**, *2*. [CrossRef] [PubMed]
51. Miguel-Alvarez, M.; Santos-Lozano, A.; Sanchis-Gomar, F.; Fiuza-Luces, C.; Pareja-Galeano, H.; Garatachea, N.; Lucia, A. Non-steroidal anti-inflammatory drugs as a treatment for Alzheimer's disease: A systematic review and meta-analysis of treatment effect. *Drugs Aging* **2015**, *32*, 139–147. [CrossRef] [PubMed]
52. Varvel, N.H.; Bhaskar, K.; Kounnas, M.Z.; Wagner, S.L.; Yang, Y.; Lamb, B.T.; Herrup, K. NSAIDs prevent, but do not reverse, neuronal cell cycle reentry in a mouse model of Alzheimer disease. *J. Clin. Investig.* **2009**, *119*, 3692–3702. [CrossRef] [PubMed]
53. Wyss-Coray, T.; Mucke, L. Ibuprofen, inflammation and Alzheimer disease. *Nat. Med.* **2000**, *6*, 973–974. [CrossRef] [PubMed]
54. Ano, Y.; Kutsukake, T.; Hoshi, A.; Yoshida, A.; Nakayama, H. Identification of a novel dehydroergosterol enhancing microglial anti-inflammatory activity in a dairy product fermented with *Penicillium candidum*. *PLoS ONE* **2015**, *10*, e0116598. [CrossRef] [PubMed]
55. Awasthi, N.P.; Singh, R.P. Lipase-catalyzed synthesis of fatty acid amide (erucamide) using fatty acid and urea. *J. Oleo Sci.* **2007**, *56*, 507–509. [CrossRef] [PubMed]

56. Slotema, W.F.; Sandoval, G.; Guieysse, D.; Straathof, A.J.; Marty, A. Economically pertinent continuous amide formation by direct lipase-catalyzed amidation with ammonia. *Biotechnol. Bioeng.* **2003**, *82*, 664–669. [CrossRef] [PubMed]
57. Cravatt, B.F.; Giang, D.K.; Mayfield, S.P.; Boger, D.L.; Lerner, R.A.; Gilula, N.B. Molecular characterization of an enzyme that degrades neuromodulatory fatty-acid amides. *Nature* **1996**, *384*, 83–87. [CrossRef] [PubMed]
58. Boger, D.L.; Henriksen, S.J.; Cravatt, B.F. Oleamide: An endogenous sleep-inducing lipid and prototypical member of a new class of biological signaling molecules. *Curr. Pharm. Des.* **1998**, *4*, 303–314. [PubMed]
59. Prospero-Garcia, O.; Amancio-Belmont, O.; Becerril Melendez, A.L.; Ruiz-Contreras, A.E.; Mendez-Diaz, M. Endocannabinoids and sleep. *Neurosci. Biobehav. Rev.* **2016**, *71*, 671–679. [CrossRef] [PubMed]
60. Moon, S.M.; Lee, S.A.; Hong, J.H.; Kim, J.S.; Kim, D.K.; Kim, C.S. Oleamide suppresses inflammatory responses in LPS-induced RAW264.7 murine macrophages and alleviates paw edema in a carrageenan-induced inflammatory rat model. *Int. Immunopharmacol.* **2018**, *56*, 179–185. [CrossRef] [PubMed]
61. Cabral, G.A.; Griffin-Thomas, L. Emerging role of the cannabinoid receptor CB2 in immune regulation: Therapeutic prospects for neuroinflammation. *Expert Rev. Mol. Med.* **2009**, *11*, e3. [CrossRef] [PubMed]
62. Mecha, M.; Feliu, A.; Carrillo-Salinas, F.J.; Rueda-Zubiaurre, A.; Ortega-Gutierrez, S.; de Sola, R.G.; Guaza, C. Endocannabinoids drive the acquisition of an alternative phenotype in microglia. *Brain Behave. Immun.* **2015**, *49*, 233–245. [CrossRef] [PubMed]
63. Aso, E.; Andres-Benito, P.; Carmona, M.; Maldonado, R.; Ferrer, I. Cannabinoid Receptor 2 Participates in Amyloid-β Processing in a Mouse Model of Alzheimer's Disease but Plays a Minor Role in the Therapeutic Properties of a Cannabis-Based Medicine. *J. Alzheimer Dis. JAD* **2016**, *51*, 489–500. [CrossRef] [PubMed]
64. Ehrhart, J.; Obregon, D.; Mori, T.; Hou, H.; Sun, N.; Bai, Y.; Klein, T.; Fernandez, F.; Tan, J.; Shytle, R.D. Stimulation of cannabinoid receptor 2 (CB2) suppresses microglial activation. *J. Neuroinflamm.* **2005**, *2*, 29. [CrossRef] [PubMed]
65. Tolon, R.M.; Nunez, E.; Pazos, M.R.; Benito, C.; Castillo, A.I.; Martinez-Orgado, J.A.; Romero, J. The activation of cannabinoid CB2 receptors stimulates in situ and in vitro β-amyloid removal by human macrophages. *Brain Res.* **2009**, *1283*, 148–154. [CrossRef] [PubMed]
66. Navarro, G.; Morales, P.; Rodriguez-Cueto, C.; Fernandez-Ruiz, J.; Jagerovic, N.; Franco, R. Targeting Cannabinoid CB2 Receptors in the Central Nervous System. Medicinal Chemistry Approaches with Focus on Neurodegenerative Disorders. *Front. Neurosci.* **2016**, *10*, 406. [CrossRef] [PubMed]
67. Mecha, M.; Carrillo-Salinas, F.J.; Feliu, A.; Mestre, L.; Guaza, C. Microglia activation states and cannabinoid system: Therapeutic implications. *Pharmacol. Ther.* **2016**, *166*, 40–55. [CrossRef] [PubMed]
68. Cassano, T.; Calcagnini, S.; Pace, L.; De Marco, F.; Romano, A.; Gaetani, S. Cannabinoid Receptor 2 Signaling in Neurodegenerative Disorders: From Pathogenesis to a Promising Therapeutic Target. *Front. Neurosci.* **2017**, *11*, 30. [CrossRef] [PubMed]
69. Wustner, D. Fluorescent sterols as tools in membrane biophysics and cell biology. *Chem. Phys. Lipids* **2007**, *146*, 1–25. [CrossRef] [PubMed]
70. Tachibana, Y. Synthesis and structure-activity relationships of bioactive compounds using sterols. *Yakugaku Zasshi* **2006**, *126*, 1139–1154. [CrossRef] [PubMed]
71. Wu, Y.; Dissing-Olesen, L.; MacVicar, B.A.; Stevens, B. Microglia: Dynamic Mediators of Synapse Development and Plasticity. *Trends Immunol.* **2015**, *36*, 605–613. [CrossRef] [PubMed]
72. Amor, S.; Peferoen, L.A.; Vogel, D.Y.; Breur, M.; van der Valk, P.; Baker, D.; van Noort, J.M. Inflammation in neurodegenerative diseases—An update. *Immunology* **2014**, *142*, 151–166. [CrossRef] [PubMed]
73. Griffin, W.S. Inflammation and neurodegenerative diseases. *Am. J. Clin. Nutr.* **2006**, *83*, 470S–474S. [CrossRef] [PubMed]
74. Miller, A.H.; Raison, C.L. The role of inflammation in depression: From evolutionary imperative to modern treatment target. *Nat. Rev. Immunol.* **2016**, *16*, 22–34. [CrossRef] [PubMed]
75. Kohler, O.; Krogh, J.; Mors, O.; Benros, M.E. Inflammation in Depression and the Potential for Anti-Inflammatory Treatment. *Curr. Neuropharmacol.* **2016**, *14*, 732–742. [CrossRef] [PubMed]
76. Salim, S.; Chugh, G.; Asghar, M. Inflammation in anxiety. *Adv. Protein Chem. Struct. Boil.* **2012**, *88*, 1–25.
77. Komaroff, A.L. Inflammation correlates with symptoms in chronic fatigue syndrome. *Proc. Natl. Acad. Sci. USA* **2017**, *114*, 8914–8916. [CrossRef] [PubMed]

78. Kruk-Slomka, M.; Michalak, A.; Biala, G. Antidepressant-like effects of the cannabinoid receptor ligands in the forced swimming test in mice: Mechanism of action and possible interactions with cholinergic system. *Behav. Brain Res.* **2015**, *284*, 24–36. [CrossRef] [PubMed]
79. Kruk-Slomka, M.; Budzynska, B.; Slomka, T.; Banaszkiewicz, I.; Biala, G. The Influence of the CB1 Receptor Ligands on the Schizophrenia-Like Effects in Mice Induced by MK-801. *Neurotox. Res.* **2016**, *30*, 658–676. [CrossRef] [PubMed]

8

The Viral Hypothesis in Alzheimer's Disease: Novel Insights and Pathogen-Based Biomarkers

Sean X Naughton [1], Urdhva Raval [1] and Giulio M. Pasinetti [1,2,*]

[1] Department of Neurology, Icahn School of Medicine at Mount Sinai, New York, NY 10029, USA; sean.naughton@mssm.edu (S.X.N.); Urdhva.Raval@mssm.edu (U.R.)
[2] James J. Peters Veterans Affairs Medical Center, Bronx, NY 10468, USA
* Correspondence: giulio.pasinetti@mssm.edu

Abstract: Early diagnosis of Alzheimer's disease (AD) and the identification of significant risk factors are necessary to better understand disease progression, and to develop intervention-based therapies prior to significant neurodegeneration. There is thus a critical need to establish biomarkers which can predict the risk of developing AD before the onset of cognitive decline. A number of studies have indicated that exposure to various microbial pathogens can accelerate AD pathology. Additionally, several studies have indicated that amyloid-β possess antimicrobial properties and may act in response to infection as a part of the innate immune system. These findings have led some to speculate that certain types of infections may play a significant role in AD pathogenesis. In this review, we will provide an overview of studies which suggest pathogen involvement in AD. Additionally, we will discuss a number of pathogen-associated biomarkers which may be effective in establishing AD risk. Infections that increase the risk of AD represent a modifiable risk factor which can be treated with therapeutic intervention. Pathogen-based biomarkers may thus be a valuable tool for evaluating and decreasing AD risk across the population.

Keywords: Alzheimer's disease; virus; bacteria; dementia

---

1. Introduction

Alzheimer's disease (AD) is an age-related neurodegenerative disorder. AD results in progressive cognitive decline, and is the most common form of dementia in older adults. This incurable disorder is predicted to affect approximately 100 million people globally by 2050 [1,2]. The characteristic hallmarks of AD pathology are amyloid-beta (Aβ) peptide plaques, tau hyperphosphorylation, and neuroinflammation. Currently, a clinical diagnosis of AD is only possible after disease onset through post-mortem detection of amyloid plaques and neurofibrillary tangles [3]. Cognitive testing can aid in the diagnosis of dementia, but strong cognitive impairments are usually only present at a time point when successful therapeutic intervention is unlikely. Early diagnosis of AD is only possible in rare cases in which the autosomal dominant early onset form of the disease is genetically inherited [4]. Considering the impact and prevalence of AD globally, there is an increasing need to understand and identify biomarkers, in order to detect AD in individuals before the onset of disease and provide mitigating therapeutics. Preclinical detection of biomarkers of Aβ, tau, and other neurodegenerative effects have been extensively studied. Aβ and tau have been detected in cerebrospinal fluid and blood plasma. Neuroimaging via magnetic resonance imaging (MRI) and positron emission tomography (PET), specifically, FDG-PET, amyloid PET and structural MRI can also serve diagnostic roles in AD [1,5]. Interestingly, there is some indication of microbial and viral involvement in AD pathology. Given the relatively high prevalence of certain pathogens, they can serve as biomarkers for preclinical AD. In this review, we explore the role of microbes in AD pathology and the potential of various pathogens as novel biomarkers for AD. This review is based on literature generated from searches conducted between

1 April and 25 July 2020, using standard databases and search engines for scientific literature (PubMed and Google Scholar), using the following keywords: "Alzheimer's Disease", "Pathogen Hypothesis" "Viruses", "Bacteria". Additional references were collected from those discussed in the literature generated through the search.

Amyloid-Beta

The Aβ peptide is integral to AD pathology. Aβ misfolding and the resultant Aβ plaques are thought to be the root cause of cognitive decline in AD. Aβ aggregates are formed from the proteolytic cleavage of a larger type 1 membrane glycoprotein, named amyloid precursor protein (APP). APP is involved in maintaining neuronal homeostasis, neuronal development, signaling, and intracellular transport [6]. APP is cleaved by β-secretases and γ-secretases, to produce an Aβ peptide ranging from 37 to 49 amino acid residues [7]. Aβ aggregates are found in the hippocampus, neocortex, and cerebrovasculature [8]. Aβ exists in different forms, including soluble Aβ, Aβ oligomers, and Aβ plaque forms. These different forms are involved in neurodegeneration at different stages of AD [6]. Aβ plaques induce tau protein hyperphosphorylation and formation neurofibrillary tangles and synaptic dysfunction. These plaques also generate the production of 4-hydroxynonenal, a toxic aldehyde involved in lipid peroxidation, and disruption of cellular homeostasis [9]. Aβ aggregation also leads to DNA damage and the release of inflammatory responses which result in the loss of neuronal synapses and ultimately neuronal death [10]. Intriguingly, Aβ acts as an antimicrobial peptide (AMP) and has been demonstrated to be effective against viruses, bacteria, and fungi. AMPs are a group of defensins, histatins, and cathelicidins that primarily serve to defend the host against a wide variety of pathogens. AMPs can also modulate cytokine release and adaptive immune responses. Aβ has been demonstrated to function like the cathelicidin AMP LL-37. Aβ was shown to be effective against the bacteria Streptococcus pneumoniae and fungus Candida albicans, which are the causative agents of bacterial meningitis and neurocandidiasis, respectively. Aβ also inhibits certain other bacterial species of the genera Pseudomonas, Escherichia, Streptococcus, Staphylococcus, Salmonella, and Enterococcus [11,12]. There is also evidence indicating that Aβ can also inhibit replication of seasonal and pandemic strains of the influenza A and herpes simplex virus 1 (HSV-1) viruses [13]. In fact, Aβ has been shown to be as effective as the antiviral drug Acyclovir at inhibiting HSV-1 neuropathology [14].

2. Pathogens and AD

2.1. Viral Pathogens in Neurodegeneration and AD

The idea that infections may play a role in Alzheimer's disease (AD) pathogenesis dates back nearly 30 years and has been a subject of debate in the field of AD (Figure 1) [15]. Previous studies have suggested that amyloid-β (Aβ) may act as a part of the innate immune system to aggregate around infectious particles. Eimer and colleagues showed that 5XFAD mice infected with herpes simplex virus 1 (HSV-1) showed increased survival rates compared to infected non-transgenic littermates. Moreover, Aβ was found to bind to and entrap HSV1, in a process mediated by fibrillization. Aβ deposition could be triggered by HSV1 infection in young 5XFAD mice, prior to the ordinary development of Aβ deposits [16]. Additionally, brains from Alzheimer's disease patients have been shown to have increased levels of human herpesvirus 6 and human herpesvirus 7 in several key areas [17]. HSV-1 infection has also been shown to drive the development of amyloid fibrillar plaque-like formations in human-induced neural stem cells and 3D human brain-like tissue cultures [18]. While different types of herpesvirus have been associated with AD pathology and detected in the brains of AD patients, there is also evidence to suggest that other viruses (and other types of pathogens) may also play a role in AD. For example, Nimgaonkar and colleagues found that exposure to HSV-2, cytomegalovirus (CMV), or the parasite Toxoplasma gondii (TOX) was associated with cognitive decline in individuals aged 65 and older [19]. Additionally, Ljungan virus (LV) has been detected in the hippocampus of AD brains, but not in age-matched controls [20]. The detection of different viral strains in the brains of different cohorts of patients hints at the idea that viral infection may play a role in AD or that AD may increase susceptibility to neuroinvasion by viruses. It is currently unclear if one or more pathogenic infections might directly stimulate (or accelerate) AD, or if AD creates an environment which facilitates the accumulation of infections in the brain through altered immune function. In this regard, it is interesting to consider the case of HIV, in which immune function is compromised in the presence of a persistent viral infection. In particular, HIV-associated neurocognitive disorders (HAND) have been associated with the presence of β-amyloid, and HAND patients have been shown to have similar cerebrospinal fluid levels of β-amyloid 1-42 when compared to patients with Alzheimer's associated dementia [21,22] Compromised immune function may thus be a critical driver of neurodegeneration by allowing infectious pathogens such as viruses to enter the brain at levels which exceed the capacity of the innate immune system within the brain. A number of different viruses have been shown to enter the brain and cause neurodegeneration, often with accompanying protienopathy. For example, the family of H5N1 avian influenza A viruses responsible for a previous epidemic in Asia have been shown to produce Parkinsonian-like neurodegeneration in mice. H5N1 induced neurodegeneration was accompanied by α-synuclein phosphorylation and neuroinflammation. Interestingly, microgliosis persisted long after the infection resolved and was observable at a time point 90 days from the initial infection [23].

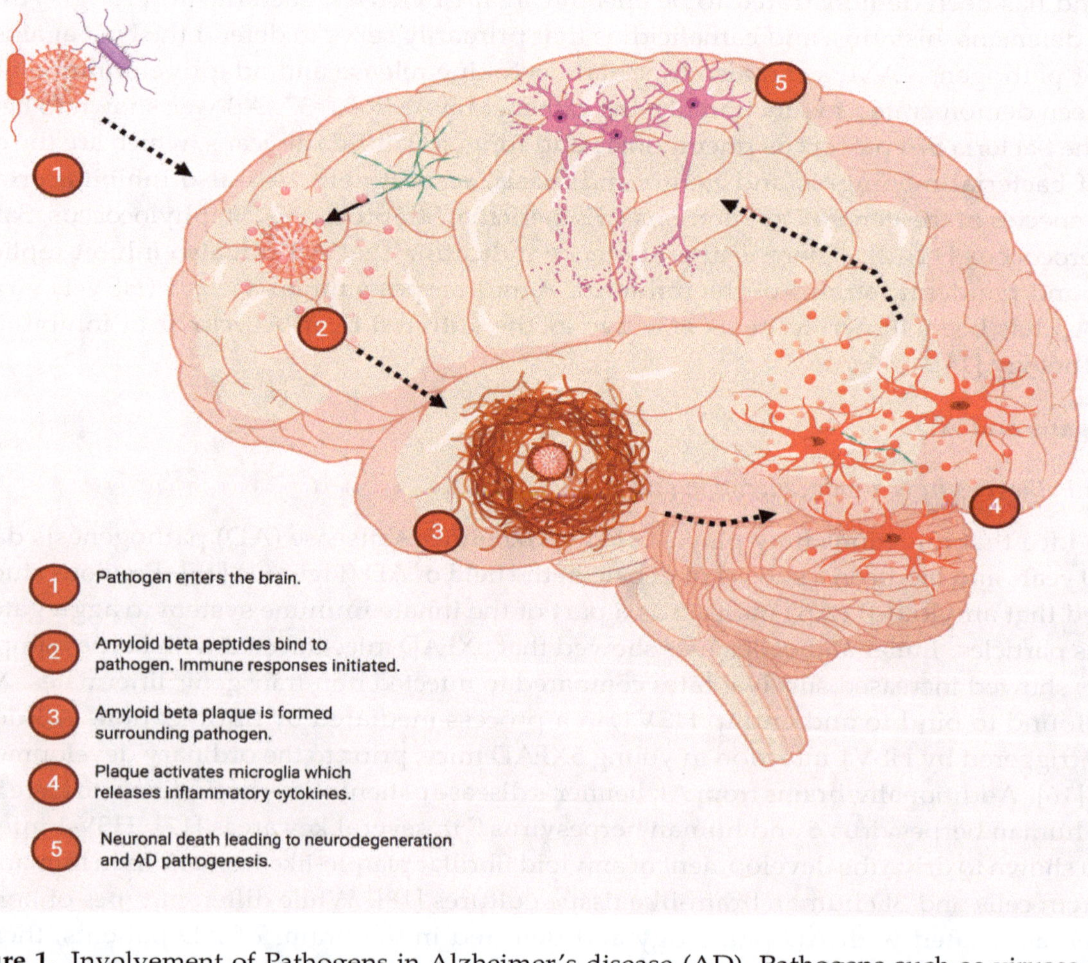

Figure 1. Involvement of Pathogens in Alzheimer's disease (AD). Pathogens such as viruses and bacteria can become entrapped by amyloid-β after entering the brain. Amyloid fibrils form in response to certain pathogens, and infection may play a role in accelerating AD pathology by stimulating inflammation and neurodegeneration.

An intriguing idea which has emerged regarding viral infection and neurodegeneration is the "multi-hit" or "hit and run" hypothesis. This notion is supported by a study from Sadasivan and colleagues, who showed that infection with influenza H1N1 virus 30 days prior to MPTP administration markedly enhanced neurodegeneration in the substantia nigra pars compacta (SNpc) of mice. Furthermore, this enhancement of MPTP induced neurodegeneration could be alleviated by prior vaccination [24]. Thus, it is possible that a viral infection at one time point may later synergize with other factors (i.e., environmental toxins, lifestyle choices, genetic background), to cause or accelerate neurodegeneration. The above-mentioned studies regarding influenza viruses and Parkinsonian like neurodegeneration provide additional insight as to the potential role of viral pathogens in stimulating neurodegeneration independent of β-amyloid. Persistent inflammation stimulated by viral infection may be a critical component in predisposing individuals to AD. Neuroinflammation and neuro-immune interactions have gained attention in recent years as potential driving factors of neurodegeneration [25]. Thus, the pathological effects of increased neuroinflammation paired with its ability to inhibit amyloid clearance may create a bi-directional relationship, whereby viruses (or other pathogens) are able to both increase amyloid activity through direct interactions, while preventing amyloid clearance through stimulation of inflammation.

2.2. Bacterial Pathogens and AD

In addition to the above-mentioned viruses, bacterial pathogens have also been associated with AD. In particular, there is mounting evidence linking periodontal disease and AD. Periodontitis, commonly known as gum disease, is an oral infection resulting in the release of proinflammatory cytokines into the bloodstream and the increase of C-reactive protein. It is caused by the gram-negative anaerobic bacterium Porphyromonas gingivalis [26]. P. gingivalis and its associated toxins, referred to collectively as gingipains, have been identified in 96% of postmortem brain tissue samples of AD patients and are thought to exacerbate AD pathology [27]. Gingipains play a key role in P. gingivalis mediated aggravation of AD. Gingipains are a group of cysteine proteases secreted by P. gingivalis that cause neuronal damage, increased tau production, and increased production of neuro-toxic APOE fragments. Additionally, P. gingivalis induces neuroinflammation, inflammasome activation, and other immune system multiprotein complexes in the brain that result in neurodegeneration and Aβ plaque formation [27,28]. In animal models, P. gingivalis has been demonstrated to travel to the brain following oral inoculation. Interestingly, in mouse models, Aβ1-42 was found to act as an antimicrobial peptide against P. gingivalis. Aβ1-42 inhibited P. gingivalis by disrupting its cell membrane. Notably, P. gingivalis can be detected in the CSF of AD patients and can thus potentially be used as a biomarker for AD [27]. Other bacteria involved in periodontitis include Aggregatibacter actinomycetemcomitans, Prevotella intermedia, Fusobacterium nucleatum, Tannerella forsythensis, Eikenella corrodens, and Treponema denticola. These various bacteria induce inflammation and thus promote neurodegeneration, though there is some evidence alluding to their presence in the brain [26]. The spirochete Borrelia burgdorferi (B. burgdorferi) is the causative agent of Lyme disease, and has also been linked with AD. B. burgdorferi has been detected in the brains of AD patients and is known for its neurodegenerative effects [29,30]. Additionally, Chlamydia pneumoniae (C. pneumoniae) has been detected in the brains of AD patients and may be another factor driving AD pathology [31]. Infection with Helicobacter pylori (H. pylori) has also been associated with increased risk of AD. Infection with H.pylori has been associated with lower cognitive abilities, as well as increased levels of CSF tau and phosphorylated tau among AD patients [32]. Gut microbiome dysbiosis and altered microbiome composition have been implicated in AD and various other neurodegenerative disorders [33]. The gut microbiome produces lipopolysaccharides, neurotoxins, and microbial amyloid. These bacterial products are involved with amyloid plaque formation, neurofibrillary tangles, and neuroinflammation. The gut microbiome composition is also altered in individuals with AD, with the increased relative abundance of bacteria of the genera Verrucomicrobia and Proteobacteria and decreased abundance of Ruminococcus and Butyricicoccus genera [33]. Interestingly, gut microbiota have also been found in the brains of AD patients [34]. The penetrance of gut bacteria into the brain could represent a potential trigger of amyloidosis, that could occur independently of traditional pathogen infection (Figure 2). This could potentially represent a potential mechanism similar to the association between gingivitis and AD, whereby dysregulation of the microbiome could render the host susceptible to amyloidosis and neurodegeneration.

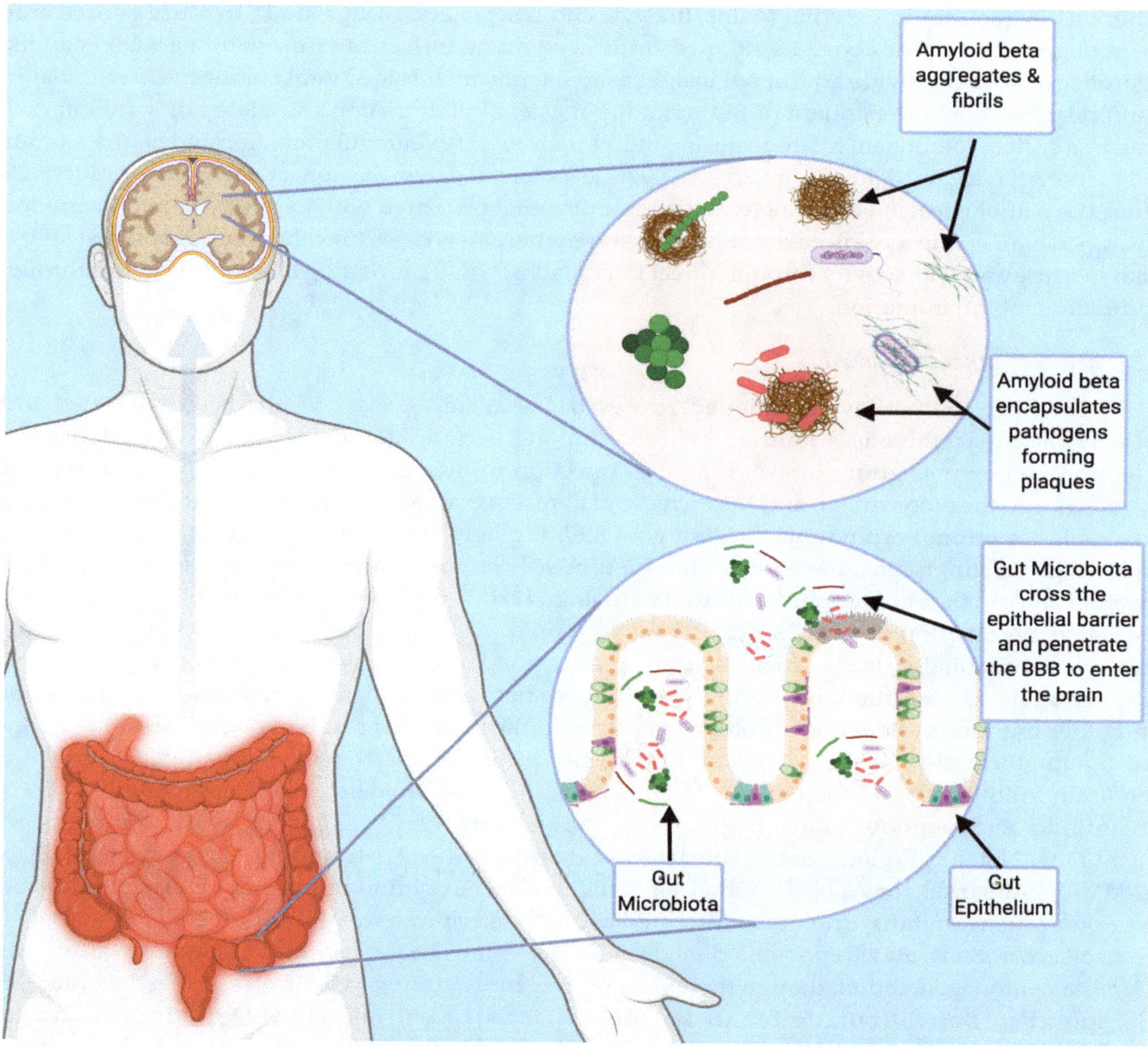

Figure 2. Potential Role of Gut Bacteria in Neurodegeneration. Age-related changes in intestinal permeability and blood brain barrier integrity may allow for penetrance of gut bacteria into the brain and promote the formation of amyloid fibrils. Future studies should focus on the role of gut bacteria as a potential trigger to the amyloid cascade.

2.3. Other Pathogens and AD

Fungal infection may also play a role in the pathology of AD. Fungal proteins and DNA have been detected in the brains of AD patients [35]. Additional studies have revealed that fungal proteins and DNA can also be detected peripherally and may make suitable biomarkers (see below for further discussion). The protozoan parasite T. gondii, which is thought to infect up to 50% of the world's population, is known to cause encephalitis and neurological dysfunction. It is thought that T. gondii may be involved with neuroinflammation and olfactory dysfunction in AD pathology [36].

3. Pathogen-Based Biomarkers

Based on the above-mentioned studies linking various pathogens with AD and age-related cognitive decline, it may be rational to use biomarkers based on pathogen exposure to assess the risk for developing AD in elderly individuals. In cases of active infection, intervention with antimicrobial treatments may be a suitable method of reducing AD risk, particularly in patients with advanced age. We discuss below a number of biomarkers based on pathogens which have been linked to AD and cognitive decline (Table 1).

3.1. Antimicrobial Peptides as Biomarkers in AD

Defensins are a family of disulfide knotted antimicrobial peptides that entrap pathogens as a part of the innate immune system [37]. Moreover, α-Defensins 1 and 2 were shown to be elevated in the blood of AD patients and may make a suitable biomarker for detecting AD status [38]. Another anti-microbial protein that might make a suitable biomarker for AD is lactoferrin. Lactoferrin is an antimicrobial peptide that is present in saliva and correlates with AD status. Saliva samples from amnesiac mild cognitive impairment (aMCI) and AD patients showed decreased levels of lactoferrin when compared with controls, and a significant negative correlation was found between lactoferrin and aMCI and AD patients. These results suggest the potential usage of lactoferrin as a non-invasive salivary biomarker for AD [39]. Tears contain a number of antimicrobial proteins that act as part of the innate immune system. Several proteins present in tears have been shown to be differentially expressed in AD patients and may serve as suitable biomarkers. In particular, changes in the expression of the antimicrobial proteins lipocalin-1, dermcidin, lysozyme-C and lacritin have been reported using tear samples of AD patients [40].

Table 1. Pathogen-Based Biomarkers in AD. Numerous pathogens have been associated with AD pathogenesis and the onset of cognitive decline. Biomarkers are listed along with their source and relationship to AD.

	Biomarker	Source	Description	Reference
Antimicrobial Peptides				
	α-Defensin 1	Blood	Increased in blood of AD patients.	[39]
	α-Defensin 2	Blood	Increased in blood of AD patients.	[39]
	Lactoferrin	Saliva	Decreased with AD and aMCI.	[40]
	Lipocalin-1	Tears	Decreased in AD.	[41]
	Dermcidin	Tears	Increased in AD.	[41]
	Lysozyme-C	Tears	Decreased in AD.	[41]
	Lacritin	Tears	Decreased in AD.	[41]
Antibodies				
	IgG against Epstein-Barr Virus	Blood	Correlates with development of aMCI.	[42]
	IgG and IgA against *C. pneumoniae*	Blood	Detectable in patients with vascular dementia.	[43]
	IgG against HSV-2	Blood	Correlates with cognitive decline.	[25]

Table 1. *Cont.*

	Biomarker	Source	Description	Reference
	IgG against CMV	Blood	Correlates with cognitive decline.	[25]
	IgG against *T. gondii*	Blood	Correlates with cognitive decline.	[25]
	IgM against HSV-1	Blood	Associated with increased risk of AD.	[44,45]
	IgG against *H. Pylori*	Blood	Associated with lower MMSE scores.	[35]
Other				
	Fungal Proteins and DNA	CSF, Blood	Detectable in AD patients.	[36,46]
	Gut Microbiome composition	fecal matter	Correlates to gut dysbiosis and cognitive decline.	[6,47]
	Porphyromonas gingivalis	CSF	Identified in 96% of postmortem brain tissue samples of AD patients.	[30]

3.2. Antibodies as Biomarkers for AD

Antibodies against pathogens associated with AD are readily detectable in blood, and may be a reasonable way of establishing AD risk in the elderly. A number of studies have shown correlations between antibodies against various pathogens and cognitive decline. For example, elevated levels of IgG against Epstein–Barr Virus (EBV) have been shown to correlate with the development of aMCI [41]. The presence of C. pneumoniae in AD patients has been well documented (see discussion above), and IgG and IgA antibodies against C. pneumoniae have been detected in patients with vascular dementia [42]. Additionally, IgG antibodies against HSV-2, CMV, and TOX have been shown to correlate with cognitive decline in individuals over the age of 65 and may also serve as rational biomarkers. While the study by [19] did not find any significant correlation between HSV-1 antibodies and cognitive decline, other groups have reported on the possibility of HSV-1 antibodies as potential biomarkers for AD [43,44]. In a study by Roubaud-Baudron et al., the presence of IgG antibodies against H.Pylori was associated with lower scores on the mini-mental state examination (MMSE) and increased CSF tau levels, among AD patients [32]. AD has also been linked with increased T. gondii IgG antibodies. These antibodies can serve as potential AD biomarkers, given the high prevalence of T. gondii infection globally [36].

3.3. Other Potential Biomarkers

Additional pathogens such as fungi may also serve as potential biomarkers in AD. Fungal proteins and DNA have been detected in the CSF for AD patients [45]. Furthermore, fungal polysaccharides, proteins, and DNA have all been detected in blood samples drawn from AD patients [35]. The relationship between the gut microbiome and various neurological diseases has been an area of growing interest in recent years, and may be another option to consider for monitoring the progression of AD. Variation in gut microbiome composition detected from stool samples can also be a preclinical biomarker for AD, given the increased relative abundance of bacteria of the genera Verrucomicrobia and Proteobacteria found in AD. Gut microbiome products such as microbial amyloids and neurotoxin BMAA play a role in neurodegeneration, and can also potentially serve as AD biomarkers [33,46].

4. Conclusions

While the presence of pathogens or antibodies against certain pathogens may not directly indicate a positive diagnosis of AD per se, it is important to note that these biomarkers may be appropriate for determining at-risk cohorts of elderly individuals. The potential to identify at risk individuals and administer prophylactic treatments is of great value to the field of AD research. In particular, the administration of antimicrobial treatments (antiviral, antifungal, antibacterial, anti-parasitic) after positive confirmation of an infection carries little risk, and could be neuroprotective. A recent analysis of data from Taiwan's National Health Insurance Research Database found that treatment with antiherpetic medications was associated with a decreased risk of developing dementia [47]. Furthermore, a clinical trial is currently underway to evaluate the antiviral therapy valacyclovir in the treatment of AD [48].

As it stands, there is currently preclinical evidence to suggest that β-amyloid can directly bind pathogens, and that pathogenic infection can accelerate amyloid pathology in transgenic animal models of AD. Additionally, multiple preclinical studies have demonstrated the neurodegenerative properties of certain pathogens. In terms of clinical data, there are a number of studies providing correlational evidence between the presence of various pathogens and the diagnosis of AD. There is thus a critical missing link between amyloid entrapment of pathogenic microbes, and widespread neurodegeneration. Some insight as to the potential mechanism by which infection may stimulate neurodegeneration can be taken from a recent study examining interferon signaling in response to β-amyloid. Roy and colleagues showed that soluble oligomers interact with nucleic acids (DNA and RNA) or glycosaminoglycans (i.e., heparin), and that these interactions promote the formation of amyloid fibrils. Interestingly, only amyloid fibrils containing nucleic acids promote type 1 interferon response, inflammation, and synaptic loss. Type 1 interferon response was observed across several different transgenic mouse lines, indicating that self-DNA or self-RNA may trigger this response. Additionally, wild type mice that received a hippocampal injection of amyloid fibrils containing RNA showed an inflammatory profile similar to that observed in transgenic models of AD [49]. These findings are very exciting when viewed in the context of other studies, which have shown that amyloid fibrils can form after binding to viral particles such as herpes simplex virus (a double stranded DNA virus). Type 1 interferon response usually occurs as a part of the innate immune response to viral infection; thus, the finding that nucleic acid containing amyloid fibrils stimulates type 1 interferon suggests that Aβ may be an integral component of antiviral defense in the brain. Blocking type 1 interferon response and other immune-related signaling pathways which occur after Aβ entrapment of pathogens may thus be a rational therapeutic strategy in treating AD.

A critical question also becomes whether AD is directly stimulated by one or more pathogens entering the brain, or if AD can occur as a result of dysfunction of Aβ driven anti-viral defenses. Thus, future studies investigating both the function and dysfunction of innate immune responses in the brain will be critical to our understanding and diagnosis of AD. In particular, it is necessary to understand how other factors, such as diet, genetic background, and exposure to environmental toxins may confer susceptibility to neuroinvasion by pathogenic microbes. It is also possible that the reason why so many different pathogens are readily detected in the brains and blood of AD patients is that AD may fundamentally weaken the immune system. Decreased activity or dysfunction of the peripheral immune system may force the innate immune system of the brain to bear a heavy burden when faced with pathogenic infections during AD. Thus, increased reliance on the antimicrobial activity of Aβ during AD may force an already burdened system to a "breaking point", in which severe neurodeneration is facilitated by excessive amyloidosis, microglial activation, and immune dysfunction in the brain.

There is still a great deal of research that needs to be done to establish a direct causal link between AD and pathogenic infection. In particular, several key areas need to be addressed. One critical consideration is that AD may merely increase susceptibility of infection, thus allowing various pathogens to enter brain and making their detection either a secondary occurrence or an artifact. To address this possibility, it will be critical to examine the brains of patients with familial AD to determine if pathogens can be detected that are not present in age-matched controls. This would help one to better understand if AD fundamentally facilitates pathogenic infections in the brain, which would provide insight as to whether infection is a primary or secondary occurrence in sporadic AD. If no pathogens are present in the brains of patients with familial AD, it might suggest that AD is primarily caused by the brain's innate immune system behaving in a dysfunctional manner (i.e., amyloid entrapment of host DNA/RNA as opposed to pathogen DNA/RNA). Another critical area which must be addressed is the high detection rate of different pathogens in various cohorts of AD patients. For example, differing studies have found P. gingivalis, LV, or human herpesvirus (as well as other pathogens) in all or nearly all of the brains from AD patients observed in the respective cohorts of each study [17,20,27]. This would imply that, if we were to extrapolate the findings of each individual cohort to the broader AD population, then all AD patients would be expected to present with multiple pathogenic infections simultaneously. Thus, it is crucial to determine if multiple pathogens can indeed be detected within the same brains of AD patients. If multiple pathogens cannot be detected within a single AD brain, it might imply that geographical differences in exposure to various pathogens might cause a specific pathogen to be overrepresented in one particular cohort. This would also suggest the possibility that multiples pathogens might be independently capable of stimulating the same pathogenic processes within AD. While the underlying mechanisms linking specific infections and AD are not explicitly known, the consistent association of various pathogens in AD cannot be ignored. It is thus critical to evaluate the presence of pathogen related biomarkers in elderly individuals, to aid in the construction of an AD risk profile.

Author Contributions: S.X.N., U.R., and G.M.P. all contributed to the writing—review and editing of this manuscript. All authors have read and agreed to the published version of the manuscript.

Acknowledgments: Figures 1 and 2 were made using Biorender.com.

References

1. Nguyen, T.T.; Ta, Q.T.H.; Nguyen, T.K.O.; Nguyen, T.T.D.; Vo, V.G. Role of Body-Fluid Biomarkers in Alzheimer's Disease Diagnosis. *Diagnostics* **2020**, *10*, 326. [CrossRef]
2. Prince, M.J.; Wu, F.; Guo, Y.; Robledo, L.M.G.; O'Donnell, M.; Sullivan, R.; Yusuf, S. The burden of disease in older people and implications for health policy and practice. *Lancet* **2015**, *385*, 549–562. [CrossRef]
3. Perl, D.P. Neuropathology of Alzheimer's Disease. *Mt. Sinai J. Med. J. Transl. Pers. Med.* **2010**, *77*, 32–42. [CrossRef]
4. Giau, V.V.; Bagyinszky, E.; An, S.S.A.; Kim, S. Clinical genetic strategies for early onset neurodegenerative diseases. *Mol. Cell. Toxicol.* **2018**, *14*, 123–142. [CrossRef]
5. Zetterberg, H.; Bendlin, B.B. Biomarkers for Alzheimer's disease-preparing for a new era of disease-modifying therapies. *Mol. Psychiatry* **2020**. [CrossRef]
6. Chen, G.; Xu, T.; Yan, Y.; Zhou, Y.; Jiang, Y.; Melcher, K.; Xu, H.E. Amyloid beta: Structure, biology and structure-based therapeutic development. *Acta Pharmacol. Sin.* **2017**, *38*, 1205–1235. [CrossRef] [PubMed]
7. Nunan, J.; Small, D.H. Regulation of APP cleavage by α-, β- and γ-secretases. *FEBS Lett.* **2000**, *483*, 6–10. [CrossRef]
8. Viswanathan, A.; Greenberg, S.M. Cerebral amyloid angiopathy in the elderly. *Ann. Neurol.* **2011**, *70*, 871–880. [CrossRef] [PubMed]
9. Mattson, M.P. Pathways towards and away from Alzheimer's disease. *Nature* **2004**, *430*, 631–639. [CrossRef] [PubMed]
10. Heneka, M.T.; Golenbock, D.T.; Latz, E. Innate immunity in Alzheimer's disease. *Nat. Immunol.* **2015**, *16*, 229–236. [CrossRef] [PubMed]

11. Soscia, S.J.; Kirby, J.E.; Washicosky, K.J.; Tucker, S.M.; Ingelsson, M.; Hyman, B.; Burton, M.A.; Goldstein, L.E.; Duong, S.; Tanzi, R.E.; et al. The Alzheimer's Disease-Associated Amyloid β-Protein Is an Antimicrobial Peptide. *PLoS ONE* **2010**, *5*, e9505. [CrossRef] [PubMed]
12. Gosztyla, M.L.; Brothers, H.M.; Robinson, S.R. Alzheimer's Amyloid-β is an Antimicrobial Peptide: A Review of the Evidence. *J. Alzheimers Dis.* **2018**, *62*, 1495–1506. [CrossRef] [PubMed]
13. Bourgade, K.; Dupuis, G.; Frost, E.H.; Fülöp, T., Jr. Anti-Viral Properties of Amyloid-β Peptides. *J. Alzheimers Dis.* **2016**, *54*, 859–878. [CrossRef] [PubMed]
14. Lukiw, W.J.; Cui, J.G.; Yuan, L.Y.; Bhattacharjee, P.S.; Corkern, M.; Clement, C.; Kammerman, E.M.; Ball, M.J.; Zhao, Y.; Sullivan, P.M.; et al. Acyclovir or Aβ42 peptides attenuate HSV-1-induced miRNA-146a levels in human primary brain cells. *NeuroReport* **2010**, *21*, 922–927. [CrossRef]
15. Itzhaki, R.F.; Golde, T.E.; Heneka, M.T.; Readhead, B. Do infections have a role in the pathogenesis of Alzheimer disease? *Nat. Rev. Neurol.* **2020**, *16*, 193–197. [CrossRef]
16. Eimer, W.A.; Vijaya Kumar, D.K.; Navalpur Shanmugam, N.K.; Rodriguez, A.S.; Mitchell, T.; Washicosky, K.J.; György, B.; Breakefield, X.O.; Tanzi, R.E.; Moir, R.D. Alzheimer's Disease-Associated β-Amyloid Is Rapidly Seeded by Herpesviridae to Protect against Brain Infection. *Neuron* **2018**, *99*, 56–63.e3. [CrossRef]
17. Readhead, B.; Haure-Mirande, J.-V.; Funk, C.C.; Richards, M.A.; Shannon, P.; Haroutunian, V.; Sano, M.; Liang, W.S.; Beckmann, N.D.; Price, N.D.; et al. Multiscale Analysis of Independent Alzheimer's Cohorts Finds Disruption of Molecular, Genetic, and Clinical Networks by Human Herpesvirus. *Neuron* **2018**, *99*, 64–82.e7. [CrossRef]
18. Cairns, D.M.; Rouleau, N.; Parker, R.N.; Walsh, K.G.; Gehrke, L.; Kaplan, D.L. A 3D human brain–like tissue model of herpes-induced Alzheimer's disease. *Sci. Adv.* **2020**, *6*, eaay8828. [CrossRef]
19. Nimgaonkar, V.L.; Yolken, R.H.; Wang, T.; Chang, C.-C.H.; McClain, L.; McDade, E.; Snitz, B.E.; Ganguli, M. Temporal Cognitive Decline Associated With Exposure to Infectious Agents in a Population-based, Aging Cohort. *Alzheimer Dis. Assoc. Disord.* **2016**, *30*, 216–222. [CrossRef]
20. Niklasson, B.; Lindquist, L.; Klitz, W.; Bank, N.B.; Englund, E. Picornavirus Identified in Alzheimer's Disease Brains: A Pathogenic Path? *J. Alzheimers Dis. Rep.* **2020**, *4*, 141–146. [CrossRef]
21. Canet, G.; Dias, C.; Gabelle, A.; Simonin, Y.; Gosselet, F.; Marchi, N.; Makinson, A.; Tuaillon, E.; Van de Perre, P.; Givalois, L.; et al. HIV Neuroinfection and Alzheimer's Disease: Similarities and Potential Links? *Front. Cell. Neurosci.* **2018**, *12*. [CrossRef] [PubMed]
22. Clifford, D.B.; Fagan, A.M.; Holtzman, D.M.; Morris, J.C.; Teshome, M.; Shah, A.R.; Kauwe, J.S.K. CSF biomarkers of Alzheimer disease in HIV-associated neurologic disease. *Neurology* **2009**, *73*, 1982–1987. [CrossRef] [PubMed]
23. Jang, H.; Boltz, D.; Sturm-Ramirez, K.; Shepherd, K.R.; Jiao, Y.; Webster, R.; Smeyne, R.J. Highly pathogenic H5N1 influenza virus can enter the central nervous system and induce neuroinflammation and neurodegeneration. *Proc. Natl. Acad. Sci. USA* **2009**, *106*, 14063–14068. [CrossRef] [PubMed]
24. Sadasivan, S.; Sharp, B.; Schultz-Cherry, S.; Smeyne, R.J. Synergistic effects of influenza and 1-methyl-4-phenyl-1,2,3,6-tetrahydropyridine (MPTP) can be eliminated by the use of influenza therapeutics: Experimental evidence for the multi-hit hypothesis. *NPJ Park. Dis.* **2017**, *3*, 1–3. [CrossRef]
25. Kinney, J.W.; Bemiller, S.M.; Murtishaw, A.S.; Leisgang, A.M.; Salazar, A.M.; Lamb, B.T. Inflammation as a central mechanism in Alzheimer's disease. *Alzheimers Dement. Transl. Res. Clin. Interv.* **2018**, *4*, 575–590. [CrossRef]
26. Abbayya, K.; Puthanakar, N.Y.; Naduwinmani, S.; Chidambar, Y.S. Association between periodontitis and Alzheimer's disease. *North Am. J. Med. Sci.* **2015**, *7*, 241. [CrossRef]
27. Dominy, S.S.; Lynch, C.; Ermini, F.; Benedyk, M.; Marczyk, A.; Konradi, A.; Nguyen, M.; Haditsch, U.; Raha, D.; Griffin, C.; et al. Porphyromonas gingivalis in Alzheimer's disease brains: Evidence for disease causation and treatment with small-molecule inhibitors. *Sci. Adv.* **2019**, *5*, eaau3333. [CrossRef]
28. Venegas, C.; Kumar, S.; Franklin, B.S.; Dierkes, T.; Brinkschulte, R.; Tejera, D.; Vieira-Saecker, A.; Schwartz, S.; Santarelli, F.; Kummer, M.P.; et al. Microglia-derived ASC specks cross-seed amyloid-β in Alzheimer's disease. *Nature* **2017**, *552*, 355–361. [CrossRef]
29. MacDonald, A.B.; Miranda, J.M. Concurrent neocortical borreliosis and Alzheimer's disease. *Hum. Pathol.* **1987**, *18*, 759–761. [CrossRef]
30. MacDonald, A.B. Alzheimer's neuroborreliosis with trans-synaptic spread of infection and neurofibrillary tangles derived from intraneuronal spirochetes. *Med. Hypotheses* **2007** *68*, 822–825. [CrossRef]

31. Hammond, C.J.; Hallock, L.R.; Howanski, R.J.; Appelt, D.M.; Little, C.S.; Balin, B.J. Immunohistological detection of Chlamydia pneumoniae in the Alzheimer's disease brain. *BMC Neurosci.* **2010**, *11*, 121. [CrossRef] [PubMed]
32. Roubaud-Baudron, C.; Krolak-Salmon, P.; Quadrio, I.; Mégraud, F.; Salles, N. Impact of chronic Helicobacter pylori infection on Alzheimer's disease: Preliminary results. *Neurobiol. Aging* **2012**, *33*, 1009-e11. [CrossRef]
33. Raval, U.; Harary, J.; Zeng, E.; Pasinetti, G.M. The dichotomous role of the gut microbiome in exacerbating and ameliorating neurodegenerative disorders. *Expert Rev. Neurother.* **2020**. [CrossRef] [PubMed]
34. Westfall, S.; Dinh, D.M.; Pasinetti, G.M. Investigation of Potential Brain Microbiome in Alzheimer's Disease: Implications of Study Bias. *J. Alzheimers Dis. JAD* **2020**, *75*, 559–570. [CrossRef] [PubMed]
35. Alonso, R.; Pisa, D.; Marina, A.I.; Morato, E.; Rábano, A.; Carrasco, L. Fungal Infection in Patients with Alzheimer's Disease. *J. Alzheimers Dis.* **2014**, *41*, 301–311. [CrossRef] [PubMed]
36. Prandota, J. Possible Link Between Toxoplasma Gondii and the Anosmia Associated With Neurodegenerative Diseases. *Am. J. Alzheimers Dis. Dementiasr* **2014**, *29*, 205–214. [CrossRef]
37. Zhao, X.; Wu, H.; Lu, H.; Li, G.; Huang, Q. LAMP: A Database Linking Antimicrobial Peptides. *PLoS ONE* **2013**, *8*, e66557. [CrossRef]
38. Watt, A.D.; Perez, K.A.; Ang, C.-S.; O'Donnell, P.; Rembach, A.; Pertile, K.K.; Rumble, R.L.; Trounson, B.O.; Fowler, C.J.; Faux, N.G.; et al. Peripheral α-Defensins 1 and 2 are Elevated in Alzheimer's Disease. *J. Alzheimers Dis.* **2015**, *44*, 1131–1143. [CrossRef]
39. Carro, E.; Bartolomé, F.; Bermejo-Pareja, F.; Villarejo-Galende, A.; Molina, J.A.; Ortiz, P.; Calero, M.; Rabano, A.; Cantero, J.L.; Orive, G. Early diagnosis of mild cognitive impairment and Alzheimer's disease based on salivary lactoferrin. *Alzheimers Dement. Amst. Neth.* **2017**, *8*, 131–138. [CrossRef]
40. Kalló, G.; Emri, M.; Varga, Z.; Ujhelyi, B.; Tőzsér, J.; Csutak, A.; Csősz, É. Changes in the Chemical Barrier Composition of Tears in Alzheimer's Disease Reveal Potential Tear Diagnostic Biomarkers. *PLoS ONE* **2016**, *11*, e0158000. [CrossRef]
41. Shim, S.-M.; Cheon, H.-S.; Jo, C.; Koh, Y.H.; Song, J.; Jeon, J.-P. Elevated Epstein-Barr Virus Antibody Level is Associated with Cognitive Decline in the Korean Elderly. *J. Alzheimers Dis.* **2017**, *55*, 293–301. [CrossRef] [PubMed]
42. Yamamoto, H.; Watanabe, T.; Miyazaki, A.; Katagiri, T.; Idei, T.; Iguchi, T.; Mimura, M.; Kamijima, K. High Prevalence of Chlamydia Pneumoniae Antibodies and Increased High-Sensitive C-Reactive Protein in Patients with Vascular Dementia. *J. Am. Geriatr. Soc.* **2005**, *53*, 583–589. [CrossRef] [PubMed]
43. Lövheim, H.; Gilthorpe, J.; Johansson, A.; Eriksson, S.; Hallmans, G.; Elgh, F. Herpes simplex infection and the risk of Alzheimer's disease: A nested case-control study. *Alzheimers Dement.* **2015**, *11*, 587–592. [CrossRef] [PubMed]
44. Lövheim, H.; Gilthorpe, J.; Adolfsson, R.; Nilsson, L.-G.; Elgh, F. Reactivated herpes simplex infection increases the risk of Alzheimer's disease. *Alzheimers Dement.* **2015**, *11*, 593–599. [CrossRef] [PubMed]
45. Alonso, R.; Pisa, D.; Rábano, A.; Rodal, I.; Carrasco, L. Cerebrospinal Fluid from Alzheimer's Disease Patients Contains Fungal Proteins and DNA. *J. Alzheimers Dis.* **2015**, *47*, 873–876. [CrossRef]
46. Roy Sarkar, S.; Banerjee, S. Gut microbiota in neurodegenerative disorders. *J. Neuroimmunol.* **2019**, *328*, 98–104. [CrossRef]
47. Tzeng, N.-S.; Chung, C.-H.; Lin, F.-H.; Chiang, C.-P.; Yeh, C.-B.; Huang, S.-Y.; Lu, R.-B.; Chang, H.-A.; Kao, Y.-C.; Yeh, H.-W.; et al. Anti-herpetic Medications and Reduced Risk of Dementia in Patients with Herpes Simplex Virus Infections—A Nationwide, Population-Based Cohort Study in Taiwan. *Neurotherapeutics* **2018**, *15*, 417–429. [CrossRef]
48. Devanand, D.P.; Andrews, H.; Kreisl, W.C.; Razlighi, Q.; Gershon, A.; Stern, Y.; Mintz, A.; Wisniewski, T.; Acosta, E.; Pollina, J.; et al. Antiviral therapy: Valacyclovir Treatment of Alzheimer's Disease (VALAD) Trial: Protocol for a randomised, double-blind, placebo-controlled, treatment trial. *BMJ Open* **2020**, *10*, e032112. [CrossRef]
49. Roy, E.R.; Wang, B.; Wan, Y.; Chiu, G.; Cole, A.; Yin, Z.; Propson, N.E.; Xu, Y.; Jankowsky, J.L.; Liu, Z.; et al. Type I interferon response drives neuroinflammation and synapse loss in Alzheimer disease. *J. Clin. Investig.* **2020**, *130*, 1912–1930. [CrossRef]

9

Presenilin-2 and Calcium Handling: Molecules, Organelles, Cells and Brain Networks

Paola Pizzo [1,2,*], Emy Basso [1,2], Riccardo Filadi [1,2], Elisa Greotti [1,2], Alessandro Leparulo [1], Diana Pendin [1,2], Nelly Redolfi [1], Michela Rossini [1], Nicola Vajente [1,2], Tullio Pozzan [1,2,3] and Cristina Fasolato [1,*]

1 Department of Biomedical Sciences, University of Padua, Via U. Bassi 58/B, 35131 Padua, Italy; emy.basso@cnr.it (E.B.); riccardo.filadi@unipd.it (R.F.); elisa.greotti@cnr.it (E.G.); alessandro.leparulo@unipd.it (A.L.); diana.pendin@unipd.it (D.P.); nelly.redolfi@unipd.it (N.R.); michela.rossini@studenti.unipd.it (M.R.); nicola.vajente@studenti.unipd.it (N.V.); tullio.pozzan@unipd.it (T.P.)
2 Neuroscience Institute, Italian National Research Council (CNR), Via U. Bassi 58/B, 35131 Padua, Italy
3 Venetian Institute of Molecular Medicine (VIMM), Via G. Orus 2B, 35131 Padua, Italy
* Correspondence: paola.pizzo@unipd.it (P.P.); cristina.fasolato@unipd.it (C.F.)

Abstract: Presenilin-2 (PS2) is one of the three proteins that are dominantly mutated in familial Alzheimer's disease (FAD). It forms the catalytic core of the γ-secretase complex—a function shared with its homolog presenilin-1 (PS1)—the enzyme ultimately responsible of amyloid-β (Aβ) formation. Besides its enzymatic activity, PS2 is a multifunctional protein, being specifically involved, independently of γ-secretase activity, in the modulation of several cellular processes, such as Ca^{2+} signalling, mitochondrial function, inter-organelle communication, and autophagy. As for the former, evidence has accumulated that supports the involvement of PS2 at different levels, ranging from organelle Ca^{2+} handling to Ca^{2+} entry through plasma membrane channels. Thus FAD-linked PS2 mutations impact on multiple aspects of cell and tissue physiology, including bioenergetics and brain network excitability. In this contribution, we summarize the main findings on PS2, primarily as a modulator of Ca^{2+} homeostasis, with particular emphasis on the role of its mutations in the pathogenesis of FAD. Identification of cell pathways and molecules that are specifically targeted by PS2 mutants, as well as of common targets shared with PS1 mutants, will be fundamental to disentangle the complexity of memory loss and brain degeneration that occurs in Alzheimer's disease (AD).

Keywords: presenilin-2; calcium signalling; Alzheimer's disease mouse models; SOCE; mitochondria; autophagy; brain networks; oscillations; slow-waves; functional connectivity

1. Presenilin-2 in Physiology and Pathology

Presenilin-2 (PS2)—and its homolog presenilin-1 (PS1)—is a 50-kDa multi-pass membrane protein with nine helical transmembrane (TM) domains, and in humans it is encoded by a gene present on chromosome 1 (*PSEN2*) [1]. Both presenilins (PSs) mainly localize to the endoplasmic reticulum (ER) and Golgi apparatus (GA) membranes but also, although less abundantly, in plasma membrane (PM) and endosomes [2]. Their mRNAs are expressed in different human and mouse tissues, with the highest levels in the hippocampus and cerebellum [3].

Both PSs represent the catalytic core of the γ-secretase complex, the enzyme ultimately responsible for generation of Aβ peptides; they were both discovered in genetic analyses of families in which Alzheimer's disease (AD) is transmitted as an autosomal dominant trait. In fact, as of now, about 300 mutations in *PSEN1* and 58 mutations in *PSEN2* have been described (https://www.alzforum.org/mutations), the majority of which are dominant, mostly missense, and have been associated with the inherited forms of the disease (familial Alzheimer's disease (FAD)) [4,5]. Mutations in the gene for one of the substrate of the γ-secretase complex, the amyloid precursor protein (APP), are also responsible for FAD cases [6]. It has been proposed that FAD-PS mutations lead to a less precise γ-secretase cleavage of APP, in some cases decreasing the total production of Aβ but increasing the relative amount of the more amyloidogenic Aβ42 peptide, the seeding core of extracellular amyloid plaques, over the more soluble Aβ40 peptide [7,8].

The γ-secretase complex is part of the family of intramembrane-cleaving proteases (I-CliPs), which perform hydrolysis of protein domains embedded in the hydrophobic environment of the membrane. The family includes SP2 metalloproteases, serine proteases of the rhomboid family, and the aspartyl proteases to which γ-secretase belongs.

The γ-secretase has a central role in cellular biology, with about 150 different integral membrane proteins recognized as substrates [9]; the most studied are the Notch family of receptors, with a crucial role in signalling and cell differentiation, and APP [4,9]. The γ-secretase complex is composed of four subunits: PS1 or PS2; nicastrin, an integral membrane protein concerned with substrate recognition and selection [10]; PS enhancer-2 (PEN-2) that stabilizes the PS complex and has a role in its endoproteolytic cleavage [11–13]; and anterior pharynx defective 1 (APH1), which interacts with nicastrin, providing the initial scaffold to which PS1/2 and PEN-2 are added [14,15]. In humans, APH1 is encoded by two paralogous genes (APH1A and APH1B), and each protein can interact with either PS, resulting in the existence of four different γ-secretase complexes that might have slightly different specificities [16]. After its enclosure within the complex, PS undergoes an endoproteolytic cleavage that produces N- and C-terminal fragments; the two fragments remain associated and represent the biologically active form of the complex, each carrying one of the two key aspartic acid residues on TM6 and TM7, respectively [17,18].

PS1 and PS2 share about 66% of amino acidic sequence; one key difference is a motif in PS2 that interacts with activating protein-1 (AP-1) complexes in a phosphorylation-dependent manner and targets PS2 to the late endosome/lysosome compartment, leading to a different subcellular distribution of PS2 and perhaps to subtly different functions [19,20]. For example, it has been demonstrated that PS2-containing γ-secretase complexes are involved in the processing of premelanosome (PMEL) protein, which is involved in melanosome maturation and melanin deposition [19]. Indeed, PS2-null zebrafish showed defects in skin pigmentation [21]. Importantly, melanosome biogenesis seems to be Ca^{2+}-dependent [22] (see also below).

Several γ-secretase-independent functions of PSs have emerged in the recent years, enriching the overall importance of these proteins in cell biology. For example, PSs bind to glycogen synthase kinase 3β (GSK3β), a key protein of the Wnt signalling pathway, and to its substrate β-catenin, a transcription regulator [23,24]. The interaction of PSs with GSK3β and β-catenin is independent of γ-secretase activity [25] and influences β-catenin phosphorylation and turnover [26], as well as the activity of kinesin-1 and dynein and thus axonal transport of type 1 transmembrane receptors [27]. PSs have been implicated also in autophagy (see below) and protein trafficking [28].

Last, but not least, the regulation of cellular Ca^{2+} homeostasis has emerged as a key PS function, independent of γ-secretase activity, with relevant implications in multiple Ca^{2+}-regulated cell processes. In the present review, we summarize the central role played by PS2 in cellular Ca^{2+} homeostasis, highlighting divergent and convergent aspects of PS2 vs. PS1 pathophysiology.

2. PS2 and Ca^{2+} Homeostasis

2.1. Alterations of Ca^{2+} Homeostasis in FAD-PS2 Cell Models

According to the so-called "Ca^{2+} overload" hypothesis for AD, FAD-PS mutations increase the ER Ca^{2+} content and cause excessive cytosolic Ca^{2+} release upon cell stimulations that, in turn, alters APP processing and sensitizes neurons to Ca^{2+}-dependent cell death mechanisms [29]. Indeed, an excessive release of Ca^{2+} from the ER has been reported in different cell models expressing various FAD-PS mutations, as well as in neurons from transgenic (Tg) mice carrying FAD-PS1 mutations [30–35]. FAD-linked mutations in PS2 have also been reported to potentiate ER Ca^{2+} release from both ryanodine receptors (RyRs) [36] and inositol trisphosphate (IP3) receptors (IP3Rs) in *Xenopus* oocytes [30] and neurons from Tg mice expressing the PS2-N141I mutation [37]. Moreover, it has been proposed that wild type (WT) PSs form constitutively active ER Ca^{2+} leak channels whereas FAD-PS mutations disrupt the channel functionality; as a result of the reduced leak, the ER Ca^{2+} level increases and more Ca^{2+} is released upon stimulation [38].

In contrast, we showed that FAD patient-derived fibroblasts carrying the PS2-M239I mutation, as well as HeLa and HEK293 cells stably or transiently expressing the same PS2 mutant, show a decreased ER Ca^{2+} release when stimulated by IP3-generating agonists [39] (Figure 1); this result was confirmed in FAD patient-derived fibroblasts carrying another PS2 mutation (T122R) [40]. Of note, in this study, we analysed two monozygotic twins, one with overt signs of disease at the time of biopsy, whereas the other one was still asymptomatic; nevertheless, both cell samples shared a similar Ca^{2+} handling defect, strongly suggesting that Ca^{2+} dysregulation represents an early event in the pathogenesis of AD [40].

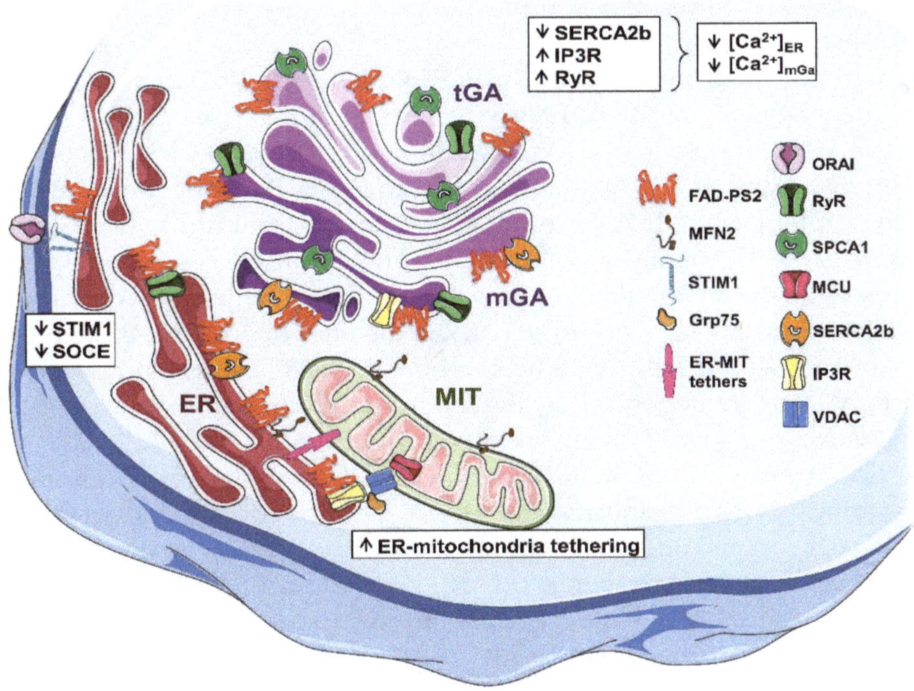

Figure 1. Familial Alzheimer's disease (FAD)-presenilin-2 (PS2) alters multiple Ca^{2+} signalling pathways. The cartoon represents different intracellular membrane localizations of FAD-PS2, its interactions with several components of the molecular Ca^{2+} toolkit, and multiple Ca^{2+} signalling pathways that are altered by its action. See text for details. ER, endoplasmic reticulum; mGA, medial-Golgi apparatus; tGA, trans-Golgi apparatus; MIT, mitochondrion.

To clarify the divergent results, we directly monitored Ca^{2+} dynamics within intracellular stores. We employed aequorin-based Ca^{2+} probes targeted to ER and GA in cells expressing different PS1 and PS2 mutants. In several cell lines [SH-SY5Y, HeLa, HEK293 and Mouse Embryonic Fibroblast (MEF) cells], expressing the ER (or GA)-targeted aequorin together with a number of PS1 (P117L, M146L, L286V, and A246E) or PS2 (M239I, T122R, and N141I) mutants, we analysed Ca^{2+} concentrations and dynamics in the two organelles. By this more specific approach, we confirmed lower ER and GA Ca^{2+} levels in the presence of all the analysed FAD-PS2 mutants, and unchanged or slightly decreased ER/GA Ca^{2+} concentrations when PS1 mutants were expressed [41]. Similar results were obtained in FAD patient-derived fibroblasts and rat primary neurons, expressing either PS1 or PS2 mutants and loaded with the Ca^{2+} sensor fura-2, confirming the capability of PS to modify Ca^{2+} homeostasis, but questioning the "Ca^{2+} overload" hypothesis for AD [41,42]. Indeed, it was also shown that FAD-PS are associated with IP3R hyperactivity [43,44], providing an alternative explanation to the "Ca^{2+} overload" hypothesis based on increased ER Ca^{2+} release findings previously reported in FAD-PS-expressing cells. In particular, Foskett and co-workers showed that FAD-PS1/2 mutants, by physically interacting with the IP3R, modulate the channel gating, causing an exaggerated ER Ca^{2+} release regardless of its Ca^{2+} content [43,44]. Furthermore, by employing ER- and GA-targeted Ca^{2+} indicators, the same group subsequently confirmed that cells expressing FAD-PS1 mutants do not present ER Ca^{2+} overload, arguing against the previously proposed role of PS as ER Ca^{2+} leak channels [45].

Similarly, by using newly developed genetically encoded Ca^{2+} indicators, the Förster resonance energy transfer (FRET)-based probe targeted to ER (D4ER [46]), medial-GA [47], and trans-GA [48], we showed that (i) in SH-SY5Y and Baby Hamster Kidney (BHK) cells, expressing the FAD-PS2-T122R mutant, and in PS2-N141I patient-derived fibroblasts, there is a clear reduction in ER Ca^{2+} concentration; (ii) in cells expressing the FAD-PS1-A246E mutant, instead, no change was observed [46,49]; (iii) the expression of FAD-PS2 mutants induced a selective decrease in the medial-GA Ca^{2+} content, but not in that of the trans-GA; (iv) in contrast, the expression of the FAD-PS1 mutant was ineffective on both GA sub-compartments [49] (Figure 1).

Concerning the molecular mechanism through which FAD-PS2 alters intracellular Ca^{2+} store dynamics, researchers have shown that the Ca^{2+} phenotype is caused by the holoprotein and that it is independent of γ-secretase activity [38,39,42,44,49–51]. Moreover, it has been shown that the protein directly interacts with the IP3R, sensitizing it to lower IP3 concentrations [43], the RyR [36], the RyR-regulating protein sorcin [52], and the SERCA2b [34], inhibiting its activity [51]. This latter result is consistent with the differential effect of FAD-PS2 mutants on GA sub-compartments (see above), given that the trans-GA, where FAD-PS2 mutants are ineffective, relies only on the secretory pathway Ca^{2+} ATPase 1 (SPCA1) for Ca^{2+} uptake [48]. Finally, in the presence of FAD-PS1/2 mutations, increased expression levels and activity of RyRs have been reported [53–55], suggesting a RyR-dependent Ca^{2+} hyperexcitability in AD that is antagonized by the channel inhibitor dantrolene (see [56] for an extensive discussion of this issue; see also [57] for the involvement of IP3Rs).

Intracellular Ca^{2+} stores, mainly the ER, are functionally and physically coupled to mitochondria with which they jointly operate modulating several cell functionalities, such as lipid synthesis and Ca^{2+} homeostasis. Specific ER membrane domains tightly juxtaposed to mitochondria, called mitochondria-associated membranes (MAM; [58]), represent signalling platforms and play a key role in these processes [59]. Interestingly, MAM appear to be altered in AD samples [42,54,59–64]; in addition PS1/2, as well as the other components of the γ-secretase complex and APP, are enriched in these domains [63,65,66]. Only FAD-PS2 mutants, however, are able to increase the interaction between the two organelles, facilitating ER–mitochondria Ca^{2+} transfer [42,54,63] by binding to mitofusin-2 [63] and thus removing its negative modulation on organelle tethering [67] (Figure 1).

The other Ca^{2+} signalling pathway affected by FAD-PS2 is the store-operated Ca^{2+} entry (SOCE) [68,69]. In particular, it has been shown that several FAD-PS2 mutants reduce SOCE activity in different cell types [40,41,49,70]. Interestingly, this effect is shared with FAD-PS1 mutants, which similarly reduce this Ca^{2+} influx [41,49,70,71] (Figure 1). Accordingly, SOCE is potentiated in cells where PS levels are reduced [70,72]. In PS double knock out (KO) MEFs and in B-lymphocytes derived from patients expressing FAD-PS mutants [73], researchers have found that the levels of the key SOCE components Stromal interaction molecule (STIM) STIM1 and STIM2 [68,69] are reduced. Of note, alterations in SOCE and STIM1 protein level have also been reported in sporadic AD (SAD) patients [74]. It has been proposed that SOCE is regulated by a γ-secretase-dependent mechanism, with STIM1 being a substrate of PS1-containing γ-secretase complexes [71]. Nevertheless, we found lower SOCE and STIM1 protein levels in both FAD-PS1- and FAD-PS2-expressing cells treated with the γ-secretase inhibitor DAPT [49] (Figure 1).

Of note, the overexpression of WT-PS2 often mimics the effect of its FAD mutants on Ca^{2+} homeostasis, although higher levels of WT-PS2 are required to obtain the alterations in Ca^{2+} homeostasis elicited by FAD-PS2 mutants [40]. This latter finding could be relevant for SAD forms of the disease, where an upregulation of the endogenous PS2 has been reported in brain AD samples due to the loss of repressor element 1-silencing transcription factor (REST) [75]. It can be speculated that an abnormal accumulation of PS2 holoprotein could cause Ca^{2+} signalling dysregulation, also typically observed in SAD cases.

2.2. Calcium Handling in AD Mouse Models Expressing PS2-N141I

The findings reported above led us to investigate Ca^{2+} handling and brain network functionality in Tg mouse lines based on FAD-PS2 mutants by means of in vitro and in vivo approaches. We took advantage of two homozygous mouse lines expressing the PS2-N141I mutant, as described in detail in Box 1: the double Tg line B6.152H, also known as B6.PS2APP, and the single Tg line PS2.30H [76]. Here, we simply refer to these two lines as 2TG and TG, respectively.

We were firstly interested to verify whether the same Ca^{2+} changes found in FAD-PS2-expressing cell lines were also detectable in primary neuronal cultures and in acute hippocampal slices from 2-week-old animals. At this age, total brain Aβ levels in 2TG mice are still very low, but are already detectable and higher when compared to WT and TG mice [54]. Both TG and 2TG neurons, in culture or in situ, show a reduction in the ER Ca^{2+} content, when estimated indirectly, through Ca^{2+} release induced by IP3-generating agonists, or directly, with the Cameleon probe D4ER [46,54].

In acute hippocampal slices, upon stimulation with IP3-generating agonists, Ca^{2+} release was dramatically reduced not only in neurons but also in astrocytes of TG and 2TG mice, suggesting defective store Ca^{2+} content, as well as Ca^{2+} entry, in these latter cell types [54]. Importantly, these changes occur precociously and independently of APP overexpression and brain Aβ load, being found equally in TG and 2TG mice; thus, they reflect the intrinsic capability of modulating Ca^{2+} handling of FAD-PS2 mutants.

Studying neurons in vitro and in situ allowed us to also highlight relevant network properties brought about by the PS2 mutant. In both conditions, neuronal cells, when exposed to picrotoxin, a γ-aminobutyric acid (GABA)-A receptor antagonist, showed synchronous Ca^{2+} spiking activity that was higher in TG and 2TG mice with respect to WT [54]. This type of Ca^{2+} spiking is independent of Ca^{2+} stores and likely due to an imbalance between excitatory and inhibitory inputs that represent an early sign of network dysfunction [77,78].

3. Functional Effects of Ca^{2+} Dysregulation by FAD-PS2

3.1. Autophagy

Macroautophagy (hereafter autophagy) is a process in which double-membrane vesicles (called autophagosomes) engulf different cellular components (including misfolded proteins, portions of cytosol, and damaged organelles) and target them to lysosomes, where they are degraded into simpler molecular constituents.

In 2004, two seminal papers firstly suggested that PSs might be involved in autophagy modulation [79,80]. Specifically, Esselens and co-workers reported telencephalin accumulation within autophagosomes in PS1-KO hippocampal neurons as a result of a defective fusion of these vesicles with lysosomes. Similarly, Wilson and colleagues observed that PS1 deficiency, in fibroblasts and primary cortical neurons, resulted in the formation of enlarged lysosomes, with accumulation of α- and β-synuclein. Importantly, this phenomenon was likely associated with SOCE augmentation, suggesting that altered Ca^{2+} signalling may underpin the effect of PSs on the autophagy pathway [79]. Additional investigations, mostly focused on PS1, consistently reported that PSs modulate autophagosome-lysosome fusion. Nevertheless, consensus has not been reached on the underlying mechanism. Indeed, either a defective lysosomal acidification [81], a reduced lysosomal Ca^{2+} content [82], or altered expression of key genes belonging to the coordinated lysosomal expression and regulation (CLEAR) network [83,84] have been suggested as possible mechanisms (reviewed in [85]).

As far as FAD-PS mutants are concerned, some of the discrepancies might be linked to mutation-specific effects. Nevertheless, most studies converge on the lack of involvement of the γ-secretase activity, whereas Ca^{2+} signalling dysregulation has been frequently reported as a common feature among different FAD-PS mutants [85]. Recently, we observed that the reduced ER Ca^{2+} content, consistently observed in different FAD-PS2 cell models, affects the fusion of autophagosomes with lysosomes, thus inducing autophagosome accumulation [86] (Figure 2). Specifically, the phenomenon appears linked to the generation of lower cytosolic Ca^{2+} rises upon IP3-induced release of ER Ca^{2+}, given that it can be mimicked by increasing the cytosolic Ca^{2+}-buffering capacity (loading cells with the permeable forms of Ca^{2+} chelating agents). Mechanistically, we found that alterations of cytosolic Ca^{2+} dynamics affect the recruitment to autophagosomes of Ras-associated binding protein RAB7, a small GTPase whose association with both autophagosomes and lysosomes tunes their fusion in the final steps of the autophagy pathway [87]. Importantly, at variance with previous studies focused on FAD-PS1 [81,82,88], neither the pH of lysosomes nor their Ca^{2+} content were found to be affected by FAD-PS2 mutants [86]. Taken together these observations suggest that slightly different mechanisms might underlie the effects of FAD-PS1 and FAD-PS2 on the autophagy flux, with an altered Ca^{2+} signalling (though by distinct pathways) being a common feature.

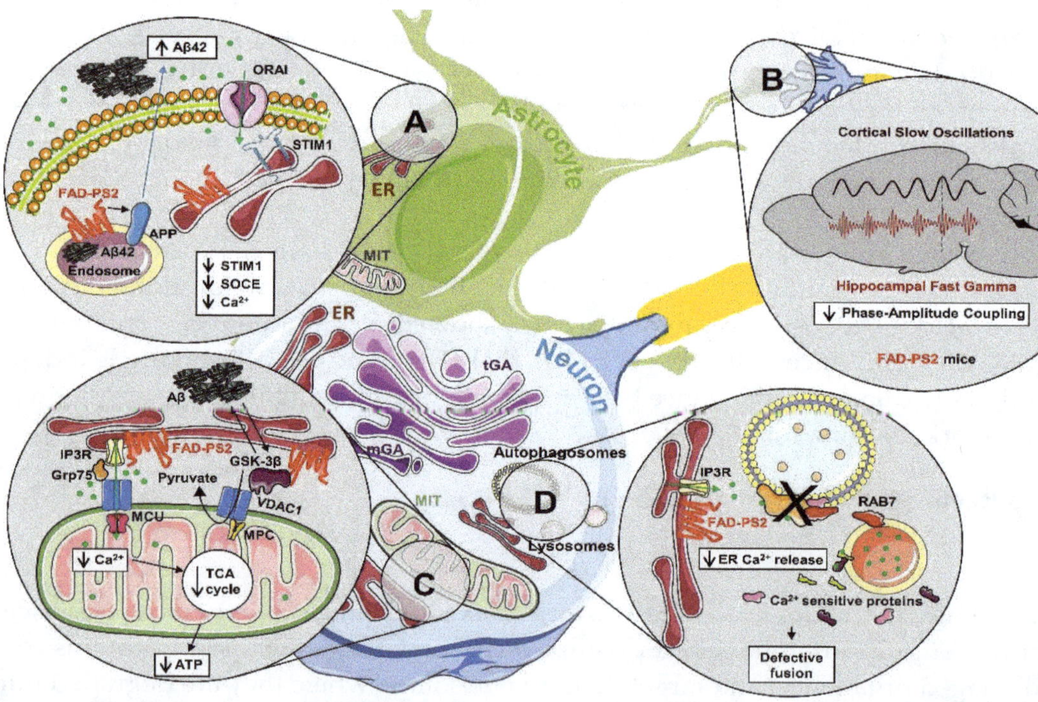

Figure 2. Functional consequences of dysregulated Ca^{2+} signalling induced by FAD-PS2. The cartoon represents the major dysfunctions linked to the expression of FAD-PS2 mutants at both the cellular and brain network levels. (**A**) Decreased store-operated Ca^{2+} entry (SOCE) potentiates amyloid precursor protein (APP) processing and Aβ42 production. (**B**) FAD-PS2-N141I-based mice show altered neuronal circuits (decreased phase-amplitude coupling between cortical slow oscillations and hippocampal fast gamma frequencies). (**C**) Decreased mitochondrial Ca^{2+} signalling and pyruvate uptake impair mitochondrial metabolism and cell bioenergetics. (**D**) Reduced endoplasmic reticulum (ER) Ca^{2+} release blocks the recruitment to autophagosomes of the Ras-associated binding protein RAB7 and their subsequent fusion with lysosomes. See text for details.

3.2. Cell Metabolism and Bioenergetics

The first piece of evidence that WT-PS2 modulates mitochondrial metabolism was found in 2006, when lower mitochondrial respiration and decreased mitochondrial membrane potential ($\Delta\psi m$) were observed in *PSEN2*$^{-/-}$, but not in *PSEN1*$^{-/-}$ MEFs [89]. Later, similar results were obtained by Contino and co-investigators [90], who found reduced basal and maximal mitochondrial oxygen consumption in *PSEN2*$^{-/-}$ and PS double KO MEFs (but not in *PSEN1*$^{-/-}$ MEFs), associated with an altered morphology of the mitochondrial cristae and a dampened expression of different subunits of the mitochondrial respiratory chain. Interestingly, in both studies, the ATP/ADP ratio was not significantly altered by *PSEN2* ablation, likely because of a compensatory upregulation of the glycolytic flux [90]. Recently, we obtained data suggesting that, in primary cortical neurons from PS2$^{-/-}$ mice (see Box 1), reduced mitochondrial respiration is associated with a defective mitochondrial Ca^{2+} signal (Rossi et al., in preparation). This finding suggests that the Ca^{2+}-mediated modulation of mitochondrial metabolism has a key role in the effects reported above [91].

It is well established that mitochondrial activity is critical for brain health—not only is the majority of neuronal ATP synthesized by mitochondria, but also the rate of ATP synthesis matches synaptic activity [92]. Therefore, the effects of FAD-PS on mitochondria metabolism might be relevant to FAD pathogenesis.

Alterations of mitochondrial activity have been reported in different AD models, mostly in Tg mouse models harboring FAD-PS1 and FAD-APP mutations. However, consensus has not been reached on the underlying molecular mechanisms. Indeed, either defective assembly/expression/activity of different subunits of the mitochondrial respiratory chain [93], altered mitochondrial Ca^{2+} signals [94,95], or organelle positioning/transport [96] have been suggested to contribute to the observed alterations. In contrast, only a few studies have focused on FAD-PS2 mutants. In primary cortical neurons from 2TG mice (see Box 1), we observed a reduced mitochondrial respiratory capacity [97]. This defect is not due to any intrinsic alteration of the respiratory chain, but rather depends on an impaired glycolytic flux, in turn affecting nutrient supply to mitochondria and thus organelle metabolism. However, considering that 2TG mice also express the FAD-APP mutant, it is not clear to what extent FAD-PS2 contributes to this phenotype. Recently, however, in different FAD-PS2-expressing cells, we observed a lower mitochondrial activity associated with a reduced ATP synthesis [98]. Mechanistically, these alterations depend in part on reduced mitochondrial Ca^{2+} signalling (due to partial depletion of ER Ca^{2+} content; see above), and in part on defective mitochondrial pyruvate uptake, caused by alterations in a signalling pathway driven by hyperactive GSK3β [98] (Figure 2), a feature commonly reported in AD [99]. Importantly, when compared to WT, in primary cortical neurons from TG mice (see Box 1), basal ATP levels are not significantly affected, whereas a faster ATP decrease is observed in cells exposed to ATP-consuming stimuli. In addition, we found that these metabolic alterations are associated with an increased susceptibility of FAD-PS2-N141I neurons to excitotoxicity induced by glutamate at physiological concentrations [98]. Overall, these results suggest that subtle mitochondrial alterations may be tolerated for a long time until specific stress conditions, imposing a high energy-demand, unveil their pathological potential. This might be relevant in neurological disorders characterized by a late onset, such as AD.

3.3. Brain Network Activity

Ca^{2+} dysregulation and altered APP processing, the two major hits linked to PS2-N141I expression, could affect neural circuit dynamics during the progression of amyloidosis. By studying brain oscillatory activity of adult 2TG mice under anesthesia, we observed that these mice develop a condition of hippocampal hyperactivity, with increased power in the gamma frequency range (45–90 Hz), as measured by spontaneous local field potential (LFP) signals. Curiously, age-matched TG mice also show a similar increase in the gamma power [100]. This hyperactivity is thus independent of Aβ production given that TG mice, unlike the 2TG animals, show neither plaque deposition nor gliosis, and Aβ42 levels are not significantly different from those found in WT mice [100]. This also suggests that, in 2TG mice, network hyperactivity is not due to compensatory, protective mechanisms and likely exerts a pathogenic role in the disease [78]. Of note, in humans, mild cognitive impairment (MCI) is marked by hyperactivity in the hippocampus, as well as in other cortical regions, that disappears with overt AD [101]. 2TG mice also present hyper-synchronicity, which is detectable as early as 3 months of age [100]. This aspect is likely attributable to the early phase of Aβ accumulation and represents a common feature in AD, often in the form of silent seizures, especially in FAD cases that show a higher incidence of epilepsy [102–104].

Studies on the brain electrical activity of both AD patients and mouse models have recently been focused on slow oscillations, which are directly involved in memory consolidation during sleep and unconsciousness [105]. By detecting mesoscale Ca^{2+} signals at the mouse brain level, Busche and coworkers elegantly demonstrated that functional connectivity in the slow-wave range (0.1–3 Hz) is severely reduced in the neocortex, thalamus, and hippocampus of different AD mouse models, also on the basis of PS1 [106]. Interestingly, slow-wave manipulation restores the functionality of brain circuits, rescues neuronal Ca^{2+} [107], and enhances memory consolidation in both types of mice [106,107].

Given that PS2-N141I alters neuronal and astrocytic Ca^{2+} homeostasis, it might also disturb hippocampal and cortical oscillatory activity in the slow-wave range. In mice under anesthesia, the oscillatory activity of different brain depths can be measured by simultaneously recording LFP signals with a multi-site linear probe. We used this approach to study brain rhythmicity at the cortical and hippocampal levels. In both TG and 2TG mice, the total power, which mostly reflects spontaneous activity in the low frequency range (0.1–5 Hz), is reduced, particularly at the hippocampal level, suggesting that the PS2 mutant by itself alters the brain electrical activity [108].

Another interesting feature shared by both TG and 2TG mice is the disruption of cortico-hippocampal oscillation coupling (Figure 2, [108]). The phenomenon, also known as phase-amplitude coupling (PAC), occurs when the phase of slower rhythms influences the amplitude of faster ones, and it has been found to be involved in memory consolidation and information transfer [105,109].

Unique features of 2TG mice help to mark the progression of Aβ accumulation and deposition—loss of functional connectivity in the slow-wave range marks the onset of Aβ accumulation, similarly to what reported in PS1-based AD mice [106], whereas low/high power imbalances characterize Aβ deposition in plaque-seeding mice [108]. Since Aβ42 oligomers are associated with Ca^{2+} homeostasis dysregulation [110–113], it is tempting to speculate that, in 2TG mice, Ca^{2+} handling alterations, due to PS2-N141I, sum up or synergize with defects linked to Aβ accumulation.

4. Concluding Remarks and Possible Therapeutic Targets

At the brain circuit level, the FAD-linked PS2-N141I mutant increases excitability [54,100] and disrupts the coupling of cortical slow-waves to hippocampal fast gamma frequencies [108]. Altogether, these findings are consistent with the high frequency of seizures and behavioral changes found in both FAD-PS2-N141I patients [1] and other mouse models expressing PS2-N141I [114,115]. From an pathogenic point of view, major alterations are expected in subpopulations of fast spiking interneurons that control the excitability of neuronal microcircuits, as reported in AD mouse models [103,116–118]. These highly active cells are likely more susceptible to the metabolic failure brought about by the aforementioned defective mitochondrial function [97,98]. One should also consider that, in these mouse models, only the PS2 mutant is expressed in both neurons and glial cells. In particular, astrocytes are good candidates to explain circuit dysfunctions given that, through spontaneous Ca^{2+} oscillations and intercellular Ca^{2+} waves, they can control the excitability of large neuronal networks [119,120], as well as modulate neighboring neurons by glio-transmission [121,122]. Furthermore, Ca^{2+} dysregulation and metabolic impairment in a cell type can also affect the closest cells, thus necessitating their investigation at the in situ and in vivo level.

It can be speculated that defects in metabolic and autophagic pathways, directly dependent on Ca^{2+} dysregulation (see above), are responsible for the described network hyperexcitability and excitation/inhibition imbalances, which has also been reported in other AD models [77,103,123].

As for Ca^{2+} dysregulation, a common denominator between FAD-PS1 and -PS2 mutations is SOCE. Nevertheless, up until now, only a few studies have addressed the role of this Ca^{2+} pathway in neurons, mainly because of technical problems, i.e., the difficulty of distinguishing between activation of SOCE and voltage-operated Ca^{2+} channels (VOCCs) [124,125]. Recently, STIM2 and ORAI2, two key players in SOCE machinery, have emerged as key components of neuronal SOCE, being implicated in SOCE impairment in mushroom spines of hippocampal neurons from FAD-PS1-M146V knock-in mice [126–128]. Although the role of SOCE in neurons is still unclear, it is important to stress that, in excitable cells, STIM and ORAI components might also play non-canonical roles—STIM1 binds to L-type VOCCs, inhibits their gating, and induces channel internalization [129,130] while ORAI1 increases neuronal excitability [131,132]. At variance with neuronal cells, it is now largely accepted that SOCE is crucial for the Ca^{2+}-based excitability that characterizes glial cells both in vitro [133,134] and in vivo [135]. Nonetheless, studies that specifically address the role of FAD-PS2 in glial SOCE modulation are still lacking. Considering also the complexity of microglia involvement in the onset and progression of AD [113,136], it is conceivable that these cells might also be primarily affected in the SOCE pathway, given that PS2 is the major core component of γ-secretase complexes expressed in this cell type [137].

We have recently shown that there is an inverse relationship between SOCE level and Aβ42 accumulation [138], consistent with data obtained in neurons [70] and other model cells [139]. These observations suggest the possibility of rescuing the SOCE defect in neural cells while antagonizing Aβ42 production. It has been demonstrated that, in mouse lymphocytes, SOCE is increased by knockout of ORAI2, a channel subunit and a negative modulator of SOCE that is responsible for the Ca^{2+} release-activated Ca^{2+} current [140]. In Aβ42-secreting neuroglioma cells, ORAI2 downregulation also increases SOCE and reduces the Aβ42/Aβ40 ratio [138] (Figure 2). Of note, astrocytes actively participate in Aβ production and clearance [141]. We do not know yet whether ORAI2 can play a similar role in neurons; up until now, it looks unlikely, given that recent data by Betzprozvanny's group favor the hypothesis that ORAI2 is a component of a specific type of neuronal SOCE that is based on transient receptor potential canonical 6 (TRPC6) channel and regulated by diacylglycerol [127]. What is clear is that investigating Ca^{2+} dysregulation in AD allows the design of alternative therapeutic approaches to this devastating disease.

Additional therapeutic approaches could be suggested on the basis of altered bioenergetic and autophagy pathways. Impaired mitochondria, unable to supply cellular ATP demand, cause alterations in neuronal excitability, eventually leading to Ca^{2+} overload and cell death [142]. Moreover, the accumulation of damaged mitochondria (and misfolded proteins), due to defective autophagy, further contributes to dysfunctional neurons, causing, over the long term, neurodegeneration. Indeed, mitochondrial alterations, and in particular defects in bioenergetic pathways, have been widely reported to be key factors not only in AD but also in other neurodegenerative diseases [142,143]. Importantly, bioenergetic alterations are reported in different SAD and FAD samples, appearing at the early stage of the disease, before Aβ plaque formation [144].

The bioenergetic state of neurons is a crucial determinant of their response to glutamate, with cells containing defective mitochondria undergoing bioenergetic crises, Ca^{2+} mishandling, and excitotoxicity. The Food and Drug Administration (FDA)-approved molecule memantine targets glutamate receptors and is among the few pharmacological treatments that provide modest benefits in AD patients, in addition to cholinesterase inhibitors [145]. Targeting Ca^{2+} defects, at multiple levels, was suggested as a possible therapeutic strategy, especially in the form of drug repurposing. Among the best candidates, there are dantrolene, a RyR modulator [146], and isradipine, a VOCC inhibitor, as reviewed by Chakraborty and Stutzmann [147]. Attention has to be payed to the fact that dihydropyridines, especially nimodipine, also increase Aβ42 secretion [148]. None of these drugs are in the pipeline yet, and thus additional interventions aiming at supporting other pathways, such as mitochondrial performance, are desirable. In line with this, we showed that GSK3β inhibition rescues the FAD-PS2-linked bioenergetic defect [98]. Interestingly, both PS and Aβ oligomers have been reported to interact with the kinase, favoring its activity [99]. Considering the fact that GSK3β activity has been observed at MAM [149], where PSs are also enriched and Aβ peptides are generated [63,65,66], a MAM-targeted intervention might represent a useful therapeutic strategy [98].

Finally, the impairment in mitochondrial bioenergetics described in AD models is likely linked to a metabolic rewiring, possibly resulting in systemic alterations in the concentration of specific metabolites. Thus, the detailed metabolic profiling of AD patient-derived peripheral samples (blood and cerebrospinal fluid) might offer the possibility to discover new biomarkers that are helpful for early AD diagnosis, as has been previously suggested [150,151].

5. Box 1: AD Mouse Models Based on PS2

Several mouse models have been developed to understand the pathogenesis of AD, however, none of them are capable of reproducing the full spectrum of the human disease. The large majority of the most used AD models are double-Tg mice based on human FAD-APP and -PS1 mutations, both required to obtain fast amyloid accumulation, plaque deposition, and gliosis between 2 and 8 months of age. These Tg mice are widely considered to be adequate models of Aβ amyloidosis and its inflammatory process; they allow us to study the initial stages of the disease, according to the vision that places Aβ toxicity among the first hits in the AD cascade [6,152,153]. Nonetheless, the latter appears necessary but not sufficient in terms of causing neurodegeneration, with other concomitant and downstream factors playing a key role [7]. Neurodegeneration, linked to tau aggregation, is in fact mainly present in 3xTg-AD mice, which host three human mutant genes encoding PS1, APP, and tau [154].

Curiously, only the PS2-N141I mutation has been used to generate AD mouse models based on *PSEN2*. In terms of the latter, we used two homozygous lines: the double Tg (2TG) B6.152H, also known as B6.PS2APP, and the single Tg (TG) PS2.30H [76]. The latter line expresses the human PS2-N141I under the *prion protein* promoter, with background C57Bl/6 > 90% [155]. The B6.152H line was instead obtained by co-injection of human *PSEN2*, carrying the N141I mutation—under the mouse *prion protein* promoter—and the human *APP* isoform 751, carrying the APP-KM670/671NL Swedish mutation—under the *Thy1.2* promoter—into zygotes of the C57Bl/6 strain (background C57Bl/6 100%) [76].

The PS2.30H line was originally used to obtain hemizygous PS2APP mice by crossing PS2.30H females with APP-Swedish males of the BD.AD147.71H line, with background C57Bl/6 > 90% [155]. Up to 12 months of age, TG mice show neither plaques nor Aβ accumulation in the brain [100]. The histopathological traits of PS2APP and B6.PS2APP are very similar, showing an exponential growth of Aβ accumulation and plaques at 3 and 6 months of age, respectively [76,155]. Plaque deposition starts in the frontal cortex, subiculum, and hippocampus; increases for up to 12–16 months of age; and correlates with the level of human APP transcript [76,155]. Behavioral deficits have only been characterized thoroughly in PS2APP mice, with spatial learning (Morris water maze) and memory defects appearing at 8 months [155]. Biochemical and functional differences between the two closely related models are also present [156,157]. In our studies, TG and 2TG mice are maintained and used in homozygosity, a condition that allows for the reduction of the variability of APP expression [76]. The two lines express PS2 at a similar level, about twice that found in C57Bl/6 WT mice, used as controls [54].

B6.152H mice have also been used in hemizygosity (B6.152) to study different aspects of the AD phenotype [158], or to generate TauPS2APP triple Tg mice, upon crossing the B6.152H line with the Tau-overexpressing pR5 line [159,160] that expresses the human tau-40 isoform under the *Thy1.2* promoter [161]. Of note, a PS2-/- mouse line has been obtained by neomycin insertion in the C57Bl/6 × 129Sv genetic background [162,163]. This line does not show alterations of the endogenous APP processing and it is useful in terms of studying the physiological role of PS2 and possible loss-of-function defects associated with PS2-N141I expression [100,108]. It was also used to produce

PSEN conditional double KO mice and study neurodegeneration and memory impairments due to PS deficiency [164].

Other AD mouse models, based on PS2-N141I, have been generated under different promoters and genetic backgrounds. Comparison of their histopathological, functional, and behavioral properties is beyond the scope of this review. The latest generation of AD mouse models avoids the overexpression of FAD mutations and is focused on risk genes, such as Triggering receptor expressed on myeloid cells 2 (*TREM2*) [165] and Apolipoprotein E4 (*APOE4*) [166]. More than 200 AD mouse models are now available; detailed information about these AD animal models is available at the Alzforum website (https://www.alzforum.org/). It is also necessary to mention that doubts have recently been raised on the use of Tg mice to study human AD, given that, at variance with the trascriptomic profiles of physiological human and rodent brain aging, which appear very similar, those of AD brains are largely different between humans and rodents, and even between different Tg AD mouse lines [167].

Author Contributions: Writing—original draft preparation, P.P., E.B., R.F., E.G., A.L., D.P., N.R., M.R., N.V., T.P., C.F. Review and editing P.P., T.P., C.F. All authors have read and agreed to the published version of the manuscript.

Acknowledgments: PS2.30H and B6.152H mouse lines used for the authors' research were kindly donated by L. Ozmen and F. Hoffmann-La Roche Ltd. (Basel, Switzerland).

References

1. Jayadev, S.; Leverenz, J.B.; Steinbart, E.; Stahl, J.; Klunk, W.; Yu, C.E.; Bird, T.D. Alzheimer's disease phenotypes and genotypes associated with mutations in presenilin 2. *Brain* **2010**, *133*, 1143–1154. [CrossRef] [PubMed]
2. Brunkan, A.L.; Goate, A.M. Presenilin function and gamma-secretase activity. *J. Neurochem.* **2005**, *93*, 769–792. [CrossRef] [PubMed]
3. Lee, M.K.; Slunt, H.H.; Martin, L.J.; Thinakaran, G.; Kim, G.; Gandy, S.E.; Seeger, M.; Koo, E.; Price, D.L.; Sisodia, S.S. Expression of presenilin 1 and 2 (PS1 and PS2) in human and murine tissues. *J. Neurosci.* **1996**, *16*, 7513–7525. [CrossRef] [PubMed]
4. Chévez-Gutiérrez, L.; Bammens, L.; Benilova, I.; Vandersteen, A.; Benurwar, M.; Borgers, M.; Lismont, S.; Zhou, L.; Van Cleynenbreugel, S.; Esselmann, H.; et al. The Mechanism of γ-Secretase Dysfunction in Familial Alzheimer Disease. *EMBO J.* **2012**, *31*, 2261–2274. [CrossRef]
5. Chávez-Gutiérrez, L.; Szaruga, M. Mechanisms of neurodegeneration-insights from familial alzheimer's disease. In *Seminars in Cell and Developmental Biology*; Elsevier Ltd.: Amsterdam, The Netherlands, 2020; pp. 75–85.
6. Selkoe, D.J.; Hardy, J. The amyloid hypothesis of alzheimer's disease at 25years. *EMBO Mol. Med.* **2016**, *8*, 595–608. [CrossRef]
7. Long, J.M.; Holtzman, D.M. Alzheimer disease: An update on pathobiology and treatment strategies. *Cell* **2019**, *179*, 312–339. [CrossRef]
8. Walker, E.S.; Martinez, M.; Brunkan, A.L.; Goate, A. Presenilin 2 familial alzheimer's disease mutations result in partial loss of function and dramatic changes in abeta 42/40 ratios. *J. Neurochem.* **2005**, *92*, 294–301. [CrossRef]
9. Güner, G.; Lichtenthaler, S.F. The substrate repertoire of γ-secretase/presenilin. In *Seminars in Cell and Developmental Biology*; Elsevier Ltd.: Amsterdam, The Netherlands, 2020; pp. 27–42.
10. Bolduc, D.M.; Montagna, D.R.; Gu, Y.; Selkoe, D.J.; Wolfe, M.S. Nicastrin functions to sterically hinder γ-secretase-substrate interactions driven by substrate transmembrane domain. *Proc. Natl. Acad. Sci. USA* **2016**, *113*, E509–E518. [CrossRef]
11. Holmes, O.; Paturi, S.; Selkoe, D.J.; Wolfe, M.S. Pen-2 is essential for γ-secretase complex stability and trafficking but partially dispensable for endoproteolysis. *Biochemistry* **2014**, *53*, 4393–4406. [CrossRef]
12. Kim, S.H.; Sisodia, S.S. Evidence that the "NF" motif in transmembrane domain 4 of presenilin 1 is critical for binding with PEN-2. *J. Biol. Chem.* **2005**, *280*, 41953–41996. [CrossRef]

13. Prokop, S.; Shirotani, K.; Edbauer, D.; Haass, C.; Steiner, H. Requirement of PEN-2 for stabilization of the presenilin n-/c-terminal fragment heterodimer within the γ-secretase complex. *J. Biol. Chem.* **2004**, *279*, 23255–23261. [CrossRef] [PubMed]
14. Pardossi-Piquard, R.; Yang, S.P.; Kanemoto, S.; Gu, Y.; Chen, F.; Böhm, C.; Sevalle, J.; Li, T.; Wong, P.C.; Checler, F.; et al. APH1 polar transmembrane residues regulate the assembly and activity of presenilin complexes. *J. Biol. Chem.* **2009**, *284*, 16298–16307. [CrossRef] [PubMed]
15. Gu, Y.; Chen, F.; Sanjo, N.; Kawarai, T.; Hasegawa, H.; Duthie, M.; Li, W.; Ruan, X.; Luthra, A.; Mount, H.T.; et al. APH-1 interacts with mature and immature forms of presenilins and nicastrin and may play a role in maturation of presenilin.nicastrin complexes. *J. Biol. Chem.* **2003**, *278*, 7374–7380. [CrossRef] [PubMed]
16. Serneels, L.; Van Biervliet, J.; Craessaerts, K.; Dejaegere, T.; Horré, K.; Van Houtvin, T.; Esselmann, H.; Paul, S.; Schäfer, M.K.; Berezovska, O.; et al. γ-Secretase heterogeneity in the aph1 subunit: Relevance for alzheimer's disease. *Science* **2009**, *324*, 629–632. [CrossRef] [PubMed]
17. Wolfe, M.S.; Xia, W.; Ostaszewski, B.L.; Diehl, T.S.; Kimberly, W.T.; Selkoe, D.J. Two transmembrane aspartates in presenilin-1 required for presenilin endoproteolysis and g-secretase activity. *Nature* **1999**, *398*, 513–517. [CrossRef]
18. Wolfe, M.S. Substrate recognition and processing by γ-secretase. *Biochim. Biophys. Acta Biomembr.* **2020**, *1862*, 183016. [CrossRef]
19. Sannerud, R.; Esselens, C.; Ejsmont, P.; Mattera, R.; Rochin, L.; Tharkeshwar, A.K.; De Baets, G.; De Wever, V.; Habets, R.; Baert, V.; et al. Restricted location of PSEN2/gamma-secretase determines substrate specificity and generates an intracellular abeta pool. *Cell* **2016**, *166*, 193–208. [CrossRef]
20. Meckler, X.; Checler, F. Presenilin 1 and presenilin 2 target gamma-secretase complexes to distinct cellular compartments. *J. Biol. Chem.* **2016**, *291*, 12821–12837. [CrossRef]
21. Jiang, H.; Newman, M.; Lardelli, M. The zebrafish orthologue of familial alzheimer's disease gene PRESENILIN 2 is required for normal adult melanotic skin pigmentation. *PLoS ONE* **2018**, *13*, e0206155. [CrossRef]
22. Zhang, Z.; Gong, J.; Sviderskaya, E.V.; Wei, A.; Li, W. Mitochondrial NCKX5 regulates melanosomal biogenesis and pigment production. *J. Cell Sci.* **2019**, *132*, jcs232009. [CrossRef]
23. Murayama, M.; Tanaka, S.; Palacino, J.; Murayama, O.; Honda, T.; Sun, X.; Yasutake, K.; Nihonmatsu, N.; Wolozin, B.; Takashima, A. Direct association of presenilin-1 with β-catenin. *FEBS Lett.* **1998**, *433*, 73–77. [CrossRef]
24. Zhang, Z.; Hartmann, H.; Do, V.M.; Abramowski, D.; Sturchler-Pierrat, C.; Staufenbiel, M.; Sommer, B.; Van De Wetering, M.; Clevers, H.; Saftig, P.; et al. Destabilization of β-Catenin by mutations in Presenilin-1 potentiates neuronal apoptosis. *Nature* **1998**, *395*, 698–702. [CrossRef]
25. Soriano, S.; Kang, D.E.; Fu, M.; Pestell, R.; Chevallier, N.; Zheng, H.; Koo, E.H. Presenilin 1 negatively regulates β-Catenin/T cell factor/Lymphoid enhancer factor-1 signaling independently of β-Amyloid precursor protein and notch processing. *J. Cell Biol.* **2001**, *52*, 785–794. [CrossRef] [PubMed]
26. Kang, D.E.; Soriano, S.; Frosch, M.P.; Collins, T.; Naruse, S.; Sisodia, S.S.; Leibowitz, G.; Levine, F.; Koo, E.H. Presenilin 1 facilitates the constitutive turnover of β-Catenin: Differential activity of alzheimer's disease-linked PS1 mutants in the β-catenin-signaling pathway. *J. Neurosci.* **1999**, *19*, 4229–4237. [CrossRef] [PubMed]
27. Dolma, K.; Iacobucci, G.J.; Hong Zheng, K.; Shandilya, J.; Toska, E.; White, J.A.; Spina, E.; Gunawardena, S. Presenilin influences glycogen synthase kinase-3 beta (GSK-3beta) for Kinesin-1 and dynein function during axonal transport. *Hum. Mol. Genet.* **2014**, *23*, 1121–1133. [CrossRef] [PubMed]
28. Barthet, G.; Dunys, J.; Shao, Z.; Xuan, Z.; Ren, Y.; Xu, J.; Arbez, N.; Mauger, G.; Bruban, J.; Georgakopoulos, A.; et al. Presenilin mediates neuroprotective functions of ephrinb and brain-derived neurotrophic factor and regulates ligand-induced internalization and metabolism of EphB2 and TrkB receptors. *Neurobiol. Aging* **2013**, *34*, 499–510. [CrossRef] [PubMed]
29. LaFerla, F.M. Calcium dyshomeostasis and intracellular signalling in alzheimer's disease. *Nat. Rev. Neurosci.* **2002**, *3*, 862–872. [CrossRef]
30. Leissring, M.A.; Paul, B.A.; Parker, I.; Cotman, C.W.; LaFerla, F.M. Alzheimer's presenilin-1 mutation potentiates inositol 1,4,5-trisphosphate-mediated calcium signaling in xenopus oocytes. *J. Neurochem.* **1999**, *72*, 1061–1068. [CrossRef]

31. Chan, S.L.; Mayne, M.; Holden, C.P.; Geiger, J.D.; Mattson, M.P. Presenilin-1 Mutations increase levels of ryanodine receptors and calcium release in PC12 cells and cortical neurons. *J. Biol. Chem.* **2000**, *275*, 18195–18200. [CrossRef]
32. Leissring, M.A.; Akbari, Y.; Fanger, C.M.; Cahalan, M.D.; Mattson, M.P.; LaFerla, F.M. Capacitative calcium entry deficits and elevated luminal calcium content in mutant presenilin-1 knockin mice. *J. Cell Biol.* **2000**, *149*, 793–798. [CrossRef]
33. Smith, I.F.; Boyle, J.P.; Vaughan, P.F.; Pearson, H.A.; Cowburn, R.F.; Peers, C.S. Ca^{2+} stores and capacitative Ca^{2+} entry in human neuroblastoma (SH- SY5Y) cells expressing a familial alzheimer's disease presenilin-1 mutation. *Brain Res.* **2002**, *949*, 105–111. [CrossRef]
34. Green, K.N.; Demuro, A.; Akbari, Y.; Hitt, B.D.; Smith, I.F.; Parker, I.; LaFerla, F.M. SERCA pump activity is physiologically regulated by presenilin and regulates amyloid β production. *J. Cell Biol.* **2008**, *181*, 1107–1116. [CrossRef] [PubMed]
35. Cai, D.; Netzer, W.J.; Zhong, M.; Lin, Y.; Du, G.; Frohman, M.; Foster, D.A.; Sisodia, S.S.; Xu, H.; Gorelick, F.S.; et al. Presenilin-1 uses phospholipase d1 as a negative regulator of β-amyloid formation. *Proc. Natl. Acad. Sci. USA* **2006**, *103*, 1941–1946. [CrossRef] [PubMed]
36. Hayrapetyan, V.; Rybalchenko, V.; Rybalchenko, N.; Koulen, P. The N-terminus of presenilin-2 increases single channel activity of brain ryanodine receptors through direct protein-protein interaction. *Cell Calcium* **2008**, *44*, 507–518. [CrossRef] [PubMed]
37. Schneider, I.; Reverse, D.; Dewachter, I.; Ris, L.; Caluwaerts, N.; Kuiperi, C.; Gilis, M.; Geerts, H.; Kretzschmar, H.; Godaux, E.; et al. Mutant presenilins disturb neuronal calcium homeostasis in the brain of transgenic mice, decreasing the threshold for excitotoxicity and facilitating long-term potentiation. *J. Biol. Chem.* **2001**, *276*, 11539–11544. [CrossRef] [PubMed]
38. Tu, H.; Nelson, O.; Bezprozvanny, A.; Wang, Z.; Lee, S.F.; Hao, Y.H.; Serneels, L.; De Strooper, B.; Yu, G.; Bezprozvanny, I. Presenilins form ER Ca^{2+} leak channels, a function disrupted by familial alzheimer's disease-linked mutations. *Cell* **2006**, *126*, 981–993. [CrossRef]
39. Zatti, G.; Ghidoni, R.; Barbiero, L.; Binetti, G.; Pozzan, T.; Fasolato, C.; Pizzo, P. The presenilin 2 M239I mutation associated with familial alzheimer's disease reduces Ca^{2+} release from intracellular stores. *Neurobiol. Dis.* **2004**, *15*, 269–278. [CrossRef]
40. Giacomello, M.; Barbiero, L.; Zatti, G.; Squitti, R.; Binetti, G.; Pozzan, T.; Fasolato, C.; Ghidoni, R.; Pizzo, P. Reduction of Ca^{2+} stores and capacitative Ca^{2+} entry is associated with the familial alzheimer's disease presenilin-2 T122R mutation and anticipates the onset of dementia. *Neurobiol. Dis.* **2005**, *18*, 638–648. [CrossRef]
41. Zatti, G.; Burgo, A.; Giacomello, M.; Barbiero, L.; Ghidoni, R.; Sinigaglia, G.; Florean, C.; Bagnoli, S.; Binetti, G.; Sorbi, S.; et al. Presenilin mutations linked to familial alzheimer's disease reduce endoplasmic reticulum and golgi apparatus calcium levels. *Cell Calcium* **2006**, *39*, 539–550. [CrossRef]
42. Zampese, E.; Fasolato, C.; Kipanyula, M.J.; Bortolozzi, M.; Pozzan, T.; Pizzo, P. Presenilin 2 modulates endoplasmic reticulum (ER)-mitochondria interactions and Ca^{2+} cross-talk. *Proc. Natl. Acad. Sci. USA* **2011**, *108*, 2777–2782. [CrossRef]
43. Cheung, K.H.; Shineman, D.; Muller, M.; Cardenas, C.; Mei, L.; Yang, J.; Tomita, T.; Iwatsubo, T.; Lee, V.M.; Foskett, J.K. Mechanism of Ca^{2+} disruption in alzheimer's disease by presenilin regulation of InsP3 receptor channel gating. *Neuron* **2008**, *58*, 871–883. [CrossRef] [PubMed]
44. Cheung, K.H.; Mei, L.; Mak, D.O.; Hayashi, I.; Iwatsubo, T.; Kang, D.E.; Foskett, J.K. Gain-of-function enhancement of IP3 receptor modal gating by familial alzheimer's disease-linked presenilin mutants in human cells and mouse neurons. *Sci. Signal.* **2010**, *3*, ra22. [CrossRef] [PubMed]
45. Shilling, D.; Mak, D.O.; Kang, D.E.; Foskett, J.K. Lack of evidence for presenilins as endoplasmic reticulum Ca^{2+} leak channels. *J. Biol. Chem.* **2012**, *14*, 10933–10944. [CrossRef] [PubMed]
46. Greotti, E.; Wong, A.; Pozzan, T.; Pendin, D.; Pizzo, P. Characterization of the ER-targeted low affinity Ca^{2+} probe D4ER. *Sensors* **2016**, *16*, 1419. [CrossRef] [PubMed]
47. Lissandron, V.; Podini, P.; Pizzo, P.; Pozzan, T. Unique characteristics of Ca^{2+} homeostasis of the trans-golgi compartment. *Proc. Natl. Acad. Sci. USA* **2010**, *107*, 9198–9203. [CrossRef]
48. Wong, A.K.; Capitanio, P.; Lissandron, V.; Bortolozzi, M.; Pozzan, T.; Pizzo, P. Heterogeneity of Ca^{2+} handling among and within golgi compartments. *J. Mol. Cell Biol.* **2013**, *5*, 266–276. [CrossRef]
49. Greotti, E.; Capitanio, P.; Wong, A.; Pozzan, T.; Pizzo, P.; Pendin, D. Familial alzheimer's disease-linked presenilin mutants and intracellular Ca^{2+} handling: A single-organelle, FRET-based analysis. *Cell Calcium*

2019, *79*, 44–56. [CrossRef]

50. Nelson, O.; Tu, H.; Lei, T.; Bentahir, M.; de Strooper, B.; Bezprozvanny, I. Familial alzheimer disease-linked mutations specifically disrupt Ca^{2+} leak function of presenilin 1. *J. Clin. Investig.* **2007**, *117*, 1230–1239. [CrossRef]
51. Brunello, L.; Zampese, E.; Florean, C.; Pozzan, T.; Pizzo, P.; Fasolato, C. Presenilin-2 dampens intracellular Ca^{2+} stores by increasing Ca^{2+} leakage and reducing Ca^{2+} uptake. *J. Cell. Mol. Med.* **2009**, *13*, 3358–3369. [CrossRef]
52. Pack-Chung, E.; Meyers, M.B.; Pettingell, W.P.; Moir, R.D.; Brownawell, A.M.; Cheng, I.; Tanzi, R.E.; Kim, T.W. Presenilin 2 interacts with sorcin, a modulator of the ryanodine receptor. *J. Biol. Chem.* **2000**, *275*, 14440–14445. [CrossRef]
53. Chakroborty, S.; Goussakov, I.; Miller, M.B.; Stutzmann, G.E. Deviant ryanodine receptor-mediated calcium release resets synaptic homeostasis in presymptomatic 3×Tg-AD mice. *J. Neurosci.* **2009**, *29*, 9458–9470. [CrossRef] [PubMed]
54. Kipanyula, M.J.; Contreras, L.; Zampese, E.; Lazzari, C.; Wong, A.K.C.; Pizzo, P.; Fasolato, C.; Pozzan, T. Ca^{2+} dysregulation in neurons from transgenic mice expressing mutant presenilin 2. *Aging Cell* **2012**, *11*, 885–893. [CrossRef] [PubMed]
55. Smith, I.F.; Hitt, B.; Green, K.N.; Oddo, S.; LaFerla, F.M. Enhanced caffeine-induced Ca^{2+} release in the 3×Tg-AD mouse model of alzheimer's disease. *J. Neurochem.* **2005**, *94*, 1711–1718. [CrossRef]
56. Del Prete, D.; Checler, F.; Chami, M. Ryanodine receptors: Physiological function and deregulation in alzheimer disease. *Mol. Neurodegener.* **2014**, *9*, 21. [CrossRef] [PubMed]
57. Shilling, D.; Muller, M.; Takano, H.; Mak, D.O.; Abel, T.; Coulter, D.A.; Foskett, J.K. Suppression of InsP3 receptor-mediated Ca^{2+} signaling alleviates mutant presenilin-linked familial alzheimer's disease pathogenesis. *J. Neurosci.* **2014**, *34*, 6910–6923. [CrossRef]
58. Vance, J.E. Phospholipid synthesis in a membrane fraction associated with mitochondria. *J. Biol. Chem.* **1990**, *265*, 7248–7256.
59. Filadi, R.; Theurey, P.; Pizzo, P. The endoplasmic reticulum-mitochondria coupling in health and disease: Molecules, functions and significance. *Cell Calcium* **2017**, *62*, 1–15. [CrossRef]
60. Hedskog, L.; Pinho, C.M.; Filadi, R.; Ronnback, A.; Hertwig, L.; Wiehager, B.; Larssen, P.; Gellhaar, S.; Sandebring, A.; Westerlund, M.; et al. Modulation of the endoplasmic reticulum-mitochondria interface in alzheimer's disease and related models. *Proc. Natl. Acad. Sci. USA* **2013**, *110*, 7916–7921. [CrossRef]
61. Area-Gomez, E.; Del Carmen Lara Castillo, M.; Tambini, M.D.; Guardia-Laguarta, C.; de Groof, A.J.; Madra, M.; Ikenouchi, J.; Umeda, M.; Bird, T.D.; Sturley, S.L.; et al. Upregulated function of mitochondria-associated ER membranes in alzheimer disease. *EMBO J.* **2012**, *31*, 4106–4123. [CrossRef]
62. Sepulveda-Falla, D.; Barrera-Ocampo, A.; Hagel, C.; Korwitz, A.; Vinueza-Veloz, M.F.; Zhou, K.; Schonewille, M.; Zhou, H.; Velazquez-Perez, L.; Rodriguez-Labrada, R.; et al. Familial alzheimer's disease-associated presenilin-1 alters cerebellar activity and calcium homeostasis. *J. Clin. Investig.* **2014**, *124*, 1552–1567. [CrossRef]
63. Filadi, R.; Greotti, E.; Turacchio, G.; Luini, A.; Pozzan, T.; Pizzo, P. Presenilin 2 modulates endoplasmic reticulum-mitochondria coupling by tuning the antagonistic effect of mitofusin 2. *Cell Rep.* **2016**, *15*, 2226–2238. [CrossRef] [PubMed]
64. Liu, Y.; Zhu, X. Endoplasmic reticulum-mitochondria tethering in neurodegenerative diseases. *Transl. Neurodegener.* **2017**, *6*, 1–8. [CrossRef] [PubMed]
65. Area-Gomez, E.; de Groof, A.J.; Boldogh, I.; Bird, T.D.; Gibson, G.E.; Koehler, C.M.; Yu, W.H.; Duff, K.E.; Yaffe, M.P.; Pon, L.A.; et al. Presenilins are enriched in endoplasmic reticulum membranes associated with mitochondria. *Am. J. Pathol.* **2009**, *175*, 1810–1816. [CrossRef] [PubMed]
66. Schreiner, B.; Hedskog, L.; Wiehager, B.; Ankarcrona, M. Amyloid-beta peptides are generated in mitochondria-associated endoplasmic reticulum membranes. *J. Alzheimer's Dis.* **2015**, *43*, 369–374. [CrossRef]
67. Filadi, R.; Greotti, E.; Turacchio, G.; Luini, A.; Pozzan, T.; Pizzo, P. Mitofusin 2 ablation increases endoplasmic reticulum-mitochondria coupling. *Proc. Natl. Acad. Sci. USA* **2015**, *112*, E2174–E2181. [CrossRef]
68. Hogan, P.G.; Rao, A. Store-operated calcium entry: Mechanisms and modulation. *Biochem. Biophys. Res. Commun.* **2015**, *460*, 40–49. [CrossRef]
69. Putney, J.W. Forms and functions of store-operated calcium entry mediators, stim and orai. *Adv. Biol. Regul.* **2018**, *68*, 88–96. [CrossRef]

70. Yoo, A.S.; Cheng, I.; Chung, S.; Grenfell, T.Z.; Lee, H.; Pack-Chung, E.; Handler, M.; Shen, J.; Xia, W.; Tesco, G.; et al. Presenilin-mediated modulation of capacitative calcium entry. *Neuron* **2000**, *27*, 561–572. [CrossRef]

71. Tong, B.C.; Lee, C.S.; Cheng, W.H.; Lai, K.O.; Foskett, J.K.; Cheung, K.H. Familial alzheimer's disease-associated presenilin 1 mutants promote gamma-secretase cleavage of STIM1 to impair store-operated Ca^{2+} entry. *Sci. Signal.* **2016**, *9*, ra89. [CrossRef]

72. Herms, J.; Schneider, I.; Dewachter, I.; Caluwaerts, N.; Kretzschmar, H.; Van Leuven, F. Capacitive calcium entry is directly attenuated by mutant presenilin-1, independent of the expression of the amyloid precursor protein. *J. Biol. Chem.* **2003**, *278*, 2484–2489. [CrossRef]

73. Bojarski, L.; Pomorski, P.; Szybinska, A.; Drab, M.; Skibinska-Kijek, A.; Gruszczynska-Biegala, J.; Kuznicki, J. Presenilin-dependent expression of STIM proteins and dysregulation of capacitative Ca^{2+} entry in familial Alzheimer's disease. *Biochim. Biophys. Acta* **2009**, *1793*, 1050–1057. [CrossRef] [PubMed]

74. Pascual-Caro, C.; Berrocal, M.; Lopez-Guerrero, A.M.; Alvarez-Barrientos, A.; Pozo-Guisado, E.; Gutierrez-Merino, C.; Mata, A.M.; Martin-Romero, F.J. STIM1 deficiency is linked to Alzheimer's disease and triggers cell death in SH-SY5Y cells by upregulation of L-Type voltage-operated Ca^{2+} entry. *J. Mol. Med.* **2018**, *96*, 1061–1079. [CrossRef] [PubMed]

75. Lu, T.; Aron, L.; Zullo, J.; Pan, Y.; Kim, H.; Chen, Y.; Yang, T.H.; Kim, H.M.; Drake, D.; Liu, X.S.; et al. Rest and stress resistance in ageing and Alzheimer's disease. *Nature* **2014**, *507*, 448–454. [CrossRef] [PubMed]

76. Ozmen, L.; Albientz, A.; Czech, C.; Jacobsen, H. Expression of transgenic APP MRNA is the key determinant for beta-amyloid deposition in PS2APP transgenic mice. *Neurodegener. Dis.* **2009**, *6*, 29–36. [CrossRef]

77. Zott, B.; Busche, M.A.; Sperling, R.A.; Konnerth, A. What happens with the circuit in Alzheimer's disease in mice and humans? *Annu. Rev. Neurosci.* **2018**, *41*, 277–297. [CrossRef]

78. Stargardt, A.; Swaab, D.F.; Bossers, K. Storm before the quiet: Neuronal hyperactivity and ab in the presymptomatic stages of alzheimer's Disease. *Neurobiol. Aging* **2015**, *36*, 1–11. [CrossRef]

79. Wilson, C.A.; Murphy, D.D.; Giasson, B.I.; Zhang, B.; Trojanowski, J.Q.; Lee, V.M. Degradative organelles containing mislocalized alpha-and beta-synuclein proliferate in presenilin-1 null neurons. *J. Cell Biol.* **2004**, *165*, 335–346. [CrossRef]

80. Esselens, C.; Oorschot, V.; Baert, V.; Raemaekers, T.; Spittaels, K.; Serneels, L.; Zheng, H.; Saftig, P.; De Strooper, B.; Klumperman, J.; et al. Presenilin 1 mediates the turnover of telencephalin in hippocampal neurons via an autophagic degradative pathway. *J. Cell Biol.* **2004**, *166*, 1041–1054. [CrossRef]

81. Lee, J.H.; Yu, W.H.; Kumar, A.; Lee, S.; Mohan, P.S.; Peterhoff, C.M.; Wolfe, D.M.; Martinez-Vicente, M.; Massey, A.C.; Sovak, G.; et al. Lysosomal proteolysis and autophagy require presenilin 1 and are disrupted by alzheimer-related PS1 mutations. *Cell* **2010**, *141*, 1146–1158. [CrossRef]

82. Coen, K.; Flannagan, R.S.; Baron, S.; Carraro-Lacroix, L.R.; Wang, D.; Vermeire, W.; Michiels, C.; Munck, S.; Baert, V.; Sugita, S.; et al. Lysosomal calcium homeostasis defects, not proton pump defects, cause endo-lysosomal dysfunction in PSEN-deficient cells. *J. Cell Biol.* **2012**, *198*, 23–35. [CrossRef]

83. Zhang, X.; Garbett, K.; Veeraraghavalu, K.; Wilburn, B.; Gilmore, R.; Mirnics, K.; Sisodia, S.S. A role for presenilins in autophagy revisited: Normal acidification of lysosomes in cells lacking PSEN1 and PSEN2. *J. Neurosci.* **2012**, *32*, 8633–8648. [CrossRef] [PubMed]

84. Reddy, K.; Cusack, C.L.; Nnah, I.C.; Khayati, K.; Saqcena, C.; Huynh, T.B.; Noggle, S.A.; Ballabio, A.; Dobrowolski, R. Dysregulation of nutrient sensing and CLEARance in presenilin deficiency. *Cell Rep.* **2016**, *14*, 2166–2179. [CrossRef] [PubMed]

85. Filadi, R.; Pizzo, P. Defective autophagy and alzheimer's disease: Is calcium the key? In *Neural Regeneration Research*; Wolters Kluwer Medknow Publications: Mumbai, India, 2019; pp. 2081–2082. [CrossRef]

86. Fedeli, C.; Filadi, R.; Rossi, A.; Mammucari, C.; Pizzo, P. PSEN2 (Presenilin 2) mutants linked to familial alzheimer disease impair autophagy by altering Ca^{2+} homeostasis. *Autophagy* **2019**, 1–19. [CrossRef] [PubMed]

87. Gutierrez, M.G.; Munafo, D.B.; Beron, W.; Colombo, M.I. Rab7 is required for the normal progression of the autophagic pathway in mammalian cells. *J. Cell Sci.* **2004**, *117*, 2687–2697. [CrossRef]

88. Lee, J.H.; McBrayer, M.K.; Wolfe, D.M.; Haslett, L.J.; Kumar, A.; Sato, Y.; Lie, P.P.; Mohan, P.; Coffey, E.E.; Kompella, U.; et al. Presenilin 1 maintains lysosomal Ca^{2+} homeostasis via TRPML1 by regulating VATPase-mediated lysosome acidification. *Cell Rep.* **2015**, *12*, 1430–1444. [CrossRef]

89. Behbahani, H.; Shabalina, I.G.; Wiehager, B.; Concha, H.; Hultenby, K.; Petrovic, N.; Nedergaard, J.; Winblad, B.; Cowburn, R.F.; Ankarcrona, M. Differential role of presenilin-1 and -2 on mitochondrial

membrane potential and oxygen consumption in mouse embryonic fibroblasts. *J. Neurosci. Res.* **2006**, *84*, 891–902. [CrossRef]

90. Contino, S.; Porporato, P.E.; Bird, M.; Marinangeli, C.; Opsomer, R.; Sonveaux, P.; Bontemps, F.; Dewachter, I.; Octave, J.N.; Bertrand, L.; et al. Presenilin 2-dependent maintenance of mitochondrial oxidative capacity and morphology. *Front. Physiol.* **2017**, *8*, 796. [CrossRef]
91. Rossi, A.; Pizzo, P.; Filadi, R. Calcium, mitochondria and cell metabolism: A functional triangle in bioenergetics. *Biochim. Biophys. Acta Mol. Cell Res.* **2019**, *1866*, 1068–1078. [CrossRef]
92. Rangaraju, V.; Calloway, N.; Ryan, T.A. Activity-driven local ATP synthesis is required for synaptic function. *Cell* **2014**, *156*, 825–835. [CrossRef]
93. Weidling, I.W.; Swerdlow, R.H. Mitochondria in alzheimer's disease and their potential role in alzheimer's proteostasis. In *Experimental Neurology*; Academic Press Inc.: Cambridge, MA, USA, 2020.
94. Jadiya, P.; Kolmetzky, D.W.; Tomar, D.; Di Meco, A.; Lombardi, A.A.; Lambert, J.P.; Luongo, T.S.; Ludtmann, M.H.; Praticò, D.; Elrod, J.W. Impaired mitochondrial calcium efflux contributes to disease progression in models of alzheimer's disease. *Nat. Commun.* **2019**, *10*, 3885. [CrossRef]
95. Toglia, P.; Cheung, K.H.; Mak, D.O.D.; Ullah, G. Impaired mitochondrial function due to familial alzheimer's disease-causing presenilins mutants via Ca^{2+} disruptions. *Cell Calcium* **2016**, *59*, 240–250. [CrossRef] [PubMed]
96. Flannery, P.J.; Trushina, E. Mitochondrial dynamics and transport in alzheimer's disease. In *Molecular and Cellular Neuroscience*; Academic Press Inc.: Cambridge, MA, USA, 2019; pp. 109–120.
97. Theurey, P.; Connolly, N.M.C.; Fortunati, I.; Basso, E.; Lauwen, S.; Ferrante, C.; Moreira Pinho, C.; Joselin, A.; Gioran, A.; Bano, D.; et al. Systems biology identifies preserved integrity but impaired metabolism of mitochondria due to a glycolytic defect in alzheimer's disease neurons. *Aging Cell* **2019**, *18*, e12924. [CrossRef] [PubMed]
98. Rossi, A.; Rigotto, G.; Valente, G.; Giorgio, V.; Basso, E.; Filadi, R.; Pizzo, P. Defective mitochondrial pyruvate flux affects cell bioenergetics in alzheimer's disease-related models. *Cell Rep.* **2020**, *30*, 2332–2348. [CrossRef] [PubMed]
99. Llorens-Martin, M.; Jurado, J.; Hernandez, F.; Avila, J. GSK-3beta, a pivotal kinase in alzheimer disease. *Front. Mol. Neurosci.* **2014**, *7*, 46. [CrossRef] [PubMed]
100. Fontana, R.; Agostini, M.; Murana, E.; Mahmud, M.; Scremin, E.; Rubega, M.; Sparacino, G.; Vassanelli, S.; Fasolato, C. Early hippocampal hyperexcitability in PS2APP mice: Role of mutant PS2 and APP. *Neurobiol. Aging* **2017**, *50*, 64–76. [CrossRef]
101. Dickerson, B.C.; Salat, D.H.; Greve, D.N.; Chua, E.F.; Rand-Giovannetti, E.; Rentz, D.M.; Bertram, L.; Mullin, K.; Tanzi, R.E.; Blacker, D.; et al. Increased hippocampal activation in mild cognitive impairment compared to normal aging and AD. *Neurology* **2005**, *65*, 404–411. [CrossRef]
102. Bakker, A.; Albert, M.S.; Krauss, G.; Speck, C.L.; Gallagher, M. Response of the medial temporal lobe network in amnestic mild cognitive impairment to therapeutic intervention assessed by FMRI and memory task performance. *Neuroimage Clin.* **2015**, *7*, 688–698. [CrossRef]
103. Palop, J.J.; Mucke, L. Network abnormalities and interneuron dysfunction in alzheimer disease. *Nat. Rev. Neurosci.* **2016**, *17*, 777–792. [CrossRef]
104. Lam, A.D.; Deck, G.; Goldman, A.; Eskandar, E.N.; Noebels, J.; Cole, A.J. Silent hippocampal seizures and spikes identified by foramen ovale electrodes in alzheimer's disease. *Nat. Med.* **2017**, *23*, 678–680. [CrossRef]
105. Mitra, A.; Snyder, A.Z.; Hacker, C.D.; Pahwa, M.; Tagliazucchi, E.; Laufs, H.; Leuthardt, E.C.; Raichle, M.E. Human cortical–hippocampal dialogue in wake and slow-wave sleep. *Proc. Natl. Acad. Sci. USA* **2016**, *113*, E6868–E6876. [CrossRef]
106. Busche, M.A.; Grienberger, C.; Keskin, A.D.; Song, B.; Neumann, U.; Staufenbiel, M.; Forstl, H.; Konnerth, A. Decreased amyloid-beta and increased neuronal hyperactivity by immunotherapy in alzheimer's models. *Nat. Neurosci.* **2015**, *18*, 1725–1727. [CrossRef] [PubMed]
107. Kastanenka, K.V.; Hou, S.S.; Shakerdge, N.; Logan, R.; Feng, D.; Wegmann, S.; Chopra, V.; Hawkes, J.M.; Chen, X.; Bacskai, B.J. Optogenetic restoration of disrupted slow oscillations halts amyloid deposition and restores calcium homeostasis in an animal model of alzheimer's disease. *PLoS ONE* **2017**, *12*, e0170275. [CrossRef] [PubMed]
108. Leparulo, A.; Mahmud, M.; Scremin, E.; Pozzan, T.; Vassanelli, S.; Fasolato, C. Dampened slow oscillation connectivity anticipates amyloid deposition in the PS2APP mouse model of alzheimer's disease. *Cells* **2019**, *9*, 54. [CrossRef] [PubMed]

109. Born, J. Slow-wave sleep and the consolidation of long-term memory. *World J. Biol. Psychiatry* **2010**, *11*, 16–21. [CrossRef] [PubMed]
110. Agostini, M.; Fasolato, C. When, Where and How? Focus on neuronal calcium dysfunctions in alzheimer's disease. *Cell Calcium* **2016**, *60*, 289–298. [CrossRef]
111. Lazzari, C.; Kipanyula, M.J.; Agostini, M.; Pozzan, T.; Fasolato, C. Ab42 oligomers selectively disrupt neuronal calcium release. *Neurobiol. Aging* **2015**, *36*, 877–885. [CrossRef]
112. Tong, B.C.; Wu, A.J.; Li, M.; Cheung, K.H. Calcium signaling in alzheimer's disease & therapies. *Biochim. Biophys. Acta Mol. Cell Res.* **2018**, *1865*, 1745–1760. [CrossRef] [PubMed]
113. Brawek, B.; Garaschuk, O. Network-wide dysregulation of calcium homeostasis in alzheimer's disease. In *Cell and Tissue Research*; Springer: Berlin/Heidelberg, Germany, 2014; pp. 427–438.
114. Lee, Y.J.; Choi, I.S.; Park, M.H.; Lee, Y.M.; Song, J.K.; Kim, Y.H.; Kim, K.H.; Hwang, D.Y.; Jeong, J.H.; Yun, Y.P.; et al. 4-O-methylhonokiol attenuates memory impairment in presenilin 2 mutant mice through reduction of oxidative damage and inactivation of astrocytes and the ERK pathway. *Free Radic. Biol. Med.* **2011**, *50*, 66–77. [CrossRef]
115. Yuk, D.Y.; Lee, Y.K.; Nam, S.Y.; Yun, Y.W.; Hwang, D.Y.; Choi, D.Y.; Oh, K.W.; Hong, J.T. Reduced anxiety in the mice expressing mutant (N141I) presenilin 2. *J. Neurosci. Res.* **2009**, *87*, 522–531. [CrossRef] [PubMed]
116. Verret, L.; Mann, E.O.; Hang, G.B.; Barth, A.M.; Cobos, I.; Ho, K.; Devidze, N.; Masliah, E.; Kreitzer, A.C.; Mody, I.; et al. Inhibitory interneuron deficit links altered network activity and cognitive dysfunction in alzheimer model. *Cell* **2012**, *149*, 708–721. [CrossRef]
117. Hahn, T.T.G.; Sakmann, B.; Mehta, M.R. Phase-locking of hippocampal interneurons' membrane potential to neocortical up-down states. *Nat. Neurosci.* **2006**, *9*, 1359–1361. [CrossRef] [PubMed]
118. Hijazi, S.; Heistek, T.S.; van der Loo, R.; Mansvelder, H.D.; Smit, A.B.; van Kesteren, R.E. Hyperexcitable parvalbumin interneurons render hippocampal circuitry vulnerable to amyloid beta. *Iscience* **2020**, *23*, 101271. [CrossRef] [PubMed]
119. Fellin, T.; Halassa, M.M.; Terunuma, M.; Succol, F.; Takano, H.; Frank, M.; Moss, S.J.; Haydon, P.G. Endogenous nonneuronal modulators of synaptic transmission control cortical slow oscillations in vivo. *Proc. Natl. Acad. Sci. USA* **2009**, *106*, 15037–15042. [CrossRef] [PubMed]
120. Poskanzer, K.E.; Yuste, R. Astrocytic regulation of cortical Up states. *Proc. Natl. Acad. Sci. USA* **2011**, *108*, 18453–18458. [CrossRef] [PubMed]
121. Araque, A.; Carmignoto, G.; Haydon, P.G.; Oliet, S.H.; Robitaille, R.; Volterra, A. Gliotransmitters travel in time and space. *Neuron* **2014**, *81*, 728–739. [CrossRef]
122. Durkee, C.A.; Araque, A. Diversity and specificity of astrocyte-neuron communication. *Neuroscience* **2019**, *396*, 73–78. [CrossRef]
123. Busche, M.A.; Chen, X.; Henning, H.A.; Reichwald, J.; Staufenbiel, M.; Sakmann, B.; Konnerth, A. Critical role of soluble amyloid-beta for early hippocampal hyperactivity in a mouse model of alzheimer's disease. *Proc. Natl. Acad. Sci. USA* **2012**, *109*, 8740–8745. [CrossRef]
124. Lu, B.; Fivaz, M. Neuronal SOCE: Myth or reality? In *Trends in Cell Biology*; Elsevier Ltd.: Amsterdam, The Netherlands, 2016; pp. 890–893.
125. Majewski, L.; Kuznicki, J. SOCE in Neurons: Signaling or just refilling? In *Biochimica et Biophysica Acta-Molecular Cell Research*; Elsevier: Amsterdam, The Netherlands, 2014; pp. 1940–1952.
126. Sun, S.; Zhang, H.; Liu, J.; Popugaeva, E.; Xu, N.J.; Feske, S.; White, C.L.; Bezprozvanny, I. Reduced synaptic STIM2 expression and impaired store-operated calcium entry cause destabilization of mature spines in mutant presenilin mice. *Neuron* **2014**, *82*, 79–93. [CrossRef]
127. Zhang, H.; Sun, S.; Wu, L.; Pchitskaya, E.; Zakharova, O.; Tacer, K.F.; Bezprozvanny, I. Store-operated calcium channel complex in postsynaptic spines: A new therapeutic target for alzheimer's disease treatment. *J. Neurosci.* **2016**, *36*, 11837–11850. [CrossRef]
128. Zhang, H.; Wu, L.; Pchitskaya, E.; Zakharova, O.; Saito, T.; Saido, T.; Bezprozvanny, I. Neuronal store-operated calcium entry and mushroom spine loss in amyloid precursor protein knock-in mouse model of alzheimer's disease. *J. Neurosci.* **2015**, *35*, 13275–13286. [CrossRef]
129. Park, C.Y.; Shcheglovitov, A.; Dolmetsch, R. The CRAC channel activator STIM1 binds and inhibits L-Type voltage-gated calcium channels. *Science* **2010**, *330*, 101–105. [CrossRef] [PubMed]
130. Wang, Y.J.; Deng, X.X.; Mancarella, S.; Hendron, E.; Eguchi, S.; Soboloff, J.; Tang, X.A.D.; Gill, D.L. The calcium store sensor, STIM1, reciprocally controls orai and Ca(V)1.2 channels. *Science* **2010**, *330*, 105–109. [CrossRef] [PubMed]

131. Moccia, F.; Zuccolo, E.; Soda, T.; Tanzi, F.; Guerra, G.; Mapelli, L.; Lodola, F.; D'Angelo, E. Stim and orai proteins in neuronal Ca^{2+} signaling and excitability. *Front. Cell. Neurosci.* **2015**, *9*, 153. [CrossRef] [PubMed]
132. Dou, Y.; Ia, J.; Gao, R.; Gao, I.; Munoz, F.M.; Wei, D.; Tian, Y.; Barrett, J.E.; Ajit, S.; Meucci, O.; et al. Orai1 plays a crucial role in central sensitization by modulating neuronal excitability. *J. Neurosci.* **2018**, *38*, 887–900. [CrossRef]
133. Pizzo, P.; Burgo, A.; Pozzan, T.; Fasolato, C. Role of capacitative calcium entry on glutamate-induced calcium influx in Type-I rat cortical astrocytes. *J. Neurochem.* **2001**, *79*, 98–109. [CrossRef]
134. Okubo, Y.; Iino, M.; Hirose, K. Store-operated Ca^{2+} entry-dependent Ca^{2+} refilling in the endoplasmic reticulum in astrocytes. *Biochem. Biophys. Res. Commun.* **2020**, *522*, 1003–1008. [CrossRef]
135. Toth, A.B.; Hori, K.; Novakovic, M.M.; Bernstein, N.G.; Lambot, L.; Prakriya, M. CRAC channels regulate astrocyte Ca^{2+} signaling and gliotransmitter release to modulate hippocampal GABAergic transmission. *Sci. Signal.* **2019**, *12*, 5450. [CrossRef]
136. Verkhratsky, A.; Rodríguez-Arellano, J.J.; Parpura, V.; Zorec, R. Astroglial calcium signalling in alzheimer's disease. In *Biochemical and Biophysical Research Communications*; Elsevier, B.V.: Amsterdam, The Netherlands, 2017; pp. 1005–1012.
137. Jayadev, S.; Case, A.; Eastman, A.J.; Nguyen, H.; Pollak, J.; Wiley, J.C.; Möller, T.; Morrison, R.S.; Garden, G.A. Presenilin 2 is the predominant γ-secretase in microglia and modulates cytokine release. *PLoS ONE* **2010**, *5*, e15743. [CrossRef]
138. Scremin, E.; Agostini, M.; Leparulo, A.; Pozzan, T.; Greotti, E.; Fasolato, C. ORAI2 down-regulation potentiates SOCE and decreases Aβ42 accumulation in human neuroglioma cells. *Int. J. Mol. Sci.* **2020**, *21*, 5288. [CrossRef]
139. Zeiger, W.; Vetrivel, K.S.; Buggia-Prevot, V.; Nguyen, P.D.; Wagner, S.L.; Villereal, M.L.; Thinakaran, G. Ca^{2+} influx through store-operated Ca^{2+} channels reduces alzheimer disease b-amyloid peptide secretion. *J. Biol. Chem.* **2013**, *288*, 26955–26966. [CrossRef]
140. Vaeth, M.; Yang, J.; Yamashita, M.; Zee, I.; Eckstein, M.; Knosp, C.; Kaufmann, U.; Karoly Jani, P.; Lacruz, R.S.; Flockerzi, V.; et al. ORAI2 modulates store-operated calcium entry and T cell-mediated immunity. *Nat. Commun.* **2017**, *8*, 14714. [CrossRef] [PubMed]
141. Frost, G.R.; Li, Y.M. The role of astrocytes in amyloid production and alzheimer's disease. In *Open Biology*; Royal Society Publishing: London, UK, 2017.
142. Filadi, R.; Pizzo, P. Mitochondrial calcium handling and neurodegeneration: When a good signal goes wrong. *Curr. Opin. Physiol.* **2020**. [CrossRef]
143. Golpich, M.; Amini, E.; Mohamed, Z.; Azman Ali, R.; Mohamed Ibrahim, N.; Ahmadiani, A. Mitochondrial dysfunction and biogenesis in neurodegenerative diseases: Pathogenesis and treatment. *CNS Neurosci. Ther.* **2017**, *23*, 5–22. [CrossRef] [PubMed]
144. Swerdlow, R.H.; Burns, J.M.; Khan, S.M. The alzheimer's disease mitochondrial cascade hypothesis: Progress and perspectives. *Biochim. Biophys. Acta* **2014**, *1842*, 1219–1231. [CrossRef] [PubMed]
145. Bazzari, F.H.; Abdallah, D.M.; El-Abhar, H.S. Pharmacological interventions to attenuate alzheimer's disease progression: The story so far. *Curr. Alzheimer Res.* **2019**, *16*, 261–277. [CrossRef]
146. Oules, B.; Del Prete, D.; Greco, B.; Zhang, X.; Lauritzen, I.; Sevalle, J.; Moreno, S.; Paterlini-Brechot, P.; Trebak, M.; Checler, F.; et al. Ryanodine receptor blockade reduces amyloid-b load and memory impairments in Tg2576 mouse model of alzheimer disease. *J. Neurosci.* **2012**, *32*, 11820–11834. [CrossRef]
147. Chakroborty, S.; Stutzmann, G.E. Calcium channelopathies and alzheimer's disease: Insight into therapeutic success and failures. *Eur. J. Pharmacol.* **2014**, *739*, 83–95. [CrossRef]
148. Facchinetti, F.; Fasolato, C.; Del Giudice, E.; Burgo, A.; Furegato, S.; Fusco, M.; Basso, E.; Seraglia, R.; D'Arrigo, A.; Leon, A. Nimodipine selectively stimulates b-amyloid 1-42 secretion by a mechanism independent of calcium influx blockage. *Neurobiol. Aging* **2006**, *27*, 218–227. [CrossRef]
149. Bantug, G.R.; Fischer, M.; Grahlert, J.; Balmer, M.L.; Unterstab, G.; Develioglu, L.; Steiner, R.; Zhang, L.; Costa, A.S.H.; Gubser, P.M.; et al. Mitochondria-endoplasmic reticulum contact sites function as immunometabolic hubs that orchestrate the rapid recall response of memory CD8(+) T cells. *Immunity* **2018**, *48*, 542–555. [CrossRef]
150. Trushina, E.; Dutta, T.; Persson, X.M.; Mielke, M.M.; Petersen, R.C. Identification of altered metabolic pathways in plasma and CSF in mild cognitive impairment and alzheimer's disease using metabolomics. *PLoS ONE* **2013**, *8*, e63644. [CrossRef]

151. Parnetti, L.; Gaiti, A.; Polidori, M.C.; Brunetti, M.; Palumbo, B.; Chionne, F.; Cadini, D.; Cecchetti, R.; Senin, U. Increased cerebrospinal fluid pyruvate levels in alzheimer's disease. *Neurosci. Lett.* **1995**, *199*, 231–233. [CrossRef]
152. Sasaguri, H.; Nilsson, P.; Hashimoto, S.; Nagata, K.; Saito, T.; De Strooper, B.; Hardy, J.; Vassar, R.; Winblad, B.; Saido, T.C. APP mouse models for alzheimer's disease preclinical studies. *EMBO J.* **2017**, *36*, 2473–2487. [CrossRef] [PubMed]
153. Jankowsky, J.L.; Zheng, H. Practical considerations for choosing a mouse model of alzheimer's disease. *Mol. Neurodegener.* **2017**, *12*, 1–22. [CrossRef] [PubMed]
154. Oddo, S.; Caccamo, A.; Shepherd, J.D.; Murphy, M.P.; Golde, T.E.; Kayed, R.; Metherate, R.; Mattson, M.P.; Akbari, Y.; LaFerla, F.M. Triple-transgenic model of alzheimer's disease with plaques and tangles: Intracellular abeta and synaptic dysfunction. *Neuron* **2003**, *39*, 409–421. [CrossRef]
155. Richards, J.G.; Higgins, G.A.; Ouagazzal, A.M.; Ozmen, L.; Kew, J.N.; Bohrmann, B.; Malherbe, P.; Brockhaus, M.; Loetscher, H.; Czech, C.; et al. PS2APP transgenic mice, coexpressing HPS2mut and HAPPswe, show age-related cognitive deficits associated with discrete brain amyloid deposition and inflammation. *J. Neurosci.* **2003**, *23*, 8989–9003. [CrossRef]
156. Poirier, R.; Veltman, I.; Pflimlin, M.C.; Knoflach, F.; Metzger, F. Enhanced dentate gyrus synaptic plasticity but reduced neurogenesis in a mouse model of amyloidosis. *Neurobiol. Dis.* **2010**, *40*, 386–393. [CrossRef]
157. Weidensteiner, C.; Metzger, F.; Bruns, A.; Bohrmann, B.; Kuennecke, B.; Von Kienlin, M. Cortical hypoperfusion in the B6.PS2APP mouse model for alzheimer's disease: Comprehensive phenotyping of vascular and tissular parameters by MRI. *Magn. Reson. Med.* **2009**, *62*, 35–45. [CrossRef]
158. Brendel, M.; Jaworska, A.; Grießinger, E.; Rötzer, C.; Burgold, S.; Gildehaus, F.J.; Carlsen, J.; Cumming, P.; Baumann, K.; Haass, C.; et al. Cross-sectional comparison of small animal [18f]-florbetaben amyloid-PET between transgenic AD mouse models. *PLoS ONE* **2015**, *10*, e0116678. [CrossRef]
159. Grueninger, F.; Bohrmann, B.; Czech, C.; Ballard, T.M.; Frey, J.R.; Weidensteiner, C.; von Kienlin, M.; Ozmen, L. Phosphorylation of Tau at S422 is enhanced by Aβ in TauPS2APP triple transgenic mice. *Neurobiol. Dis.* **2010**, *37*, 294–306. [CrossRef]
160. Loreth, D.; Ozmen, L.; Revel, F.G.; Knoflach, F.; Wetzel, P.; Frotscher, M.; Metzger, F.; Kretz, O. Selective degeneration of septal and hippocampal GABAergic neurons in a mouse model of amyloidosis and tauopathy. *Neurobiol. Dis.* **2012**, *47*, 1–12. [CrossRef]
161. Kins, S.; Crameri, A.; Evans, D.R.H.; Hemmings, B.A.; Nitsch, R.M.; Götz, J. Reduced protein phosphatase 2A activity induces hyperphosphorylation and altered compartmentalization of Tau in transgenic mice. *J. Biol. Chem.* **2001**, *276*, 38193–38200. [CrossRef] [PubMed]
162. Nyabi, O.; Pype, S.; Mercken, M.; Herreman, A.; Saftig, P.; Craessaerts, K.; Serneels, L.; Annaert, W.; De Strooper, B. No endogenous ab production in presenilin-deficient fibroblasts. *Nat. Cell Biol.* **2002**, *4*, E164. [CrossRef] [PubMed]
163. Herreman, A.; Hartmann, D.; Annaert, W.; Saftig, P.; Craessaerts, K.; Serneels, L.; Umans, L.; Schrijvers, V.; Checler, F.; Vanderstichele, H.; et al. Presenilin 2 deficiency causes a mild pulmonary phenotype and no changes in amyloid precursor protein processing but enhances the embryonic lethal phenotype of presenilin 1 deficiency. *Proc. Natl. Acad. Sci. USA* **1999**, *96*, 11872–11877. [CrossRef] [PubMed]
164. Lee, S.H.; Lutz, D.; Mossalam, M.; Bolshakov, V.Y.; Frotscher, M.; Shen, J. Presenilins regulate synaptic plasticity and mitochondrial calcium homeostasis in the hippocampal mossy fiber pathway. *Mol. Neurodegener.* **2017**, *12*, 48. [CrossRef] [PubMed]
165. Gratuze, M.; Leyns, C.E.G.; Sauerbeck, A.D.; St-Pierre, M.-K.; Xiong, M.; Kim, N.; Remolina Serrano, J.; Tremblay, M.-È.; Kummer, T.T.; Colonna, M.; et al. Impact of TREM2R47H variant on tau pathology-induced gliosis and neurodegeneration. *J. Clin. Investig.* **2020**. [CrossRef]
166. Balu, D.; Karstens, A.J.; Loukenas, E.; Maldonado Weng, J.; York, J.M.; Valencia-Olvera, A.C.; LaDu, M.J. The role of APOE in transgenic mouse models of AD. *Neurosci. Lett.* **2019**, *707*, 134285. [CrossRef]
167. Hargis, K.E.; Blalock, E.M. Transcriptional signatures of brain aging and alzheimer's disease: What are our rodent models telling us? *Behav. Brain Res.* **2017**, *322*, 311–328. [CrossRef]

10

Deficits in Mitochondrial Spare Respiratory Capacity Contribute to the Neuropsychological Changes of Alzheimer's Disease

Simon M. Bell, Matteo De Marco, Katy Barnes, Pamela J. Shaw, Laura Ferraiuolo, Daniel J. Blackburn, Heather Mortiboys *,† and Annalena Venneri *,†

Sheffield Institute for Translational Neuroscience (SITraN), University of Sheffield, 385a Glossop Road, Sheffield S10 2HQ, UK; s.m.bell@sheffield.ac.uk (S.M.B.); m.demarco@sheffield.ac.uk (M.D.M.); kabarnes1@sheffield.ac.uk (K.B.); pamela.shaw@sheffield.ac.uk (P.J.S.); l.ferraiuolo@shef.ac.uk (L.F.); d.blackburn@sheffield.ac.uk (D.J.B.)

* Correspondence: h.mortiboys@sheffield.ac.uk (H.M.); a.venneri@sheffield.ac.uk (A.V.)

† These two authors are joint senior authors.

Abstract: Alzheimer's disease (AD) is diagnosed using neuropsychological testing, supported by amyloid and tau biomarkers and neuroimaging abnormalities. The cause of neuropsychological changes is not clear since they do not correlate with biomarkers. This study investigated if changes in cellular metabolism in AD correlate with neuropsychological changes. Fibroblasts were taken from 10 AD patients and 10 controls. Metabolic assessment included measuring total cellular ATP, extracellular lactate, mitochondrial membrane potential (MMP), mitochondrial respiration and glycolytic function. All participants were assessed with neuropsychological testing and brain structural MRI. AD patients had significantly lower scores in delayed and immediate recall, semantic memory, phonemic fluency and Mini Mental State Examination (MMSE). AD patients also had significantly smaller left hippocampal, left parietal, right parietal and anterior medial prefrontal cortical grey matter volumes. Fibroblast MMP, mitochondrial spare respiratory capacity (MSRC), glycolytic reserve, and extracellular lactate were found to be lower in AD patients. MSRC/MMP correlated significantly with semantic memory, immediate and delayed episodic recall. Correlations between MSRC and delayed episodic recall remained significant after controlling for age, education and brain reserve. Grey matter volumes did not correlate with MRSC/MMP. AD fibroblast metabolic assessment may represent an emergent disease biomarker of AD.

Keywords: Alzheimer's disease; mitochondrial spare respiratory capacity; mitochondrial; membrane potential; glycolytic reserve; semantic memory; phonemic fluency; episodic memory; neuropsychology; neuroimaging

---

1. Background

Alzheimer's disease (AD) is the most common cause of dementia worldwide and in 2018 was estimated to cost the global economy 1 trillion US dollars [1]. The clinical symptoms of the disease are the progressive loss of different aspects of cognitive function until a patient becomes completely dependent on the care of family members and healthcare workers [2]. Median survival after diagnosis is 7 to 10 years for people in their 60s to 70s, and 3 years for people in their 90s [3].

The disease is characterized pathologically by the presence of extracellular amyloid plaques comprising mainly of the amyloid beta protein; and intracellular neurofibrillary tangles (NFT) made mainly of the cytoskeletal protein tau [4]. To date the cause of AD still remains poorly understood.

As the buildup of amyloid appears to be a key step in the development of both familial and sporadic forms of the disease, the amyloid cascade hypothesis has become the leading theory for the cause of the condition [5]. In brief, this hypothesis states that the key step in developing AD is the accumulation of amyloid beta through reduced breakdown and clearance, and/or increased production. Strategies aimed at reducing the amyloid load in the brain, however, have failed to control the disease [6] and have resulted in a large number of clinical trials that have failed to achieve primary outcome measures [7]. Even in pre-clinical carriers of dominantly inherited AD mutations, amyloid removal therapies have not slowed disease progression [8]. Furthermore, brain amyloid load does not correlate with clinical symptoms [9]. This has led researchers to investigate alternative pathophysiological mechanisms [10].

AD is clinically defined by distinctive changes in cognitive status identified by neuropsychological assessment. Brain imaging changes and amyloid and tau protein levels in the cerebrospinal fluid are used to confirm the diagnosis in vivo [11]. The changes seen in a patient's ability to perform a cognitive task are often difficult to explain from a cellular perspective. Tau deposition does explain elements of the observed neuropsychological abnormalities [12], but does not fully account for all cognitive changes observed in AD patients [13,14].

Cognitive processing, such as that required while performing memory tasks, puts an increased metabolic demand on the brain [15]. This is evidenced by neuroimaging studies of the brain which use tracers of metabolism such as 2-[18F]fluoro-2-Deoxy-D-glucose (FDG) that have shown poor glucose utilization in patients who perform poorly on memory tasks [16,17]. Positron-emission tomography (PET) imaging studies that use oxygen-15 labelled water also show reduced uptake when AD patients perform cognitive tasks [18]. These imaging studies suggest that any deficit in metabolic function, such as deficits in mitochondrial respiration or glycolysis, are likely to affect an individual's performance on cognitive tasks. It is therefore possible that mitochondrial respiration or glycolytic dysfunction might contribute to cognitive deficits in AD, making these cellular processes suitable pharmacological targets to improve the cognitive symptoms of AD.

Cellular metabolic changes within the brains of patients with AD and in peripheral cell populations are seen very early in the condition, and often precede the development of both amyloid plaques and NFT. Abnormalities have been shown in many metabolic pathways in AD [19]. Mounting evidence suggests that deficits in glycolysis and the function of mitochondria, specifically how they control oxidative phosphorylation, are likely to be key in the development and establishment of AD [20–22].

A mitochondrial cascade hypothesis has been suggested for the aetiology of AD, and states that people who inherit mitochondrial genes that predispose them to lower mitochondrial respiration rates may be more likely to develop the condition [23]. In animal models of AD, changes in mitochondrial function are seen prior to amyloid deposition [20,24], and cell models show changes in mitochondrial function and oxidative stress without the presence of amyloid [25], giving further evidence for the key role of mitochondrial dysfunction in AD.

Impairment of glycolysis is also seen early in patients with AD. A 2-[18F]fluoro-2-Deoxy-D-glucose positron-emission tomography (FDG-PET) imaging of the brain shows a reduction in glucose metabolism [26]. In particular, there is a reduction in aerobic glycolysis in brain areas susceptible to amyloid deposition [27], and in those regions where high levels of tau accumulation are seen [28].

We have previously shown that fibroblasts from sporadic AD (sAD) patients have multiple mitochondrial structural and functional abnormalities, and that these can be ameliorated by treatment with ursodeoxycholic acid (UDCA) [29]. Other studies have shown that glycyl-l-histidyl-l-lysine (GHK-Cu), by increasing gene expression, has an effect on improving mitochondrial activity and influencing cognitive decline [30]. In our previous study we showed sAD fibroblasts to have deficits in mitochondrial membrane potential (MMP) and mitochondrial spare respiratory capacity (MSRC). MSRC refers to the difference in oxidative phosphorylation rates between the basal level of mitochondrial respiration and the maximal level a cell can achieve [31]. In essence, MSRC measures the cellular reserve respiratory capacity. In animal models of AD it has been shown that deficits in MSRC cause cognitive deficits that treatment with the antioxidant pyrroloquinoline quinone can improve [32]. It has not been previously shown, however, whether changes in MSRC in human cell lines obtained from sAD patients correlate with their performance on neuropsychological tests.

As deficits in both glycolysis and mitochondrial function have been shown in AD patients and models, in this proof of concept study we explored metabolic function in fibroblasts from sporadic AD patients and its role in the cognitive decline experienced by these patients. To this end, we assessed mitochondrial functional changes in a larger cohort of patients compared to the findings described in our previous study [29]. We have then assessed additional metabolic parameters in the sAD fibroblasts including glycolytic function and cellular ATP levels, which have previously not been described. Finally, we investigated whether these metabolic abnormalities detected in sAD fibroblasts correlated with neuropsychological and neuroimaging features typical of the early stages of this disease.

2. Results

2.1. Patient Demographic Details

Skin biopsies were taken from ten sAD patients (mean age 61.3 years, 6 male) and ten controls (mean age 66.7 years, 5 male). Body mass index (BMI) did not differ significantly between the groups (sAD mean 27.8 kg/m^2 SD 5.37 kg/m^2 Controls mean 28.2 kg/m^2 SD 4.00 kg/m^2 t-test $p = 0.44$). Table 1 shows patient and control demographic data.

Table 1. Patient Demographic Information and contemporary treatment status.

Patient Number	Age (Years)	Sex	MMSE	Length of Education (Years)	AD Treatment (in Disease Cohort, at Time of Biopsy)
1	63	Male	20	16	None
2	57	Male	18	15	Donepezil
3	53	Male	14	11	Donepezil
4 *	60	Male	18	9	None
5 *	59	Female	23	11	Galantamine
6 *	63	Female	26	10	Donepezil
7 *	60	Male	18	11	Memantine
8	60	Male	18	11	None
9	79	Female	28	15	None
10	61	Female	25	11	Donepezil
Group Mean (Standard Dev)	61.33 (7.19)		20.8 (4.4)	12.0 (2.4)	
Controls					
1	66	Male	29	11	NA
2 *	54	Male	27	17	NA
3 *	53	Male	29	16	NA
4 *	56	Male	24	11	NA
5	61	Female	30	NA	NA
6	54	Female	29	17	NA
7 *	100	Female	24 #	14	NA
8	75	Female	28	18	NA
9	73	Female	26	12	NA
10	75	Male	27	10	NA
Group Mean (Standard Dev)	65.77 (14.7)		27.6 (1.8)	14 (3.1)	

For control 7 some items of the Mini Mental State Examination (MMSE) could not be tested due to sensory impairment * indicates fibroblast lines in which Mitochondrial Membrane Potential (MMP) and Mitochondrial Spare Respiratory Capacity (MRSC) values were published in our previous paper [29].

2.2. Neuropsychological Profiles

Neuropsychological profiling of controls and patients used in this study was performed as part of the VPH-DARE research project (http://www.vph-dare.eu/), (see Methods section for additional details). For the present study, a subgroup of neuropsychological tests was selected to be correlated with metabolic findings. The tests which can detect the earliest typical cognitive impairments in mild sAD were selected. These included assessment of semantic memory, immediate and delayed episodic recall. Phonemic fluency was also selected as dysfunction on this cognitive test is seen later in AD but not in its earlier stages [33]. All 10 controls and 10 patients with AD were assessed. The Mini-Mental

State Examination (MMSE) [34] was also used, as this test is useful in staging disease severity in sAD [34,35].

Patients with sAD performed at a lower level than controls on all tests (see Figure 1). The most significant differences were seen in the tests of semantic memory (mean score in controls 42.6 points, mean score in sAD 17.5 points, difference between means 25.1 points, SD 4.774 $p < 0.0001$); immediate (mean score in controls 15.8 points, mean score in sAD 6.4 points, difference between means 25.1 points, SD 1.468 $p < 0.0001$); and delayed recall of the Prose Memory test (mean score in controls 18.6 points, mean score in sAD 5.5 points, difference between means 13.4 points, SD 1.488 $p < 0.0001$). The phonemic fluency test performance was also significantly different between the 2 groups (mean score in controls 50.5 points, mean score in sAD 27.4 points, difference between means 23.1 points, SD 6.837 $p = 0.0033$), but to a lesser extent than the other neuropsychological tests. As expected, MMSE scores of sAD patients were significantly lower than those of controls (mean score in controls 27.3 points, mean score in sAD 21.3 points, mean difference 6.0 points, SD 1.54 $p = 0.0011$).

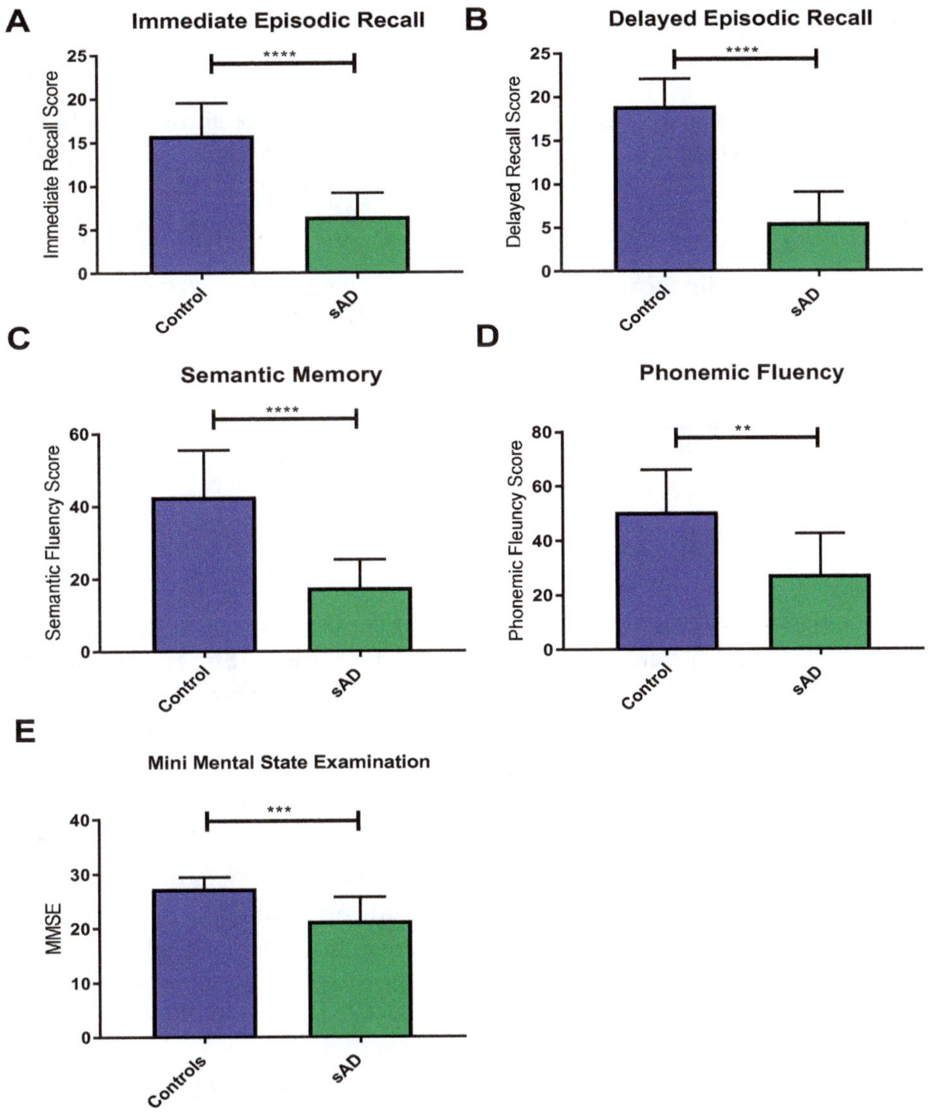

Figure 1. Mean scores of sporadic AD (sAD) patients and controls on cognitive tests included in the neuropsychological assessment. Graphs show mean with error bars indicating standard deviation. **** $p < 0.0001$; *** $p < 0.001$; ** $p < 0.01$. Controls are indicated by blue bars and sAD patients indicated by green bars. Significant reductions were seen in sAD immediate recall (**A**), delayed recall (**B**), semantic memory (**C**), phonemic fluency (**D**) and Mini Mental State Examination (**E**) when compared to controls.

2.3. Neuroimaging Profiles

Volumetric structural MRI scans were acquired on 9 controls and 10 patients with sAD. One control did not complete their MRI scan as an incidental finding (of no diagnostic significance for this study) on initial scans meant the participant could no longer take part in the VPH-DARE@IT original study. For the remaining participants, the left and right parietal lobes, anterior medial pre-frontal cortex and posterior cingulate gyrus, and left hippocampal grey matter volumes were extracted as these brain areas are affected early in AD [36].

Comparisons between the 2 groups showed no significant differences between the grey matter volumes of the preselected areas when performing a *t*-test. Brain grey matter volumes can be affected by age, education and brain reserve [37,38]. For these reasons a further analysis of the 2 groups was completed controlling for these covariates. A significant difference emerged in the volume of the left hippocampus, left parietal, right parietal and anterior medial prefrontal cortex in patients with sAD after controlling for confounding variables. Table 2 highlights the F-test and *p*-values for these differences. No significant difference was seen in the posterior cingulate cortex grey matter volume between the 2 groups.

Table 2. Differences in Control and sAD brain volumes. This table shows the significance of the differences in brain volumes between controls and patients with sAD when controlling for age, years of education and brain reserve.

Brain Volume	F-Test	p-Value
Left Hippocampal Volume	9.420	0.001
Left Parietal Volume	7.882	0.002
Right Parietal Volume	10.051	<0.0001
Anterior Medial Prefrontal Cortex	0.056	0.017
Posterior Cingulate Cortex	0.752	0.575

2.4. Fibroblast Metabolic Assessment

Mitochondrial function was investigated in both sAD patients and controls. We measured elements of both mitochondrial function and glycolysis. Five metabolic parameters were chosen that best describe different factors influencing the ability of the fibroblast to meet its energy demands. Mitochondrial parameters included: total cellular ATP, as this is a global marker of the energetic status of the cell; MMP and MSRC. MMP and MSRC were selected as these parameters are important in maintaining the rate of ATP production as cellular energy demand changes. These are also the two parameters which we have previously identified as being relevant to the mitochondrial phenotype in sAD fibroblasts [29]. Measures of glycolysis included glycolytic reserve and extracellular lactate levels. Glycolytic reserve, like MSRC and MMP for mitochondrial function, is a measure of cellular metabolic flexibility and deficits in this parameter are likely to contribute to an inability to maintain cellular energy production. Extracellular lactate is the final breakdown product of glycolysis and contributes information about how well the cell can utilize glucose as a metabolite.

First, we assessed MMP and MRSC as we have done in our previous work [29]. In this cohort, MRSC was significantly reduced (36% reduction $p < 0.0001$) in sAD when compared to controls (Figure 2A). MMP was also significantly reduced in the sAD fibroblast lines (14% reduction $p = 0.011$) (See Figure 2B). Figure 2C shows a representative oxygen consumption trace for the mitochondrial stress test experiment.

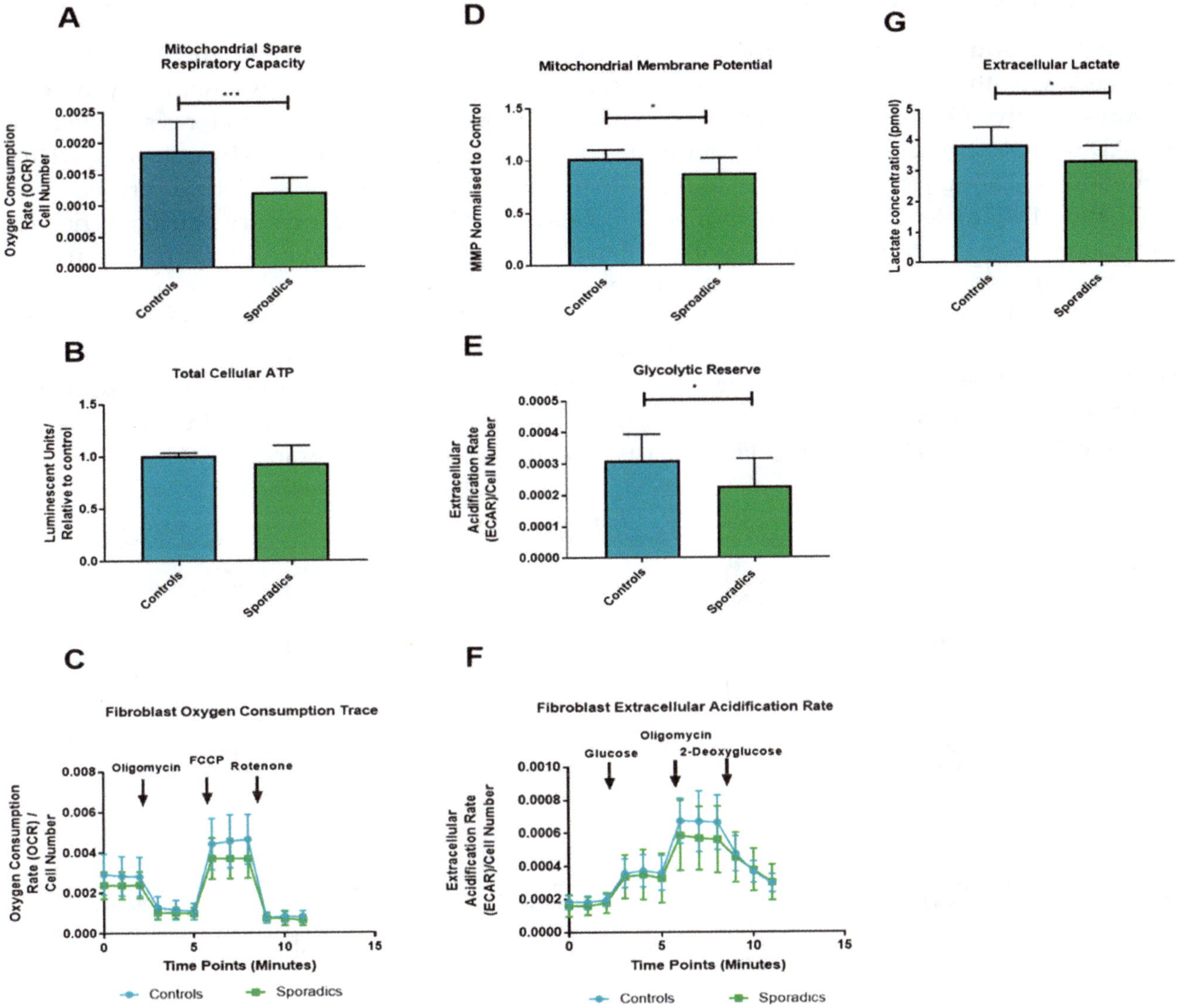

Figure 2. Oxidative phosphorylation and Glycolytic fibroblast Assessment: *** = $p < 0.001$; * = $p < 0.05$. Significant reductions in mitochondrial spare respiratory capacity (**A**), Mitochondrial Membrane potential (**D**), Glycolytic Reserve (**E**) and Extracellular lactate (**G**) was detected in sAD when compared to controls. No significant difference was seen in total cellular ATP (**B**). OCR and ECAR traces for mitochondrial stress test and glycolysis stress test are displayed in panels (**C**) and (**F**) respectively. For all panels controls are represented in blue and sAD are represented in green. Graphs represent mean with error bars indicating standard deviation.

Next, we assessed total cellular ATP, which showed no significant difference between sAD patient fibroblasts and controls when comparing mean values ($p = 0.165$, Figure 2D). The final metabolic assessment of the fibroblast lines involved assessment of glucose metabolism using the glycolysis stress test programme on the Seahorse analyzer and extracellular lactate measurement. A significantly lower glycolytic reserve was found in sAD fibroblasts when compared to controls (see Figure 1E, 25.8% reduction, $p = 0.031$). No significant differences were seen in maximum glycolytic rate ($p = 0.792$), or basal glycolytic rate ($p = 0.381$). Figure 1F shows the extracellular acidification rate (ECAR) trace for the glycolysis stress test, comparing the group of controls against the sAD fibroblast group. Measurement of extracellular lactate levels revealed significantly lower lactate levels released from sAD fibroblasts (14% reduction, $p = 0.0227$, Figure 2G).

2.5. Neuropsychological/Metabolic Correlations

Next, we sought to correlate the neuropsychological scores of the sAD patients and controls combined with their metabolic parameters measured in fibroblasts. As five neuropsychological measures and five fibroblast metabolic markers had been assessed to identify differences in the control and sAD fibroblast groups, we controlled for the effect of multiple comparisons by adjusting what we deemed to be a significant association to $p \leq 0.01$ (0.05/5). Using this new statistical threshold, only MSRC and MMP metabolic tests and immediate, delayed and semantic memory neuropsychological assessments were identified as significantly different between control and sAD groups. Correlations were, therefore, performed only for these data sets.

MSRC had a significant positive correlation with immediate episodic recall (r = 0.612, p = 0.004), delayed episodic recall (r = 0.669, p = 0.001) and semantic memory scores (r = 0.614, p = 0.003). MMP correlated only with semantic memory scores (r = 0.565, p = 0.009). Immediate episodic recall (r = 0.552, p = 0.0134) and delayed episodic recall correlated positively with MMP, but at a lower level of significance (r = 0.540, p = 0.015). Figure 3 displays these correlations graphically.

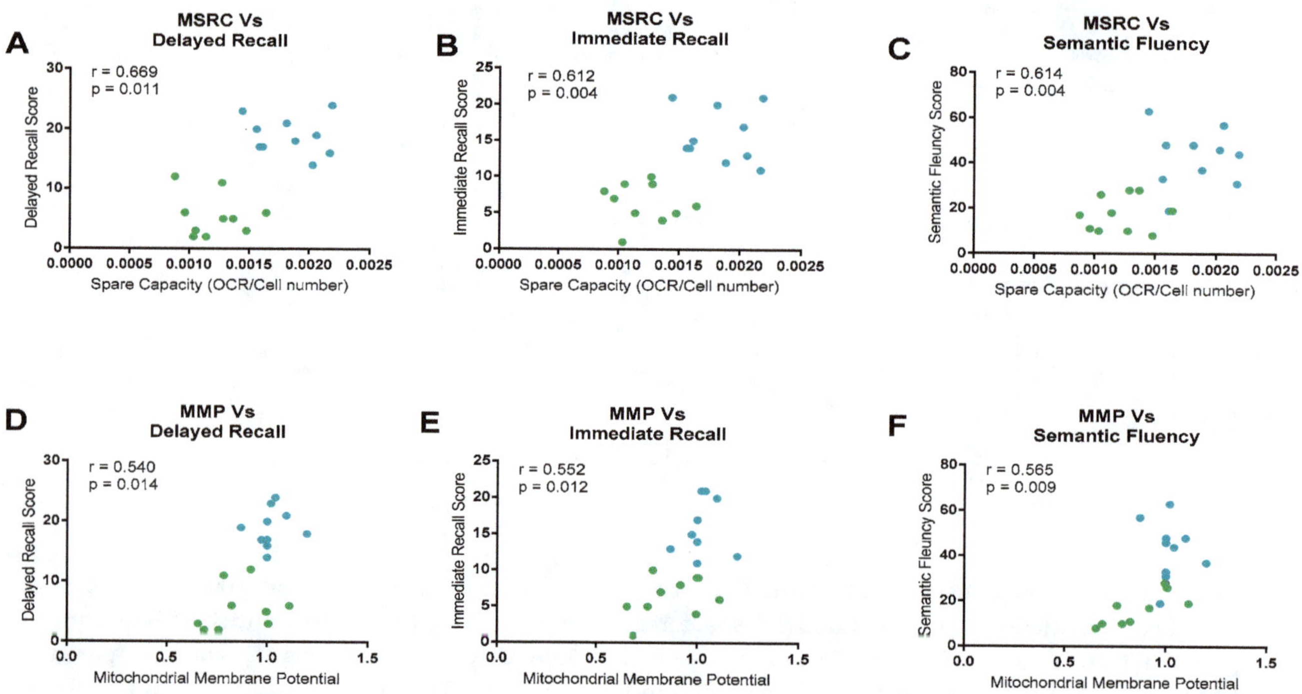

Figure 3. Neuropsychological Fibroblast Metabolism Correlations. Significant correlations were seen between mitochondrial spare respiratory capacity (MSRC) and delayed recall (**A**), Immediate recall (**B**) and semantic fluency (**C**). Mitochondrial membrane potential (MMP) correlated significantly with semantic fluency (**F**), and with delayed recall (**D**) and immediate recall (**E**) but to a lesser extent. For all panels controls are represented in blue and sAD are represented in green. Correlation coefficients and p-values for each correlation are displayed.

Age, years of education and brain reserve can potentially confound the correlations between neuropsychological measurements and the fibroblast metabolic markers, as all three factors have been shown to affect either performance on neuropsychological tests [39,40] or mitochondrial function [41]. To control for the effect of these three covariates, a further analysis was performed taking these parameters into account. This further analysis showed that the correlation between delayed episodic recall and MSRC was still significant at the more conservative significance threshold. Both immediate episodic recall (p = 0.013) and semantic memory (p = 0.012) correlations with MSRC were no longer significant once covariates were included in the analysis at the new more stringent p-value. All correlations seen between the neuropsychological tests and MMP were no longer significant after controlling for age, education and brain reserve. Table 3 displays the new correlation coefficients and p-values for the neuropsychological data.

Table 3. Neuropsychological fibroblast metabolism correlations corrected for age, years of education and grey matter reserve.

Psychological Test	Fibroblast Marker	R Value	p-Value
Immediate Episodic Recall			
	MSRC	0.605	0.013
	MMP	0.196	0.466
Delayed Episodic Recall			
	MSRC	0.695	0.003
	MMP	0.204	0.448
Semantic Memory			
	MSRC	0.610	0.012
	MMP	0.345	0.191

2.6. *Neuroimaging/Metabolic Correlations*

Volumetric imaging for areas of the brain known to be affected by AD were correlated with metabolic markers of the disease. Only the grey matter volumes that had shown significant differences between the sAD and control groups (with a p-value equal to or less than 0.01) were included. None of the grey matter volumes showed a significant correlation with changes in cellular metabolism. Table 4 shows the results of the correlations.

Table 4. Grey Matter Volume Fibroblast metabolic correlations: No significant correlations were seen between MMP nor MSRC and any grey matter volume when controlling for age, length of disease or brain reserve.

Grey Matter Volume	Fibroblast Marker	R Value	p-Value
Left Hippocampal Volume			
	MSRC	0.371	0.157
	MMP	0.041	0.881
Left Parietal Volume			
	MSRC	0.341	0.196
	MMP	−0.047	0.862
Right Parietal Volume			
	MSRC	0.418	0.107
	MMP	−0.043	0.875

3. Discussion

This proof of concept study shows that fibroblast MSRC correlates with established neuropsychological abnormalities that are affected early in AD. This is one of the first studies to show a functional biomarker of AD correlating with a marker of fibroblast mitochondrial function. MSRC is a measure of the ability of mitochondria within cells to increase the production of ATP in response to an increased energy demand. The correlation of MSRC with neuropsychological scores potentially helps to describe the cellular pathology underlying these neuropsychological changes seen in AD. This is the first study in humans to show that peripheral cell MSRC correlates with neuropsychological profiles. Correcting the abnormality in MSRC could be a future therapeutic approach in AD. The fact that this abnormality in mitochondrial function correlates with a clinical biomarker of AD also opens the avenue for monitoring drug response in future clinical trials.

MSRC has been shown to be abnormal in multiple diseases including acute myeloid leukaemia (AML) [42], Parkinson's disease [43,44] and motor neuron disease (MND) [45]. MSRC deficits may not be disease specific, but the combination of cellular metabolic changes seen here may represent a cellular metabolic profile specific to sAD. This metabolic phenotype could potentially represent a biomarker that can stratify and define a specific subset of sAD patients that might then respond to a personalised therapeutic approach. Previous research has shown that the metabolic profile identified in fibroblasts from sporadic Parkinson's disease patients differs from that identified here in fibroblasts from sAD [46,47].

Reductions in MSRC and MMP were seen in all sAD fibroblast lines when compared to controls at a group level. These data reinforce and extend the findings reported in our previous paper [29], and show that the finding of reduced MSRC and MMP is reproducible and more robust in sporadic AD fibroblasts when sample size is increased. Extracellular lactate levels and cellular glycolytic reserves, both markers of glycolytic function, were significantly reduced in all sAD fibroblasts. These measures, however, did not meet the statistical significance for correlation with neuropsychological markers of the disease. The deficits in markers of mitochondrial function and glycolysis in the fibroblasts reflect a lack of flexibility of metabolic pathways in sAD. This lack of flexibility is likely to be very important when performing cognitive tasks that depend on the coordination of multiple brain regions. Taken together, these results suggest that sAD fibroblasts may have limited ability to respond to increased cellular energy demand.

MMP did correlate with neuropsychological markers, but correlations did not survive the correction for confounding factors unlike MSRC, for which correlation with delayed episodic recall (a core feature in the clinical diagnostic criteria for sAD) remained significant. Semantic memory and immediate episodic memory did not significantly correlate with MSRC at the more conservative significance threshold after confounder consideration, but p-values for both of these correlations were less than 0.02. Potentially, these correlations would reach significance level with an increased sample size. The difference in MMP between control and sAD groups was much smaller than the difference seen in MSRC. MMP has a key role in maintaining many pathways in the mitochondria outside that of ATP generation, such as apoptosis fates [48]. It is likely that several mechanisms not affected by sAD in the fibroblast cell help to maintain MMP levels, which may explain the reduced variability seen in this parameter in sAD and the lack of a significant correlation with neuropsychological scores.

Baseline ATP levels were not significantly different between the two groups. These results suggest that, in a controlled environment when cells are not stressed, they can maintain ATP levels similar to that of controls. Interestingly though, the functional capacity of mitochondria is impaired, as described above, suggesting a potential inability to respond appropriately to increased ATP demand. The measurements of ATP we performed in this study only gives information about the total cellular ATP level. We did not investigate the rate of ATP breakdown nor how ATP levels change when the cell is under stressed conditions or the ratio of ATP/ADP in the cell. This may explain why no significant correlations were seen with ATP measurements, but were seen with the other markers of mitochondrial respiration.

It is interesting that the correlation between scores on phonemic fluency, a neuropsychological test not affected early in sAD, and cell metabolism markers did not reach significance threshold. It. The medial temporal lobe is important in semantic memory processing [49], an area of cognition that is impaired very early in sAD [50]. This is not the case for phonemic fluency which is supported by processes associated with frontal executive regions [51]. It could be that the correlations we see between neuropsychological tests and cellular metabolic function may reflect which areas of the brain are more susceptible to metabolic failure. It has been previously shown that areas of the brain that are affected early in sAD express lower levels of electron transport chain (ETC) genes when compared to controls [52], suggesting that this might be the case. Data from FDG-PET studies also support the concept of focal brain hypometabolism in sAD, with areas such as the medial temporal lobes, precuneus and lateral parietal lobes all preferentially affected [53].

We did not see a significant correlation between mitochondrial function or glycolysis and brain structural imaging markers of sAD. This may be explained by the fact that multiple factors can affect grey matter volume such as age, levels of education and brain reserve. It has been previously shown that smaller grey matter volumes in the frontal lobes associated with ageing are associated with worse performance on frontal lobe cognitive tests [54]. The neuropsychological assessment performed in this study mainly focused on temporal lobe cognitive functioning and not frontal lobe function. Potentially, the effect of brain ageing on grey matter volumes may mask any effect metabolic function may have.

The limitations of our study include a small sample size, and the fact that we have used fibroblasts to measure metabolic function. It could also be argued that a correlation between metabolic function of central nervous system cells and neuropsychological parameters would be more meaningful. This is not the first study, however, to show that the metabolism of peripheral cells outside the nervous system is affected in sAD. White blood cells [55], platelets [56] and fibroblasts have been shown to have metabolic abnormalities in multiple studies [46,47,57,58]. Identifying that fibroblast mitochondrial abnormalities correlate with neuropsychological markers of AD opens up avenues to use fibroblast metabolic parameters as biomarkers of sAD, and also as a high throughput drug screening model, as well as potential outcome measures of therapeutic efficacy. Replication of the findings of this study in larger cohorts and by other groups is needed, however, to consolidate the evidence that fibroblast metabolic function is a reliable biomarker of sAD.

Our patient cohort were selected at an early stage of sAD to try and reduce group variability. To understand the use of fibroblast metabolic abnormalities as a biomarker, further work investigating cohorts of patients with amnestic mild cognitive impairment (MCI), the prodromal stage of sAD, would be advantageous as well as investigating these parameters in more advanced sAD patients.

Future work could extend the findings of metabolic-neuropsychological correlations by creating neuronal lineage cells via cellular reprogramming methods such as that described by Takahashi et al. [59]. This type of model would allow for direct comparison between human nervous system cells and human nervous system function in a context where reprogrammed cells would maintain their ageing phenotype [60].

4. Methods

4.1. Patient Details

Skin biopsies and fibroblast metabolic assessments were performed as part of the MODEL-AD research study (Yorkshire and Humber Research and Ethics Committee number: 16/YH/0155). Due to the initial success of fibroblast metabolic assessment, the initial cohort of four controls and four patients (previously reported in [29]) with sAD was expanded to ten healthy controls (mean age: 65.77 years, SD 14.70 years) and 10 patients with sAD (mean age: 61.33 years, SD 7.19 years). All patients had been involved in the EU-funded Framework Programme 7 Virtual Physiological Human: Dementia Research Enabled by IT (VPH-DARE@IT) initiative (http://www.vph-dare.eu/). A diagnosis of sAD was made based on clinical criteria [11]. Ethical approval for the neuropsychological and neuroimaging measures collected was gained from Yorkshire and Humber Regional Ethics Committee, Reference number: 12/YH/0474. Informed written consent was obtained from each participant. Investigations were carried out following the rules of the Declaration of Helsinki of 1975 (https://www.wma.net/what-we-do/medical-ethics/declaration-of-helsinki/), revised in 2013.

4.2. Neuropsychological Testing

A battery of tests was devised to detect impaired performance in the cognitive domains most susceptible to sAD neurodegeneration. This included tests of short- and long-term memory, attention and executive functioning, language and semantics, and visuoconstructive skills. A detailed description of each task is provided elsewhere [61]. Most tests were exclusively used as part of the clinical assessment of patients and controls. Three tests were also included as part of the experimental protocol. Immediate and delayed recall on the Logical Memory test were used as measures of episodic memory, the cognitive domain centrally defined by diagnostic criteria for a diagnosis of sAD. The performance on the Category Fluency test was used as an index of semantic memory, the cognitive domain affected by the accumulation of neurofibrillary pathology in the transentorhinal cortex [50]. Finally, the Letter Fluency test (phonemic fluency) was used as a methodological control, since performance on this task is often within normal age limits in patients with mild sAD [33,62].

4.3. *MRI Acquisition and Processing*

An MRI protocol of anatomical scans was acquired on a Philips Ingenia 3 T scanner. Several acquisitions (including T1-weighted, T2-weighted, FLAIR and diffusion-weighted sequences) were used for diagnostic purposes. Three-dimensional T1-weighted images (voxel size: 0.94 mm × 0.94 mm × 1.00 mm; repetition time: 8.2 s; echo delay time: 3.8 s; field of view: 256 mm; matrix size: 256 × 256 × 170) were also used for the calculation of hippocampal volumes. These were processed with the Similarity and Truth Estimation for Propagated Segmentations routine [63]. This procedure, available at niftyweb.cs.ucl.ac.uk, allows automated segmentation of the left and right hippocampus in the brain's native space using multiple reference templates. Hippocampal volumes were then quantified using Matlab (version R2014a) and the "get totals" script (http://www0.cs.ucl.ac.uk/staff/G.Ridgway/vbm/get_totals.m). Fractional measures were also obtained dividing hippocampal volumes by the volume of the total intracranial space. The left hippocampal volume and left hippocampal ratio were chosen as structural markers of AD as evidence suggests the left hippocampus is affected early in the progression of the disease [64]. Native space maps created to extract hippocampal volume from MRI images are shown in Supplementary Figure S1. Additional regions of interest (listed in Table 2) were then defined as binary image masks. Segmented grey matter maps were registered to the Montreal Neurological Institute space, and mask-constrained volumes were extracted.

4.4. *Tissue Culture*

Fibroblasts were cultured as described previously [29]. In brief, all 10 control and all 10 sAD lines were cultured in EMEM-based media (Corning) incubated at 37 °C in a 5% carbon dioxide atmosphere. Sodium pyruvate (1%) (Sigma Aldrich), non-essential amino acids (1%) (Lonza), penicillin and streptomycin (1%) (Sigma Aldrich), multi-vitamins (1%) (Lonza), Fetal Bovine Serum (10%) (Biosera) and 50μg/mL uridine (Sigma Aldrich) were added to the media. All experiments described were performed on all 20 cell lines. Fibroblasts were plated at a density of 5000 cells per well in a white 96 well plate for ATP assays. For MMP assays fibroblasts were plated at a density of 2500 cells per well in a black 96 well plate. Each assay was performed on three separate passages of fibroblasts; cells between passages 5–10 were used. All experiments were performed on passage-matched cells.

4.5. *Intracellular ATP levels*

Cellular adenosine triphosphate (ATP) levels were measured using the ATPlite kit (Perkin Elmer) as described previously [65]. ATP levels were corrected for cell number by using CyQuant (ThermoFisher) measurements, as previously described [29]. These values were then normalised to control levels.

4.6. *Mitochondrial Membrane Potential*

MMP was measured using tetramethlyrhodamine (TMRM) staining of live fibroblasts, as previously described [29]. Cells were plated in a black 96 well plate, incubated at 37 °C for 48 h. TMRM dye was added one hour prior to imaging on an InCell Analyzer 2000 high-content imager (GE Healthcare).

4.7. *Extracellular Lactate Measurement*

Extracellular lactate was measured from confluent flasks of fibroblasts using an L-Lactate assay kit (Abcam ab65331). The assay was performed according to the manufacturer's instructions.

4.8. Metabolic Flux Assay

4.8.1. Mito Stress Test

Oxygen consumption rates (OCR) were measured using a 24-well Agilent Seahorse XF analyzer as described previously [29]. In brief, cells were plated at a density of 65,000 cells per well 48 h prior to measurement. Three measurements were taken at the basal point: after the addition of oligomycin (0.5 μM), after the addition of carbonyl cyanide-4-(trifluoromethoxy)phenylhydrazone (FCCP) (0.5 μM) and after the addition of rotenone (1 μM). OCR measurements were normalised to cell count as described in [29]. Measurements of basal mitochondrial respiration, maximal mitochondrial respiration and MSRC were also calculated.

4.8.2. Glycolysis Stress Test

Cells were plated in a Seahorse XF24 Cell Culture Microplate (Agilent) at a density of 65,000 cells per well 48 h prior to measurement. The glycolysis stress test standard protocol was used [66]. This is a completely separate assay to the mitochondrial stress test, and allows for the thorough interrogation of glycolysis via the addition of supplements and inhibitors of the glycolytic pathway. Three measurements were taken at the basal point: after the addition of glucose (10 μM), after the addition of oligomycin (1.0 μM) and after the addition of 2-deoxyglucose (50 μM). The glycolysis stress test can measure several aspects of cellular glycolysis. These include the basal glycolytic rate of the cell, the maximum level of glycolysis the cell can achieve and the glycolytic reserve which refers to the difference between maximum level of glycolysis and the basal level of glycolysis. The different aspects of glycolysis are calculated by measuring the extracellular acidification rate (ECAR). ECAR rates were normalised to cell count as described above.

4.9. Statistical Analysis

For comparing each neuropsychological, neuroimaging and metabolic functional markers, a Student's *t*-test was used, comparing the means of the control group for each parameter to the disease group. Statistics were calculated using GraphPad Prism Software (V7.02). Analyses of covariance were also used for group comparisons including confounding variables. For covariate analysis when comparing control and disease group grey matter volumes, or when correlating neuropsychological and neuroimaging sAD markers with fibroblast functional markers, the IBM SPSS Statistics suite (Version 26; https://www.ibm.com/uk-en/products/spss-statistics) was used as this function was not available in the GraphPad Prism Software. Significance levels were adjusted to account for multiple comparisons.

5. Conclusions

These data highlight how in-depth analysis of mitochondrial and glycolytic function in sAD fibroblasts identifies metabolic abnormalities that parallel changes seen in neuropsychological features distinctive of the early stages of sporadic Alzheimer's disease. This model system could be used to develop biomarkers useful in early detection as well as in the development of novel therapeutic approaches for sAD.

Author Contributions: Conceptualization, S.M.B., D.J.B., H.M., L.F., A.V., M.D.M. and P.J.S.; Methodology, S.M.B., M.D.M., K.B., H.M. and A.V.; Software, S.M.B., and M.D.M.; Validation, S.M.B., D.J.B., K.B., H.M., L.F., A.V., M.D.M. and P.J.S.; Formal Analysis, S.M.B., D.J.B., K.B., H.M., L.F., A.V., M.D.M. and P.J.S.; Investigation, S.M.B., M.D.M., and K.B.; Resources, S.M.B., D.J.B., K.B., H.M., L.F., A.V., M.D.M. and P.J.S.; Data Curation, S.M.B., D.J.B., K.B., H.M., L.F., A.V., M.D.M. and P.J.S.; Writing—Original Draft Preparation, S.M.B.; Writing—Review and Editing, S.M.B., D.J.B., K.B., H.M., L.F., A.V., M.D.M. and P.J.S.; Visualization, S.M.B., D.J.B., K.B., H.M., L.F., A.V., M.D.M. and P.J.S.; Supervision, H.M., P.J.S., A.V., L.F. and D.J.B.; Project Administration, S.M.B.; Funding Acquisition, S.M.B., D.J.B., K.B., H.M., L.F., A.V. and P.J.S. All authors have read and agreed to the published version of the manuscript.

Acknowledgments: We would like to thank all research participants involved in this study. This research was supported by the Wellcome 4ward North Academy and ARUK Yorkshire Network Centre Small Grant Scheme (to SMB), Parkinson's UK (to HM, F1301) and the NIHR Sheffield Biomedical Research Centre. This is a summary of independent research carried out at the NIHR Sheffield Biomedical Research Centre (Translational Neuroscience). The views expressed are those of the author(s) and not necessarily those of the NHS, the NIHR or the Department of Health and Social Care (DHSC). Support of the European Union Seventh Framework Programme (FP7/2007–2013) under grant agreement no. 601055, VPH-DARE@IT to AV is acknowledged. PJS is supported by an NIHR Senior Investigator award. The support of the NIHR Clinical Research Facility—Sheffield Teaching Hospital is also acknowledged.

References

1. Wimo, A.; Guerchet, M.; Ali, G.-C.; Wu, Y.-T.; Prina, A.M.; Winblad, B.; Jönsson, L.; Liu, Z.; Prince, M. The worldwide costs of dementia 2015 and comparisons with 2010. *Alzheimer's Dement.* **2017**, *13*, 1–7. [CrossRef]
2. Scheltens, P.; Blennow, K.; Breteler, M.M.B.; de Strooper, B.; Frisoni, G.B.; Salloway, S.; Van der Flier, W.M. Alzheimer's disease. *Lancet* **2016**, *388*, 505–517. [CrossRef]
3. Brookmeyer, R.; Corrada, M.M.; Curriero, F.C.; Kawas, C. Survival following a diagnosis of Alzheimer disease. *Arch. Neurol.* **2002**, *59*, 1764–1767. [CrossRef]
4. Perl, D.P. Neuropathology of Alzheimer's Disease. *Mt. Sinai J. Med.* **2010**, *77*, 32–42. [CrossRef] [PubMed]
5. Hardy, J.; Selkoe, D.J. The Amyloid Hypothesis of Alzheimer's Disease: Progress and Problems on the Road to Therapeutics. *Science* **2002**, *297*, 353. [CrossRef] [PubMed]
6. Honig, L.S.; Vellas, B.; Woodward, M.; Boada, M.; Bullock, R.; Borrie, M.; Hager, K.; Andreasen, N.; Scarpini, E.; Liu-Seifert, H.; et al. Trial of Solanezumab for Mild Dementia Due to Alzheimer's Disease. *N. Engl. J. Med.* **2018**, *378*, 321–330. [CrossRef] [PubMed]
7. Cummings, J.L.; Morstorf, T.; Zhong, K. Alzheimer's disease drug-development pipeline: Few candidates, frequent failures. *Alzheimers Res. Ther.* **2014**, *6*, 37. [CrossRef]
8. ALZFORUM. Topline Result for First DIAN-TU Clinical Trial: Negative on Primary. Available online: https://www.alzforum.org/news/research-news/topline-result-first-dian-tu-clinical-trial-negative-primary (accessed on 29 March 2020).
9. Savva, G.M.; Wharton, S.B.; Ince, P.G.; Forster, G.; Matthews, F.E.; Brayne, C. Age, neuropathology, and dementia. *N. Engl. J. Med.* **2009**, *360*, 2302–2309. [CrossRef]
10. Le Couteur, D.G.; Hunter, S.; Brayne, C. Solanezumab and the amyloid hypothesis for Alzheimer's disease. *BMJ* **2016**, *355*, i6771. [CrossRef]
11. McKhann, G.M.; Knopman, D.S.; Chertkow, H.; Hyman, B.T.; Jack, C.R., Jr.; Kawas, C.H.; Klunk, W.E.; Koroshetz, W.J.; Manly, J.J.; Mayeux, R.; et al. The diagnosis of dementia due to Alzheimer's disease: Recommendations from the National Institute on Aging-Alzheimer's Association workgroups on diagnostic guidelines for Alzheimer's disease. *Alzheimers Dement. J. Alzheimers Assoc.* **2011**, *7*, 263–269. [CrossRef]
12. Braak, H.; Braak, E. Neuropathological stageing of Alzheimer-related changes. *Acta Neuropathol.* **1991**, *82*, 239–259. [CrossRef] [PubMed]
13. Haroutunian, V.; Schnaider-Beeri, M.; Schmeidler, J.; Wysocki, M.; Purohit, D.P.; Perl, D.P.; Libow, L.S.; Lesser, G.T.; Maroukian, M.; Grossman, H.T. Role of the neuropathology of Alzheimer disease in dementia in the oldest-old. *Arch. Neurol.* **2008**, *65*, 1211–1217. [CrossRef] [PubMed]
14. Weintraub, S.; Wicklund, A.H.; Salmon, D.P. The neuropsychological profile of Alzheimer disease. *Cold Spring Harb. Perspect. Med.* **2012**, *2*, a006171. [CrossRef] [PubMed]
15. Magistretti, P.J.; Allaman, I. A Cellular Perspective on Brain Energy Metabolism and Functional Imaging. *Neuron* **2015**, *86*, 883–901. [CrossRef]
16. Ewers, M.; Brendel, M.; Rizk-Jackson, A.; Rominger, A.; Bartenstein, P.; Schuff, N.; Weiner, M.W. Alzheimer's Disease Neuroimaging I Reduced FDG-PET brain metabolism and executive function predict clinical progression in elderly healthy subjects. *NeuroImage. Clin.* **2013**, *4*, 45–52. [CrossRef]
17. Kalpouzos, G.; Eustache, F.; de la Sayette, V.; Viader, F.; Chételat, G.; Desgranges, B. Working memory and FDG–PET dissociate early and late onset Alzheimer disease patients. *J. Neurol.* **2005**, *252*, 548–558. [CrossRef]
18. Ishii, K.; Sasaki, M.; Yamaji, S.; Sakamoto, S.; Kitagaki, H.; Mori, E. Demonstration of decreased posterior cingulate perfusion in mild Alzheimer's disease by means of H215O positron emission tomography. *Eur. J. Nucl. Med.* **1997**, *24*, 670–673.

19. Morgen, K.; Frolich, L. The metabolism hypothesis of Alzheimer's disease: From the concept of central insulin resistance and associated consequences to insulin therapy. *J. Neural Transm.* **2015**, *122*, 499–504. [CrossRef]
20. Yao, J.; Irwin, R.W.; Zhao, L.; Nilsen, J.; Hamilton, R.T.; Brinton, R.D. Mitochondrial bioenergetic deficit precedes Alzheimer's pathology in female mouse model of Alzheimer's disease. *Proc. Natl. Acad. Sci. USA* **2009**, *106*, 14670. [CrossRef]
21. Blass, J.P.; Sheu, R.K.; Gibson, G.E. Inherent abnormalities in energy metabolism in Alzheimer disease. Interaction with cerebrovascular compromise. *Ann. N. Y. Acad. Sci.* **2000**, *903*, 204–221. [CrossRef]
22. Baik, S.H.; Kang, S.; Lee, W.; Choi, H.; Chung, S.; Kim, J.I.; Mook-Jung, I. A Breakdown in Metabolic Reprogramming Causes Microglia Dysfunction in Alzheimer's Disease. *Cell Metab.* **2019**, *30*, 493–507.e496. [CrossRef] [PubMed]
23. Swerdlow, R.H.; Khan, S.M. A "mitochondrial cascade hypothesis" for sporadic Alzheimer's disease. *Med. Hypotheses* **2004**, *63*, 8–20. [CrossRef]
24. Hartl, D.; Schuldt, V.; Forler, S.; Zabel, C.; Klose, J.; Rohe, M. Presymptomatic Alterations in Energy Metabolism and Oxidative Stress in the APP23 Mouse Model of Alzheimer Disease. *J. Proteome Res.* **2012**, *11*, 3295–3304. [CrossRef]
25. Gan, X.Q.; Huang, S.B.; Wu, L.; Wang, Y.F.; Hu, G.; Li, G.Y.; Zhang, H.J.; Yu, H.Y.; Swerdlow, R.H.; Chen, J.X.; et al. Inhibition of ERK-DLP1 signaling and mitochondrial division alleviates mitochondrial dysfunction in Alzheimer's disease cybrid cell. *Biochim. Biophys. Acta Mol. Basis Dis.* **2014**, *1842*, 220–231. [CrossRef] [PubMed]
26. Mosconi, L.; Tsui, W.H.; De Santi, S.; Li, J.; Rusinek, H.; Convit, A.; Li, Y.; Boppana, M.; de Leon, M.J. Reduced hippocampal metabolism in MCI and AD: Automated FDG-PET image analysis. *Neurology* **2005**, *64*, 1860–1867. [CrossRef] [PubMed]
27. Vlassenko, A.G.; Vaishnavi, S.N.; Couture, L.; Sacco, D.; Shannon, B.J.; Mach, R.H.; Morris, J.C.; Raichle, M.E.; Mintun, M.A. Spatial correlation between brain aerobic glycolysis and amyloid-beta (Abeta) deposition. *Proc. Natl. Acad. Sci. USA* **2010**, *107*, 17763–17767. [CrossRef]
28. Vlassenko, A.G.; Gordon, B.A.; Goyal, M.S.; Su, Y.; Blazey, T.M.; Durbin, T.J.; Couture, L.E.; Christensen, J.J.; Jafri, H.; Morris, J.C.; et al. Aerobic glycolysis and tau deposition in preclinical Alzheimer's disease. *Neurobiol. Aging* **2018**, *67*, 95–98. [CrossRef]
29. Bell, S.M.; Barnes, K.; Clemmens, H.; Al-Rafiah, A.R.; Al-Ofi, E.A.; Leech, V.; Bandmann, O.; Shaw, P.J.; Blackburn, D.J.; Ferraiuolo, L.; et al. Ursodeoxycholic Acid Improves Mitochondrial Function and Redistributes Drp1 in Fibroblasts from Patients with Either Sporadic or Familial Alzheimer's Disease. *J. Mol. Biol.* **2018**, *430*, 3942–3953. [CrossRef]
30. Pickart, L.; Vasquez-Soltero, J.M.; Margolina, A. The Effect of the Human Peptide GHK on Gene Expression Relevant to Nervous System Function and Cognitive Decline. *Brain Sci.* **2017**, *7*, 20. [CrossRef]
31. Desler, C.; Hansen, T.L.; Frederiksen, J.B.; Marcker, M.L.; Singh, K.K.; Juel Rasmussen, L. Is There a Link between Mitochondrial Reserve Respiratory Capacity and Aging? *J. Aging Res.* **2012**, *2012*, 192503. [CrossRef]
32. Martino Adami, P.V.; Quijano, C.; Magnani, N.; Galeano, P.; Evelson, P.; Cassina, A.; Do Carmo, S.; Leal, M.C.; Castaño, E.M.; Cuello, A.C.; et al. Synaptosomal bioenergetic defects are associated with cognitive impairment in a transgenic rat model of early Alzheimer's disease. *Off. J. Int. Soc. Cereb. Blood Flow Metab.* **2017**, *37*, 69–84. [CrossRef] [PubMed]
33. Capitani, E.; Rosci, C.; Saetti, M.C.; Laiacona, M. Mirror asymmetry of Category and Letter fluency in traumatic brain injury and Alzheimer's patients. *Neuropsychologia* **2009**, *47*, 423–429. [CrossRef] [PubMed]
34. Folstein, M.F.; Folstein, S.E.; McHugh, P.R. "Mini-mental state". A practical method for grading the cognitive state of patients for the clinician. *J. Psychiatr. Res.* **1975**, *12*, 189–198. [CrossRef]
35. Doody, R.S.; Massman, P.; Dunn, J.K. A method for estimating progression rates in Alzheimer disease. *Arch. Neurol.* **2001**, *58*, 449–454. [CrossRef] [PubMed]
36. Scahill, R.I.; Schott, J.M.; Stevens, J.M.; Rossor, M.N.; Fox, N.C. Mapping the evolution of regional atrophy in Alzheimer's disease: Unbiased analysis of fluid-registered serial MRI. *Proc. Natl. Acad. Sci. USA* **2002**, *99*, 4703–4707. [CrossRef] [PubMed]
37. Boller, B.; Mellah, S.; Ducharme-Laliberte, G.; Belleville, S. Relationships between years of education, regional grey matter volumes, and working memory-related brain activity in healthy older adults. *Brain Imaging Behav.* **2017**, *11*, 304–317. [CrossRef]

38. Rzezak, P.; Squarzoni, P.; Duran, F.L.; de Toledo Ferraz Alves, T.; Tamashiro-Duran, J.; Bottino, C.M.; Ribeiz, S.; Lotufo, P.A.; Menezes, P.R.; Scazufca, M.; et al. Relationship between Brain Age-Related Reduction in Gray Matter and Educational Attainment. *PLoS ONE* **2015**, *10*, e0140945. [CrossRef]
39. Harada, C.N.; Natelson Love, M.C.; Triebel, K.L. Normal cognitive aging. *Clin. Geriatr. Med.* **2013**, *29*, 737–752. [CrossRef]
40. Stern, Y. Cognitive reserve: Implications for assessment and intervention. *Folia Phoniatr. Logop. Off. Organ. Int. Assoc. Logop. Phoniatr. IALP* **2013**, *65*, 49–54. [CrossRef]
41. Schniertshauer, D.; Gebhard, D.; Bergemann, J. Age-Dependent Loss of Mitochondrial Function in Epithelial Tissue Can Be Reversed by Coenzyme Q10. *J. Aging Res.* **2018**, *2018*, 6354680. [CrossRef] [PubMed]
42. Sriskanthadevan, S.; Jeyaraju, D.V.; Chung, T.E.; Prabha, S.; Xu, W.; Skrtic, M.; Jhas, B.; Hurren, R.; Gronda, M.; Wang, X.; et al. AML cells have low spare reserve capacity in their respiratory chain that renders them susceptible to oxidative metabolic stress. *Blood* **2015**, *125*, 2120–2130. [CrossRef] [PubMed]
43. Yadava, N.; Nicholls, D.G. Spare Respiratory Capacity Rather Than Oxidative Stress Regulates Glutamate Excitotoxicity after Partial Respiratory Inhibition of Mitochondrial Complex I with Rotenone. *J. Neurosci.* **2007**, *27*, 7310–7317. [CrossRef] [PubMed]
44. Mortiboys, H.; Johansen, K.K.; Aasly, J.O.; Bandmann, O. Mitochondrial impairment in patients with Parkinson disease with the G2019S mutation in LRRK2. *Neurology* **2010**, *75*, 2017–2020. [CrossRef] [PubMed]
45. Tan, W.; Pasinelli, P.; Trotti, D. Role of mitochondria in mutant SOD1 linked amyotrophic lateral sclerosis. *Biochim. Biophys. Acta* **2014**, *1842*, 1295–1301. [CrossRef]
46. Carling, P.J.; Mortiboys, H.; Green, C.; Mihaylov, S.; Sandor, C.; Schwartzentruber, A.; Taylor, R.; Wei, W.; Hastings, C.; Wong, S.; et al. Deep phenotyping of peripheral tissue facilitates mechanistic disease stratification in sporadic Parkinson's disease. *Prog. Neurobiol.* **2020**, *187*, 101772. [CrossRef]
47. Milanese, C.; Payán-Gómez, C.; Galvani, M.; Molano González, N.; Tresini, M.; Nait Abdellah, S.; van Roon-Mom, W.M.; Figini, S.; Marinus, J.; van Hilten, J.J.; et al. Peripheral mitochondrial function correlates with clinical severity in idiopathic Parkinson's disease. *Mov. Disord.* **2019**, *34*, 1192–1202. [CrossRef] [PubMed]
48. Gottlieb, E.; Armour, S.M.; Harris, M.H.; Thompson, C.B. Mitochondrial membrane potential regulates matrix configuration and cytochrome c release during apoptosis. *Cell Death Differ.* **2003**, *10*, 709–717. [CrossRef]
49. Grogan, A.; Green, D.W.; Ali, N.; Crinion, J.T.; Price, C.J. Structural correlates of semantic and phonemic fluency ability in first and second languages. *Cereb. Cortex* **2009**, *19*, 2690–2698. [CrossRef]
50. Venneri, A.; Jahn-Carta, C.; De Marco, M.; Quaranta, D.; Marra, C. Diagnostic and prognostic role of semantic processing in preclinical Alzheimer's disease. *Biomark. Med.* **2018**, *12*, 637–651. [CrossRef]
51. Baldo, J.V.; Schwartz, S.; Wilkins, D.; Dronkers, N.F. Role of frontal versus temporal cortex in verbal fluency as revealed by voxel-based lesion symptom mapping. *J. Int. Neuropsychol. Soc.* **2006**, *12*, 896–900. [CrossRef]
52. Liang, W.S.; Reiman, E.M.; Valla, J.; Dunckley, T.; Beach, T.G.; Grover, A.; Niedzielko, T.L.; Schneider, L.E.; Mastroeni, D.; Caselli, R.; et al. Alzheimer's disease is associated with reduced expression of energy metabolism genes in posterior cingulate neurons. *Proc. Natl. Acad. Sci. USA* **2008**, *105*, 4441–4446. [CrossRef] [PubMed]
53. Mosconi, L. Brain glucose metabolism in the early and specific diagnosis of Alzheimer's disease. FDG-PET studies in MCI and AD. *Eur. J. Nucl. Med. Mol. Imaging* **2005**, *32*, 486–510. [CrossRef] [PubMed]
54. Ramanoël, S.; Hoyau, E.; Kauffmann, L.; Renard, F.; Pichat, C.; Boudiaf, N.; Krainik, A.; Jaillard, A.; Baciu, M. Gray Matter Volume and Cognitive Performance During Normal Aging. A Voxel-Based Morphometry Study. *Front. Aging Neurosci.* **2018**, *10*, 235. [CrossRef] [PubMed]
55. Maynard, S.; Hejl, A.M.; Dinh, T.S.T.; Keijzers, G.; Hansen, Å.M.; Desler, C.; Moreno-Villanueva, M.; Bürkle, A.; Rasmussen, L.J.; Waldemar, G.; et al. Defective mitochondrial respiration, altered dNTP pools and reduced AP endonuclease 1 activity in peripheral blood mononuclear cells of Alzheimer's disease patients. *Aging* **2015**, *7*, 793. [CrossRef]
56. Fisar, Z.; Hroudová, J.; Hansíková, H.; Lelková, P.; Wenchich, L.; Jirák, R.; Zeman, J.; Martásek, P.; Raboch, J. Mitochondrial Respiration in the Platelets of Patients with Alzheimer's Disease. *Curr. Alzheimer Res.* **2016**, *13*, 930–941. [CrossRef]
57. Martin-Maestro, P.; Gargini, R.; Garcia, E.; Perry, G.; Avila, J. Slower Dynamics and Aged Mitochondria in Sporadic Alzheimer's Disease. *Oxid. Med. Cell. Longev.* **2017**, *2017*, 9302761. [CrossRef]

58. Sonntag, K.C.; Ryu, W.I.; Amirault, K.M.; Healy, R.A.; Siegel, A.J.; McPhie, D.L.; Forester, B.; Cohen, B.M. Late-onset Alzheimer's disease is associated with inherent changes in bioenergetics profiles. *Sci. Rep.* **2017**, *7*, 14038. [CrossRef]
59. Takahashi, K.; Yamanaka, S. Induction of pluripotent stem cells from mouse embryonic and adult fibroblast cultures by defined factors. *Cell* **2006**, *126*, 663–676. [CrossRef]
60. Mertens, J.; Paquola, A.C.; Ku, M.; Hatch, E.; Böhnke, L.; Ladjevardi, S.; McGrath, S.; Campbell, B.; Lee, H.; Herdy, J.R.; et al. Directly Reprogrammed Human Neurons Retain Aging-Associated Transcriptomic Signatures and Reveal Age-Related Nucleocytoplasmic Defects. *Cell Stem Cell* **2015**, *17*, 705–718. [CrossRef]
61. Wakefield, S.J.; McGeown, W.J.; Shanks, M.F.; Venneri, A. Differentiating normal from pathological brain ageing using standard neuropsychological tests. *Curr. Alzheimer Res.* **2014**, *11*, 765–772. [CrossRef]
62. De Marco, M.; Duzzi, D.; Meneghello, F.; Venneri, A. Cognitive Efficiency in Alzheimer's Disease is Associated with Increased Occipital Connectivity. *J. Alzheimers Dis.* **2017**, *57*, 541–556. [CrossRef] [PubMed]
63. Cardoso, M.J.; Leung, K.; Modat, M.; Keihaninejad, S.; Cash, D.; Barnes, J.; Fox, N.C.; Ourselin, S. STEPS: Similarity and Truth Estimation for Propagated Segmentations and its application to hippocampal segmentation and brain parcelation. *Med. Image Anal.* **2013**, *17*, 671–684. [CrossRef] [PubMed]
64. Vijayakumar, A.; Vijayakumar, A. Comparison of hippocampal volume in dementia subtypes. *ISRN Radiol.* **2013**, *2013*, 174524. [CrossRef] [PubMed]
65. Mortiboys, H.; Thomas, K.J.; Koopman, W.J.; Klaffke, S.; Abou-Sleiman, P.; Olpin, S.; Wood, N.W.; Willems, P.H.; Smeitink, J.A.; Cookson, M.R. Mitochondrial function and morphology are impaired in parkin-mutant fibroblasts. *Ann. Neurol.* **2008**, *64*, 555–565. [CrossRef] [PubMed]
66. Agilent Technologies, Agilent Seahorse XF Glycolysis Stress Test Kit. Available online: https://www.agilent.com/cs/library/usermanuals/public/XF_Glycolysis_Stress_Test_Kit_User_Guide.pdf (accessed on 29 March 2020).

11

Alterations of the Endoplasmic Reticulum (ER) Calcium Signaling Molecular Components in Alzheimer's Disease

Mounia Chami * and Frédéric Checler

Team Labelled "Laboratory of Excellence (LABEX) DistAlz", INSERM, CNRS, IPMC, Université Côte d'Azur, 660 route des Lucioles, Sophia-Antipolis, 06560 Valbonne, France; checler@ipmc.cnrs.fr

* Correspondence: mchami@ipmc.cnrs.fr

Abstract: Sustained imbalance in intracellular calcium (Ca^{2+}) entry and clearance alters cellular integrity, ultimately leading to cellular homeostasis disequilibrium and cell death. Alzheimer's disease (AD) is the most common cause of dementia. Beside the major pathological features associated with AD-linked toxic amyloid beta (Aβ) and hyperphosphorylated tau (p-tau), several studies suggested the contribution of altered Ca^{2+} handling in AD development. These studies documented physical or functional interactions of Aβ with several Ca^{2+} handling proteins located either at the plasma membrane or in intracellular organelles including the endoplasmic reticulum (ER), considered the major intracellular Ca^{2+} pool. In this review, we describe the cellular components of ER Ca^{2+} dysregulations likely responsible for AD. These include alterations of the inositol 1,4,5-trisphosphate receptors' (IP_3Rs) and ryanodine receptors' (RyRs) expression and function, dysfunction of the sarco-endoplasmic reticulum Ca^{2+} ATPase (SERCA) activity and upregulation of its truncated isoform (S1T), as well as presenilin (PS1, PS2)-mediated ER Ca^{2+} leak/ER Ca^{2+} release potentiation. Finally, we highlight the functional consequences of alterations of these ER Ca^{2+} components in AD pathology and unravel the potential benefit of targeting ER Ca^{2+} homeostasis as a tool to alleviate AD pathogenesis.

Keywords: calcium; Alzheimer's disease; endoplasmic reticulum; SERCA; IP_3R; RyR; S1T; presenilin

---

1. Introduction

1.1. Ca^{2+} Signaling

As a signal transduction molecule, calcium (Ca^{2+}) regulates a large number of neuronal processes including growth and differentiation, neurotransmitter release and synaptic function, activity-dependent changes in gene expression and apoptosis [1]. Cytosolic Ca^{2+} ($[Ca^{2+}]$cyt) signals are regulated in a spatiotemporal-dependent manner underlined by an intricate interplay between Ca^{2+} entry through the plasma membrane, storage in the internal stores (i.e., the endoplasmic reticulum (ER), considered the major dynamic Ca^{2+} intracellular pool), Ca^{2+} mobilization from the ER and its buffering by Ca^{2+}-binding proteins (CaBP) (Figure 1). Ca^{2+} entry through the plasma membrane occurs through ligand-dependent Ca^{2+} receptors (i.e., *N*-methyl-D-aspartate receptor (NMDA) and Alpha7 nicotinic acetylcholine receptors (nAChRs)) and through voltage-gated Ca^{2+} channels (VGCC) (Figure 1). Ca^{2+} mobilization from the ER occurs through activation of the inositol 1,4,5-trisphosphate receptors (IP_3R) downstream of metabotropic receptors (Figure 1), or through the activation of ryanodine receptors (RyRs) that are activated by a slight increase in $[Ca^{2+}]$cyt, a mechanism known as Ca^{2+}-induced Ca^{2+} release (CICR) (Figure 1). Elevations of cytosolic Ca^{2+} signals are "shut down" through the plasma membrane Na^+/Ca^{2+} exchanger (NCX) and two Ca^{2+} ATPases which consume ATP to actively extrude Ca^{2+} out of the cells (i.e., the plasma membrane

Ca^{2+} ATPase (PMCA)) or to actively sequester Ca^{2+} into the ER lumen (i.e., the sarco-endoplasmic reticulum Ca^{2+} ATPase (SERCA)) (Figure 1). Intriguingly, coupling between ER Ca^{2+} depletion and Ca^{2+} influx through the plasma membrane occurs through a canonical store-operated Ca^{2+} entry (SOCE) pathway [2] mainly consisting of a direct physical interaction between the Ca^{2+}-sensing stromal interacting molecules (STIM1/2) oligomers within the ER membrane and the pore-forming ORAI proteins in the plasma membrane [3–5] (Figure 1). Several lines of evidence indicate that Ca^{2+} homeostasis could be disrupted upon cellular challenges as well as in neurodegenerative conditions.

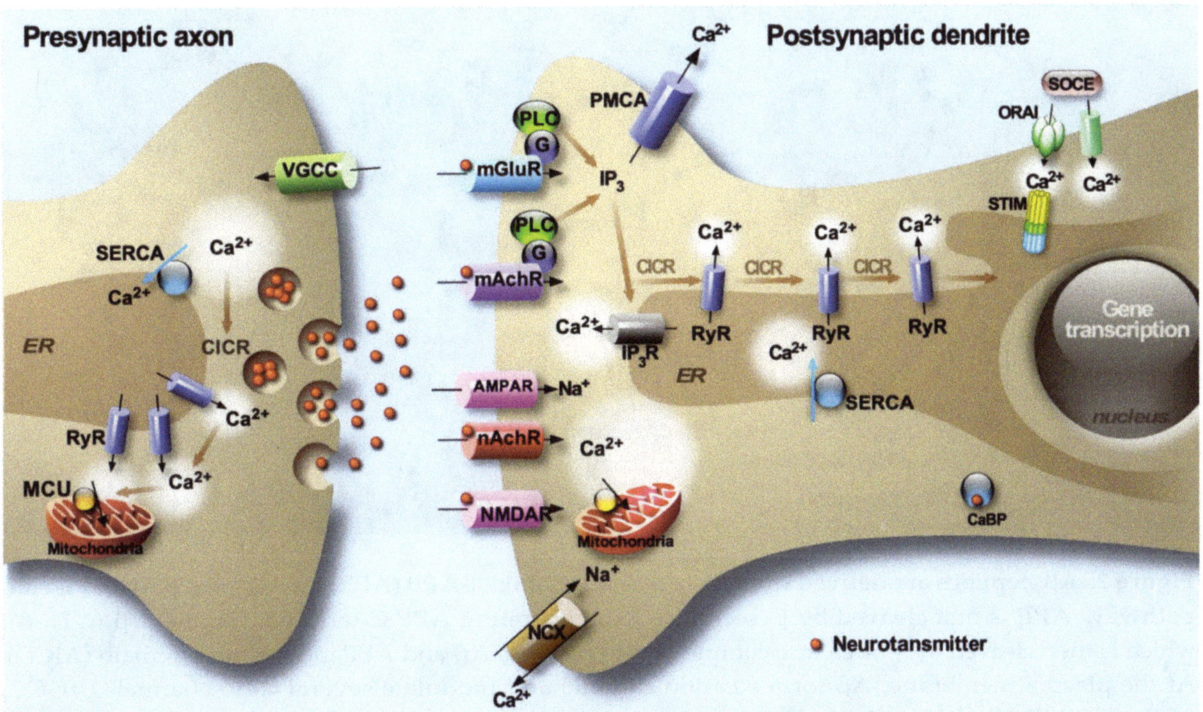

Figure 1. Elevations of intraneuronal [Ca^{2+}] are the result of an influx across the plasma membrane and the release from the ER through various channels and receptors. The low intraneuronal Ca^{2+} level is then maintained by the activity of Ca^{2+}-binding proteins (CaBP) and involves the sodium-Ca^{2+} exchanger (Na^+/Ca^{2+}) acting in concert with the ATP-dependent Ca^{2+} pumps located at the plasma membrane and the ER. Depletion of ER Ca^{2+} content activates the store-operated Ca^{2+} entry (SOCE) pathway.

1.2. *Alzheimer's Disease*

Alzheimer's disease (AD) is an age-associated dementia disorder characterized by the accumulation of extracellular amyloid-beta (Aβ) peptides in the senile plaques and by the hyperphosphorylation of tau (pTau) protein, leading to intracellular protein aggregation into bundles or filaments that are deposited as neurofibrillary tangles [6–8]. Notably, Aβ peptide derives from the sequential processing of the β-amyloid precursor protein (βAPP referred to as APP hereafter) [9,10] by the β-seceretase (BACE1) and the γ–secretase complex (composed of presenilins (PSs: PS1 or PS2, the catalytic subunits of the enzyme), Nicastrin, anterior pharynx-defective-1 (APH-1) and presenilin enhancer-2 (PEN-2) [11,12])) (Figure 2). Importantly, a significant number of aggressive AD cases generally characterized by early onset are inherited in an autosomal-dominant manner (FAD: familial AD) and are caused by mutations on APP and on PS1 and PS2 [13,14] (Figure 2). These mutations either modify the nature of Aβ peptides and/or affect the levels of their production [15,16]. Besides the canonical disease-associated intracellular pTau and extracellular Aβ accumulations, recent studies unraveled additional processes that could contribute to AD progression, including: (i) the intracellular accumulation of Aβ [17,18] and other APP-derived fragments [18–24], and (ii) the spreading of both extracellular Tau and Aβ between neurons and between neurons and glial cells [25,26].

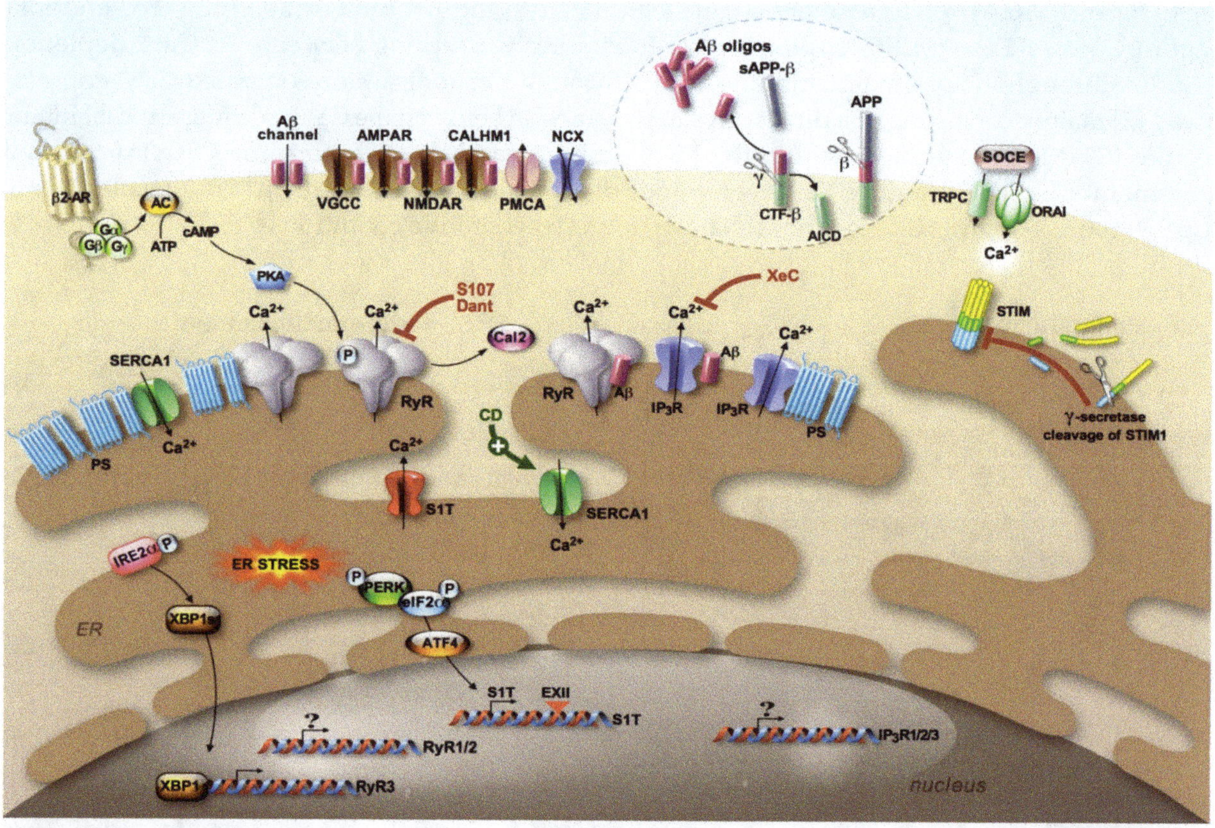

Figure 2. Aβ peptides are derived from the processing of the βAPP (APP) through the amyloidogenic pathway. APP is first cleaved by β–secretase (β), generating APP C-terminal fragment β (CTF-β), which is then cleaved by γ–secretase complex (γ) to produce Aβ and APP intracellular domain (AICD). At the plasma membrane, Aβ form a cation channel and modulate several Ca^{2+} channels (VGCC, AMPAR, NMDAR and CALHM1). ER Ca^{2+} deregulation occurs through presenilin (PS)-associated Ca^{2+} leak and/or enhanced IP_3R- and RyR-mediated Ca^{2+} release, dysfunctional Sarco-endoplasmic reticulum Ca^{2+} ATPase (SERCA) activity, enhanced expression of S1T driven by ER stress response and enhanced expression and dysfunctional IP_3Rs and RyRs. SOCE is also deregulated in AD and implicates STIM, ORAI and TRPC. RyR2 macromolecular complex destabilization (PKA phosphorylation and calstabin2 (Cal2) dissociation) is linked to β2-adrenergic receptor activation. Pharmacological stabilization of ER Ca^{2+} content by S107, Dantrolene (Dant) blocking RyRs-mediated Ca^{2+} release/leak, Xestospongin C (XeC) blocking IP_3R-mediated Ca^{2+} release and CD1163 (CD) activating SERCA provided beneficial effects in reversing several AD-related pathogenic paradigms in vitro and in vivo.

1.3. Physiology of ER Calcium Handling in Neurons

The ER forms a continuous and highly motile network distributed throughout the neuron. Within dendrites and dendritic spines, ER Ca^{2+} release is involved in modulating postsynaptic responses and synaptic plasticity [27]. In presynaptic nerve terminals, as well as in growth cones, ER is involved in vesicle fusion and neurotransmitter release [28,29]. In the soma, ER Ca^{2+} handling is coupled to the activation of Ca^{2+}-sensitive kinases and phosphatases [30]. In the perinuclear space, ER Ca^{2+} handling triggers gene transcription [31]. Ca^{2+} mobilization from the ER has been shown to be involved in growth cone activity and in the formation of new connections and/or the strengthening of preexisting connections that occur during learning and memory in the adult brain [32].

1.4. Calcium Deregulation in AD

As stated above, the tight but subtle control of intracellular Ca^{2+} homeostasis is required for neuronal health, development and function [29,30,33,34]. Therefore, persistent imbalance in Ca^{2+}

entry and clearance alters cellular integrity, leading to cellular homeostasis disequilibrium. These Ca^{2+} deregulations ultimately trigger excessive proliferation or cell death depending on the strength and the duration of the insult and in a cell-type-specific manner. Ca^{2+} signaling deregulation has a central role in AD pathophysiology [35]. The relevance of Ca^{2+} signaling in AD is supported by the fact that Ca^{2+} alterations were reported in both sporadic (SAD) and familial (FAD) forms of AD and that this can exacerbate Aβ formation and promote tau hyperphosphorylation [35–37]. As first evidence, in vitro studies have shown that Ca^{2+} may directly interact and enhance the proteolytic activity of BACE1 [38] and to stabilize γ–secretase and enhance its activity in reconstituted in vitro assay [39]. Moreover, tau hyperphosphorylation at disease-specific sites has been associated with abnormal intracellular Ca^{2+} signaling occurring upstream of Ca^{2+}/calmodulin (CaM)-dependent protein kinase II (CaMKII) and CDK5 activation [37,40–42]. The bulk of data gathered these last 30 years allows us to draw up a scenario where Ca^{2+} deregulation is not only a consequence of the disease but also participates in a feedback loop to disease progression and amplification [35,36,43–46]. These studies reported a Ca^{2+}-dependent enhancement of APP processing and the production of toxic APP-derived fragments, activation of signaling cascades through the modulation of kinases and phosphatases activities, thus affecting synaptic plasticity and cognitive function [34–36,47–49].

Several studies demonstrated a tight relationship between altered Ca^{2+} handling and the amyloidogenic cascade. These studies lead to identifying the physical or functional interaction of Aβ with several Ca^{2+} handling proteins in various AD models. At least four lines of evidence have emerged: (i) at the plasma membrane, Aβ has been shown to form a cation channel [50], or to act as a channel-modulator for the VGCCs, the nAChRs, the ionotropic glutamatereceptors NMDARs and AMPARs (α-amino-3-hydroxy-5-methyl-4-isoxazolepropionic acid receptors), the Ca^{2+} homeostasis modulator 1 (CALHM1), and more recently the store-operated Ca^{2+}channels (SOCE) (Figure 2) [51–60]; (ii) dysfunctional mitochondria were associated with Aβ-mediated Ca^{2+} toxicity [61,62] (discussed in this Special Issue [63]). Importantly, mitochondrial permeability transition pore, mitochondrial Ca^{2+} uniporter (MCU) dysfunctions and impaired mitochondrial Ca^{2+} efflux contribute to mitochondrial alteration in AD [63–65]; (iii) the autophagic failure in AD has been linked to lysosomal degradation defects [24,66] likely occurring upon lysosomal Ca^{2+} depletion [67,68]; (iv) a complex scenario of AD-associated ER Ca^{2+} dysregulation also emerged, where disturbances were linked to presenilin (PS1 and PS2)-associated ER Ca^{2+} leak and/or ER Ca^{2+} release potentiation functions [69–73], dysfunctional SERCA activity [74] and the upregulation of the recently described SERCA1 truncated isoform (S1T) [75], alterations of IP_3Rs function [56,69,70,72,76–81] and dysfunctional RyRs [44,80,82–94] (Figure 2).

Besides APP-derived amyloidogenic products, previous studies described a physiological role of APP in regulating Ca^{2+} signaling. Knockdown of endogenous APP increases the frequency and reduces the amplitude of neuronal Ca^{2+} oscillations [95]. In addition, a recent study specifically reported that APP-deficient cells exhibited elevated resting Ca^{2+} levels in the ER and reduced ER Ca^{2+} leakage rates [96]. Pathogenic tau has also been associated with nuclear Ca^{2+} deregulation [97], with increasing the ionic current of artificial membranes [98], with inducing spontaneous Ca^{2+} oscillations in the neurons [99] and with the inhibition of mitochondrial Ca^{2+} efflux via the mitochondrial Na^+/Ca^{2+} exchanger [99] (also discussed in this Special Issue [63]).

In this review, we will specifically present an update of the alterations of the molecular components controlling ER Ca^{2+} signaling in AD and discuss the potential benefit of targeting ER Ca^{2+} homeostasis as a tool to alleviate AD pathogenesis.

2. The Ryanodine Receptors: RyRs

RyRs are a family of three mammalian isoforms, RyR1, RyR2 and RyR3, mainly expressed in the skeletal muscle, heart and brain. All RyRs isoforms are expressed in the brain, with an abundance range of order as follows, RyR2 > RyR1 >> RyR3 [100,101]. RyRs activity is influenced on the one hand by Ca^{2+}, Mg^{2+} and ATP [102–105] and, on the other hand, by the integrated effects of co-proteins forming

RyR1 and RyR2 homotetramer macromolecular complexes [106–108]. These include calmodulin (CaM) [109,110], FKBP12 (12.0 kDa) and FKBP12.6 (12.6 kDa), known as Calstabin1 (Cal1) and Calstabin2 (Cal2), respectively [111]; PKA anchored to RyR1 and RyR2 via a kinase anchoring protein (mAKAP) [112,113], and Ca^{2+}/calmodulin-dependent protein kinase II (CaMKII) [114]. Other regulatory proteins were also described to interact with RYR1, thus controlling the channel gating activity [109]. RyR1/2 macromolecular complexes contain also the requisite molecular machinery allowing channel dephosphorylation (i.e., PP1 and PP2A) [113,115,116].

Enhanced RyR-mediated Ca^{2+} release was reported in primary cultured neurons derived from 3xTg-AD mice (knock in (KI) for the mutated PS1M146V and overexpressing mutated APP and microtubule-associated tau protein (PS1M146V/APPswe/tauP301L)) [85,87]. This was further confirmed in cellular models expressing wild-type or mutated APP, PS1 or PS2 [44,80,82–84,86–94,117]. Exacerbated IP_3R-evoked Ca^{2+} signals in AD mice (PS1KI and 3xTg-AD)-derived neurons were shown to be linked to RYR-associated CICR [85]. These findings were further supported by using the RyR blocker dantrolene (Dant), shown to reduce enhanced $[Ca^{2+}]$cyt level [92,93,118]. While some studies reported that RyR dysfunction in AD-related study models occurs independently of PS mutation or overexpression, namely in models expressing APP and overproducing Aβ [86,92,119–122], in many cases, PS mutation-mediated Ca^{2+} deregulation was associated with the alteration of the activity of RyRs (discussed beyond in PSs chapter). In addition, it was also reported that exogenous Aβ oligomers may directly stimulate RyR-mediated Ca^{2+} release [123] and that the application of soluble Aβ caused a marked increase in channel open probability [124].

RyR isoform expression is modified throughout AD progression and between different brain regions [125]. Exogenous application of Aβ peptide was also shown to specifically increase RyR3 isoform expression [86,123]. RyRs mRNAs increase throughout the lifetime of PS1-M146V transgenic mice and 3xTg-AD mice [84,85,87] as well as in cellular and mice AD models overexpressing wild-type or mutated APP (bearing the Swedish mutation APPswe) [92]. Conversely, neuronal conditional PS1/2 knockout (KO) (PScDKO) is associated with a downregulation of RyR2 expression, demonstrating that PS may regulate Ca^{2+} homeostasis and synaptic function via RyRs [126]. It has been proposed that the modulation of RyR expression may act as a disease promoter or a compensatory beneficial mechanism. In fact, while on the one hand, enhanced $[Ca^{2+}]$cyt response is associated with the increased expression of RyRs [127], the activation of the ER stress response factor X-box binding protein 1 spliced isoform (XBP1s) may occur upon Aβ oligomer treatment [128,129], triggering a reduction of $[Ca^{2+}]$cyt linked to the down-expression of the RyR3 isoform [130]. Accordingly, a dual role for endogenous RyR3 has been suggested in an AD mouse model. Thus, the deletion of RyR3 in young (≤ 3 mo) APPPS1 mice increased hippocampal neuronal network excitability and accelerated AD pathology, leading to mushroom spine loss and increased Aβ accumulation. Meanwhile, deletion of RyR3 in older APPPS1 mice (≥6 mo) rescued network excitability and mushroom spine loss, reduced Aβ load and reduced spontaneous seizure occurrence [131] (Figure 2).

RyRs mutations are liked to various pathologies affecting muscle and heart [132,133]. The development of transgenic mouse models (i.e., KO of RyR1, RyR2 or RyR3, or expressing RyR harboring disease mutations, or lacking exon sequence) [134] strengthens the fact that RyRs play a key role in physiology and pathophysiology. The viability of RyR3 KO mouse, in contrast to the RyR1 and RyR2 KO mice [135,136], led to the demonstration that RyR3-deficient mice exhibit decreased social behavior [137], greater locomotor activity [136,138], altered memory [138,139] associated with impaired maintenance of long-term potentiation (LTP) [140]. To date, no mutations have been reported in RYRs linked to brain disorders. Nevertheless, the role of leaky RyR2 in the pathogenesis of epilepsy has been described in the RyR2-R2474S mice model [101]. Interestingly, three single nuclear polymorphisms were significantly associated with risk for hypertension, diabetes and AD [141]. A meta-analysis based on four genome-wide association study (GWAS) also identified *RYR3* association with AD risk [142]. Another study observed a significant interaction between *RYR3* and *CACNA1C* (gene encoding for the

Ca^{2+} voltage-gated channel subunit Alpha1 C) in three independent datasets of AD Neuroimaging Initiative cohorts [143].

RyRs post-translational modifications (PTMs) shift the channel from a finely regulated state to a non-regulated Ca^{2+} leak channel. RyR PTMs were associated with different pathologies affecting skeletal muscle, heart and, recently, brain [133] [113,144–150]. Experimental transgenic mice expressing RyR harboring PKA-non-phosphorylated sites or phosphomimetic RyR mutants demonstrated the role of the PKA phosphorylation site in RyR macromolecular complex remodeling, Calstabin dissociation and ER Ca^{2+} leak [133]. In addition to phosphorylation sites, RyRs also contain a large number of amino acid residues that are potential targets for reactive oxygen species (ROS) and for reactive nitrogen species (RNS) [108,151,152]. Recently, we described a new molecular mechanism and signaling cascade underlying altered RyR-mediated intracellular Ca^{2+} release in AD [116,150,153]. We reported that the RyR2 channel undergoes PKA phosphorylation, oxidation/nitrosylation and depletion of the channel stabilizing subunit Calstabin2 in SH-SY5Y neuroblastoma cells expressing APP harboring the familial Swedish mutations (APPswe), in APP/PS1 (APPswe, PS1-M146V), as well as in 3xTg-AD, transgenic mice models and, most importantly, in human SAD brains [150,153]. We further reported that RyR2 macromolecular complex remodeling occurs through synergistic mitochondrial reactive oxygen species (ROS) production and β-adrenergic stimulation [150,153]. Notably, oxidative stress is considered a major contributor to AD pathogenesis [154,155], and β2-adrenergic receptors (β2-ARs) have also been implicated in the development of AD [51,156–161]. However, targeting β-adrenergic signaling is questionable, since both beneficial versus defective effects were described in AD mice [162–164]. In our study, we specifically targeted the downstream PKA-mediated RyR2 phosphorylation and macromolecular complex destabilization (Figure 2). We showed that pharmacological stabilization of calstabin2 on the RyR2 macromolecular complex by S107 (a benzothiazepine derivative molecule [101]) reduces elevated Ca^{2+} signals in AD cells [153], prevents ER Ca^{2+} leakage and reduces single channel open probabilities in AD mice brains [150]. Most importantly, S107 treatment reduces APP processing and Aβ production both in vitro and in vivo [150,153]. S107 administration also inhibited calpain activity and AMPK-dependent tau phosphorylation in an APP/PS1 mouse model [150]. These data agree well with previously reported studies demonstrating the beneficial effects of the pharmacological targeting of RyR with dantrolene [88,92,93,165]. In support of these findings, RyR macromolecular complex stabilization improved the hippocampal synaptic plasticity (LTP and LTD) and cognitive function of APP/PS1 and 3xTg-AD mice [150]. Importantly, we further showed that crossing APP/PS1 mice with RyR2-S2808A KI mice, harboring RyR2 channels that cannot be PKA-phosphorylated, resulted in improved cognitive function and decreased neuropathology. In contrast, phosphormimetic RyR2-S2808D KI mice exhibit early altered hippocampal synaptic plasticity (LTP and LTD) and cognitive dysfunction [150]. Overall, these results emphasize the broad implication of RyRs in ER Ca^{2+} signaling deregulation in AD occurring through the regulation of RYRs expression, CICR-dependent activity, macromolecular complex stability-linked to β2-AR signaling cascade, Aβ- and PS-mediated RyRs channel opening and likely RYR3 gene polymorphism.

3. The Inositol 1,4,5-Trisphosphate Receptors: IP_3Rs

Among the three IP_3Rs isoforms, the predominant one in neurons is IP_3R1 [166–169]. In addition to Ca^{2+} and IP_3, there are other allosteric IP_3R modulators, including ATP [170]. The activity of IP_3R can also be regulated by its phosphorylation by different kinases [166,170]. Among them are PKA, protein kinase C (PKC), cGMP-dependent protein kinase (PKG), CaMKII and different protein tyrosine kinases. Moreover, similarly to RyRs, the IP_3Rs can also be regulated by the redox status and by several interacting proteins (i.e., CaM-related Ca^{2+}-binding proteins (CaBPs), Bcl2 family members, proteases (Caspase-3 and calpain) and ER lumen-specific protein (ERp44) [170]).

IP_3Rs activity controls spine morphology, synaptic plasticity and memory consolidation [171–173]. Notably, alterations of IP_3Rs expression and function were reported to be implicated in Ca^{2+} signaling deregulation in several AD models [174]. Ca^{2+} imaging experiments demonstrated that orthologous expression of FAD PS1 mutants potentiates IP_3-mediated Ca^{2+} release [175]. These data were confirmed in cortical neurons isolated from PS1-M146V KI mice [79] and in cells expressing FAD PS1-DeltaE9 mutant [176]. PS1-DeltaE9 mutant cells harbored enhanced basal phosphoinositide hydrolysis and cyt[Ca^{2+}], which were both reversed by the PLC inhibitor neomycin. PS1-DeltaE9 mutant cells also showed high basal [Ca^{2+}] and agonist-evoked Ca^{2+} signals that were reversed by xestospongin C (XeC, a reversible IP_3R antagonist) [176]. The molecular mechanisms underlying enhanced IP_3R-mediated Ca^{2+} release have been described to be PS-dependent and/or PS-independent [73,177] (also discussed in PSs chapter below). The computational modeling of single IP_3R activity was used to analyze and quantify the pathological enhancement of IP_3R function by FAD-causing mutant PS [178]. This study revealed that the gain-of-function enhancement of IP_3R was sensitive to both IP_3 and Ca^{2+}, thus triggering a higher frequency of local Ca^{2+} signals, while enhancing the activity of the channel at extremely low ligand concentrations will lead to spontaneous Ca^{2+} signals in cells expressing FAD-causing mutant PS [178]. It has been consequently observed that the gain-of-function enhancement of IP_3R channels in cells expressing PS1-M146L leads to the opening of mitochondrial permeability transition pore (PTP) in high-conductance state, triggering a reduction in the inner mitochondrial membrane potential and in NADH and ATP levels [179]. Conversely, genetic reduction of IP_3R1 normalizes disturbed Ca^{2+} signaling in PS1-M146V KI mice and most importantly alleviates AD pathogenesis (i.e., rescues aberrant hippocampal long-term potentiation (LTP), attenuates Aβ accumulation and tau hyperphosphorylation and memory deficits) in both PS1-M146V KI and 3xTg-AD mice [72]. Accordingly, in vitro experiments showed that XeC effectively ameliorated Aβ42-induced apoptosis and intracellular Ca^{2+} overload in the primary hippocampal neurons [180]. Notably, intracerebroventricular injection of XeC reduced the number of Aβ plaques, alleviated ER stress response and significantly improved the cognitive behavior of APP/PS1 mice [180]. Exacerbated IP_3R-mediated Ca^{2+} release is also linked to Aβ, independently of PS overexpression/mutation. Jensen L.E., et al. reported that Aβ42 induced elevation of cytosolic Ca^{2+} in an IP_3R-dependent and -independent manner [91]. In addition, it was also shown that the treatment with Aβ42 significantly increased mRNA levels of $IP_3R1/2$ and mGluR5 [181]. Enhanced IP3R1 expression and ER Ca^{2+} release were also reported in astrocytes derived from the entorhinal cortex and from the hippocampus from WT mice and mice treated with Aβ42 oligomers [182]. Finally, as stated above, IP_3R function is regulated by several binding proteins. Thus, it is also conceivable that any alteration of the expression, localization, activity and binding affinity of these proteins may affect IP_3R structural/functional state, thus impacting AD development.

4. Presenilins 1 and 2: PS1/2

PS1 and PS2 are multispanning transmembrane (TM) proteins located in intracellular membranous organelles such as the ER, nuclear envelope and Golgi apparatus but also in multiple secretory and endocytic organelles as well as the plasma membrane [183]. PS1 was first cloned as a causative gene of FAD [184]. Its homologue PS2 gene was then identified, sharing an approximately 60% sequence homology as a whole and approximately 90% within the TM domains [185,186]. Accordingly, PS1 and PS2 were also shown to share similar predicted topology [187–189].

Both PS1 and PS2 are expressed in neurons [190] and are essential for embryonic development since PS1 KO mice die at birth [191] and PS1/PS2 double KO mice (PSDKO) mice die before embryonic day 9.5 [192]. Importantly, PSs were also shown to play key roles in neuronal function and survival. Therefore, conditional PSDKO mice show impaired spatial and associative memory, deficits in short- and long-term plasticity [193,194] and develop synaptic, dendritic and neuronal degeneration in an age-dependent manner [193]. Importantly, being the catalytic component of γ–secretase complex cleaving the APP [195], most of the PS mutations associated with early-onset FAD affect APP processing and, more particularly, the ratio Aβ40/42 by increasing the aggregation-prone Aβ42 species [196–198]. Several studies proposed the contribution of PSs to ER Ca^{2+} signaling deregulation in AD. It has been proposed that PSs act as ER Ca^{2+} leak channels, and FAD mutations in PSs disrupt this function, leading to ER Ca^{2+} overload [69,70,76]. Tu et al. also proposed that the full-length PSs function as ER Ca^{2+} leak channels independently of other γ–secretase components [69]. Cysteine point mutants combined with NMR studies revealed that TM7 and TM9, but not TM6, could play an important role in forming the conductance pore of mouse PS1 [77]. A recent study investigated the interaction of Ca^{2+} with both PS1 and PS2 using all-atom molecular dynamics (MD) simulations in realistic membrane models [199]. Although the Ca^{2+} leak event linked to PS1 or PS2 has been challenged in this study, the obtained data demonstrated the presence of four Ca^{2+} sites in membrane-bound PS1 and PS2 [199]. The authors speculated that Ca^{2+} may prevent PS maturation (i.e., "presenilinase" endoproteolysis generating PS N-and PS C-terminal derivatives [200]) by triggering conformational changes, thus preserving the immature Ca^{2+} regulation function. Meanwhile, conversely, PS maturation yielding a biologically active PS would abolish this Ca^{2+}-regulatory function [199]. Nevertheless, the PS-associated Ca^{2+} leak function was discussed in other studies proposing that FAD PSs directly potentiate the gating of IP_3R [81]. Exaggerated IP_3R-mediated Ca^{2+} responses were also reported in cells and neurons derived from transgenic mice expressing FAD-linked mutant PS1 or PS2 [84]. These findings agree well with data obtained in PS1-M146V KI mice neurons using whole-cell patch-clamp recording, flash photolysis and two-photon imaging [79]. Accordingly, genetic reduction of IP_3R 1 normalizes disturbed Ca^{2+} signaling in FAD PS1 mice and alleviates AD pathogenesis in PS1-M146V KI mice [72]. Other studies point to PS-linked disruptions in RyR signaling as an important ER molecular component associated with enhanced ER Ca^{2+} signals in both 3xTg-AD and PS1-M146V (KI) neurons [80]. PS1/PS2 were also shown to harbor a physical interaction with RyRs in the ER [83,117,201]. Specifically, PS2 interacts with RyR and with sorcin (a RyR regulator) in a Ca^{2+}-dependent manner in both cellular models and in the brain [201,202], thus increasing both mean currents and open probability of single brain RyR channels [203,204]. Discrepancies regarding the role of PSs in ER Ca^{2+} handling alterations were further highlighted in a recent study [205] showing that FAD PS2 mutants, but not FAD PS1, are able to partially block SERCA activity, thereby reducing ER Ca^{2+} content in either SH-SY5Y cells or FAD patient-derived fibroblasts [205]. Despite this incongruity concerning the exact molecular mechanism underlying PS-mediated ER Ca^{2+} deregulation, FAD PSs undoubtedly directly or indirectly contribute to the Ca^{2+} hypothesis in AD. However, whether PS-mediated ER Ca^{2+} deregulation is dependent on or independent of its endoproteolysis generating PS N-and PS C-terminal derivatives still remains an open question.

5. The Sarco-Endoplasmic Reticulum (SR/ER) Ca^{2+}-ATPase and Its Truncated Isoform: SERCA and S1T

SERCAs are integral ER proteins preserving low $[Ca^{2+}]$cyt by pumping free Ca^{2+} ions into the ER lumen, utilizing ATP hydrolysis. The SERCA pumps are encoded by three distinct genes (SERCA1-3), resulting in 12 known protein isoforms, with tissue-specific expression patterns. SERCA2b is the most expressed isoform in neurons [206]. Despite the well-established structure and function of the SERCA pumps, their role in the central nervous system and whether it could be affected in brain diseases remain to be definitely established. Interestingly, SERCA-mediated Ca^{2+} dyshomeostasis has been associated with neuropathological conditions, such as bipolar disorder, schizophrenia, Parkinson's disease but also AD [207]. An initial study showed that SERCA activity is reduced in fibroblasts isolated from PSDKO. Immunoprecipitation analyses suggested a physical interaction between SERCA and PS1 and PS2 [74] and that modulation of SERCA expression regulates Aβ levels [74]. The interaction of PS1 holoprotein was further demonstrated in cells overexpressing PS1 and subjected to tunicamycin treatment [208]. It has also been shown that overexpressed wild-type or mutated PS2 triggered ER-passive leakage through IP_3R and RyR but also potently reduced ER Ca^{2+} uptake, an effect that has been counteracted by the overexpression of SERCA2b [71]. A recent study reported that the pharmacological SERCA activation by a quinoline derivative (CD1163), discovered via high-throughput screening of small molecules library, provides some beneficial effects in APP/PS1 mice [209] (Figure 2). Overall, these studies pinpointed the potential contribution of SERCA to ER Ca^{2+} dyshomeostsis in

AD cellular study models. However, dedicated studies in mice AD models and in human-derived samples are still needed to further support the beneficial versus pathogenic role of the modulation of SERCA expression and activity in AD development.

Accumulation of unfolded proteins into the ER as well as alteration of ER Ca^{2+} homeostasis induce ER stress, eliciting an unfolded protein response (UPR) [210,211]. Several studies have reported that UPR occurs in human AD brains [212,213] and in several AD study systems [214–216]. We previously demonstrated that the human SERCA1 truncated isoform (S1T) [217] is induced under pharmacological and physiopathological ER stress through the activation of the PERK-eIF2α-ATF4-CHOP pathway [218]. In turn, S1T expression induction triggered an amplification of ER stress and mitochondrial apoptosis [218]. UPR activation has been proposed to be linked to intracellular Aβ accumulation [219]. In a recent study, we revealed that S1T is upregulated in SH-SY5Y cells expressing APPswe [75]. Importantly, biochemical data indicate that enhanced human S1T expression correlates with Aβ load in human AD-affected brains and that S1T high neuronal immunostaining is selectively observed in human AD cases harboring focal Aβ. We further demonstrated that S1T expression is induced by exogenous application of Aβ oligomers in cells [75]. Interestingly, S1T overexpression in return enhances APP processing and the production of APP-derived toxic fragments (APP C-terminal fragments and Aβ) in cells and in 3xTgAD mice. Mechanistically, we find that S1T-mediated elevation of APP proteolysis occurs through the upregulation of BACE1 expression and enhanced activity [75]. In agreement with these findings, several lines of evidence indicated that enhanced phosphorylation of PERK and eIF2α in the AD brain is associated with increased amyloidogenic APP processing [214–216] through increased BACE1 expression [220,221]. We have also to consider that BACE1 upregulation occurring downstream of $[Ca^{2+}]$cyt elevation acts in a positive feedback loop with AD progression [222]. In addition, the induction of ER stress and the activation of UPR trigger neuroinflammation [223]. Accordingly, we demonstrated that S1T overexpression, as well as tunicamycin treatment, induce the expression of proinflammatory cytokines and increase the proliferation of active microglia [75]. Altogether, our data strengthen the molecular link between ER Ca^{2+} leak, ER stress and APP processing contributing to AD setting and/or progression.

6. The Molecular Bridge between ER Ca^{2+} Depletion and Plasma Membrane Ca^{2+} Entry: STIM/ORAI

The store-operated Ca^{2+} entry (SOCE) is an essential route for Ca^{2+} uptake to replenish intracellular Ca^{2+} stores [224]. The stromal interaction molecules STIM1 and STIM2 have been identified as essential components of SOCE and major sensors of the Ca^{2+} concentration located in the ER membrane (reviewed in [225]). Both STIM homologues are ubiquitously expressed in different cell types, with a higher STIM1 level in most tissues and a predominant expression of STIM2 in the brain [226]. A decrease in ER luminal Ca^{2+} concentration results in dissociation of Ca^{2+} from the STIM EF-hand domain, which, in turn, triggers oligomerization and activation of STIM1, a process that is reversed when luminal $[Ca^{2+}]$ returns to resting level [3,4]. Active STIM oligomers translocate to ER plasma membrane junctions and recruit and interact with ORAI channels located on the plasma membrane [227]. There are three ORAI isoforms displaying tissue-specific expression and activation patterns [225]. In addition, transient receptor potential channels (TRPC) can also be recruited by the ORAI/STIM complex, constituting an additional route for Ca^{2+} entry through the plasma membrane upon ER Ca^{2+} depletion [228] (Figure 1). Several TRPC isoforms were also identified and were described to harbor tissue/cell-specific expression and activation patterns [229].

Several studies pinpointed a role for STIM/ORAI in neuronal Ca^{2+} signaling-associated synaptic function [230,231]. Thus, the maturation of dendritic spines and the formation of functional synapses in immature hippocampal neurons is facilitated by the influx of Ca^{2+} through ORAI1 [232]. STIM also interact with/and or control the activity of several Ca^{2+} channels on the plasma membrane (L-type Ca^{2+} channels ($Ca_V1.2$), L-type VGCCs and mGluR [232]). Several studies suggested that the disruption of neuronal SOCE underlies AD pathogenesis. A direct connection between Aβ-induced synaptic mushroom spine loss and the neuronal SOCE pathway was reported in two studies. Popugaeva et al.

reported that the application of exogenous Aβ42 oligomers to hippocampal cultures or injection of Aβ42 oligomers directly into the hippocampal region resulted in the reduction of mushroom spines and activity of synaptic CaMKII, which were rescued by STIM2 overexpression [224]. Accordingly, similar findings were reported in APPKI hippocampal neurons accumulating extracellular Aβ42. Thus, it was shown that Aβ triggers mGluR5 receptor overactivation, leading to elevated ER Ca^{2+} levels, compensatory downregulation of STIM2 expression, impairment of synaptic SOCE and reduced CaMKII activity [58]. Inversely, overexpression of the constitutively active STIM1-D76A mutant and ORAI1 significantly reduced Aβ secretion [55]. A link between STIM1/2 and PS1 was also reported. The STIM2–SOCE–CaMKII pathway was downregulated in a PS1-M146V KI mouse model of AD, associated with loss of hippocampal mushroom spines [233], and conversely, STIM2 overexpression rescued synaptic SOCE and mushroom spine deficit in hippocampal neurons from PS1-M146V KI mice [233]. Intriguingly, even if STIM1 expression is not altered in the AD models cited above, it has been identified as a target of PS1-containing γ–secretase activity. In particular, FAD-linked PS1 mutations enhanced γ–secretase cleavage of STIM1, reducing the activation of ORAI1 and attenuating SOCE [234]. As a consequence, the inhibition of SOCE in hippocampal neurons triggered an alteration of the dendritic spine architecture [234]. A recent study showed that the hyperactivation of SOCE channels in neurons expressing PS1-DeltaE9 mutant is mediated by the STIM1 sensor and can be attenuated by pharmacological inhibition and genetic KO STIM1 [235]. Interestingly, SOCE in PS1-DeltaE9 mutant-expressing cells is not contributed by STIM2 but involves TRPC and ORAI subunits. Importantly, transgenic Drosophila flies expressing PS1-DeltaE9 in the cholinergic neuron system showed short-term memory loss, which was reversed upon pharmacological inhibition of STIM1 [235]. Accordingly, a recent study further supports the link between FAD PSs and altered SOCE, through the demonstration of reduced STIM1 expression in SH-SY5Y cells and in patient-derived fibroblasts expressing different FAD-PS mutations [205].

TRPC may also play a role in SOCE deregulation in AD. TRPC expression is not altered in mice and human AD brains [233]. However, reduced TRPC1 expression was observed in astrocytes derived from APP KO mice [181,236]. In addition, TRPC6 was shown to specifically interact with APP, thereby blocking its cleavage by γ–secretase and reducing Aβ production independently from its ion channel activity [237]. Conversely, PS2 mutations abolish agonist-induced TRPC6 activation [238]. Importantly, activation of TRPC6 stimulates the activity of the neuronal SOCE pathway in the spines and rescues mushroom spine loss and long-term potentiation impairment in APP KI mice [58]. A review by Prikhodko, V. et al. in this Special Issue addresses the potential use of TRPC modulators as drugs to treat AD [239].

7. Conclusions

Studies demonstrating the implication of ER Ca^{2+} deregulation in AD highlight a complex picture integrating several molecular ER Ca^{2+} components. This includes enhanced ER Ca^{2+} release through IP_3R and RyR, dysfunctional ER Ca^{2+} uptake by SERCA and upregulation of the S1T truncated isoform, gain- or loss-of-function of PS components of the γ–secretase complex. Disease-associated remodeling of this Ca^{2+} machinery toolkit is also coupled to specific cellular signaling cascades modulating the activity (i.e., post-translational modifications, interactions with regulatory proteins) and/or the expression of these Ca^{2+} channels and pump (i.e., linked to ER stress). Several studies also pinpointed the direct interaction of Aβ peptide with several members of the ER Ca^{2+} machinery, thus contributing to ER Ca^{2+} dyshomeostasis. In addition, recent studies demonstrated that the failure of the SOCE molecular bridge between the ER and the plasma membrane has to be seriously considered as a major molecular mechanism controlling ER Ca^{2+} content and consequently ER-mediated Ca^{2+} release. Finally, it becomes now evident that ER Ca^{2+} dyshomeostasis is significantly associated with AD development and/or progression. The treatment options for AD remain supportive and symptomatic, without attenuation of the ultimate prognosis; thus efforts have still to be made in defining therapeutic approaches targeting ER Ca^{2+} machinery to cure AD (Figure 2). The described

ER Ca^{2+} toolkits are enriched in ER–mitochondria contact sites known as mitochondria-associated membranes (MAMs) [240]. Importantly, besides Ca^{2+} tunneling from ER to mitochondria, MAMs impact various cellular housekeeping functions such as phospholipid, glucose, cholesterol and fatty acid metabolism, which are all altered in AD [240,241]. This may further highlight the potential relevance of targeting ER Ca^{2+} handling proteins as an attempt to alleviate both ER and mitochondria dysfunctions associated with AD.

Acknowledgments: We thank Franck Aguila for figure drawing.

References

1. Berridge, M.J.; Bootman, M.D.; Roderick, H.L. Calcium signalling: Dynamics, homeostasis and remodelling. *Nat. Rev. Mol. Cell Biol.* **2003**, *4*, 517–529. [PubMed]
2. Bootman, M.D.; Collins, T.J.; Peppiatt, C.M.; Prothero, L.S.; MacKenzie, L.; De Smet, P.; Travers, M.; Tovey, S.C.; Seo, J.T.; Berridge, M.J.; et al. Calcium signalling—An overview. *Semin. Cell Dev. Biol.* **2001**, *12*, 3–10. [PubMed]
3. Cahalan, M.D. STIMulating store-operated Ca(2+) entry. *Nat. Cell Biol.* **2009**, *11*, 669–677. [PubMed]
4. Putney, J.W., Jr. New molecular players in capacitative Ca2+ entry. *J. Cell Sci.* **2007**, *120*, 1959–1965.
5. Smyth, J.T.; Hwang, S.Y.; Tomita, T.; DeHaven, W.I.; Mercer, J.C.; Putney, J.W. Activation and regulation of store-operated calcium entry. *J. Cell Mol. Med.* **2010**, *14*, 2337–2349.
6. Gulisano, W.; Maugeri, D.; Baltrons, M.A.; Fa, M.; Amato, A.; Palmeri, A.; D'Adamio, L.; Grassi, C.; Devanand, D.P.; Honig, L.S.; et al. Role of Amyloid-beta and Tau Proteins in Alzheimer's Disease: Confuting the Amyloid Cascade. *J. Alzheimer's Dis* **2018**, *64*, S611–S631. [CrossRef]
7. Selkoe, D.J.; Hardy, J. The amyloid hypothesis of Alzheimer's disease at 25 years. *EMBO Mol. Med.* **2016**, *8*, 595–608. [CrossRef]
8. Jones, D.T.; Graff-Radford, J.; Lowe, V.J.; Wiste, H.J.; Gunter, J.L.; Senjem, M.L.; Botha, H.; Kantarci, K.; Boeve, B.F.; Knopman, D.S.; et al. Tau, amyloid, and cascading network failure across the Alzheimer's disease spectrum. *Cortex* **2017**, *97*, 143–159. [CrossRef]
9. Checler, F. Processing of the beta-amyloid precursor protein and its regulation in Alzheimer's disease. *J. Neurochem.* **1995**, *65*, 1431–1444.
10. Zhang, Y.W.; Thompson, R.; Zhang, H.; Xu, H. APP processing in Alzheimer's disease. *Mol. Brain* **2011**, *4*, 3. [CrossRef]
11. Edbauer, D.; Winkler, E.; Regula, J.T.; Pesold, B.; Steiner, H.; Haass, C. Reconstitution of gamma-secretase activity. *Nat. Cell Biol.* **2003**, *5*, 486–488. [CrossRef] [PubMed]
12. Kimberly, W.T.; LaVoie, M.J.; Ostaszewski, B.L.; Ye, W.; Wolfe, M.S.; Selkoe, D.J. Gamma-secretase is a membrane protein complex comprised of presenilin, nicastrin, Aph-1, and Pen-2. *Proc. Natl. Acad. Sci. USA* **2003**, *100*, 6382–6387. [CrossRef] [PubMed]
13. Tanzi, R.E.; Bertram, L. Twenty years of the Alzheimer's disease amyloid hypothesis: A genetic perspective. *Cell* **2005**, *120*, 545–555. [PubMed]
14. Van Cauwenberghe, C.; Van Broeckhoven, C.; Sleegers, K. The genetic landscape of Alzheimer disease: Clinical implications and perspectives. *Genet. Med.* **2015**, *18*, 421–430. [CrossRef] [PubMed]
15. Golde, T.E.; Cai, X.D.; Shoji, M.; Younkin, S.G. Production of amyloid beta protein from normal amyloid beta-protein precursor (beta APP) and the mutated beta APPS linked to familial Alzheimer's disease. *Ann. N.Y. Acad. Sci.* **1993**, *695*, 103–108. [PubMed]
16. Wolfe, M.S. When loss is gain: Reduced presenilin proteolytic function leads to increased Abeta42/Abeta40. Talking Point on the role of presenilin mutations in Alzheimer disease. *EMBO Rep.* **2007**, *8*, 136–140.
17. Billings, L.M.; Oddo, S.; Green, K.N.; McGaugh, J.L.; LaFerla, F.M. Intraneuronal Abeta causes the onset of early Alzheimer's disease-related cognitive deficits in transgenic mice. *Neuron* **2005**, *45*, 675–688.
18. Del Prete, D.; Suski, J.M.; Oules, B.; Debayle, D.; Gay, A.S.; Lacas-Gervais, S.; Bussiere, R.; Bauer, C.; Pinton, P.; Paterlini-Brechot, P.; et al. Localization and Processing of the Amyloid-beta Protein Precursor in Mitochondria-Associated Membranes. *J. Alzheimer's Dis.* **2017**, *55*, 1549–1570. [CrossRef]
19. Pardossi-Piquard, R.; Petit, A.; Kawarai, T.; Sunyach, C.; Alves da Costa, C.; Vincent, B.; Ring, S.; D'Adamio, L.; Shen, J.; Muller, U.; et al. Presenilin-dependent transcriptional control of the Abeta-degrading enzyme

neprilysin by intracellular domains of betaAPP and APLP. *Neuron* **2005**, *46*, 541–554. [CrossRef]
20. Nhan, H.S.; Chiang, K.; Koo, E.H. The multifaceted nature of amyloid precursor protein and its proteolytic fragments: Friends and foes. *Acta Neuropathol.* **2015**, *129*, 1–19. [CrossRef]
21. Baranger, K.; Marchalant, Y.; Bonnet, A.E.; Crouzin, N.; Carrete, A.; Paumier, J.M.; Py, N.A.; Bernard, A.; Bauer, C.; Charrat, E.; et al. MT5-MMP is a new pro-amyloidogenic proteinase that promotes amyloid pathology and cognitive decline in a transgenic mouse model of Alzheimer's disease. *Cell Mol. Life Sci.* **2016**, *73*, 217–236. [CrossRef] [PubMed]
22. Willem, M.; Tahirovic, S.; Busche, M.A.; Ovsepian, S.V.; Chafai, M.; Kootar, S.; Hornburg, D.; Evans, L.D.; Moore, S.; Daria, A.; et al. eta-Secretase processing of APP inhibits neuronal activity in the hippocampus. *Nature* **2015**, *526*, 443–447. [CrossRef] [PubMed]
23. Lauritzen, I.; Pardossi-Piquard, R.; Bauer, C.; Brigham, E.; Abraham, J.D.; Ranaldi, S.; Fraser, P.; St-George-Hyslop, P.; Le Thuc, O.; Espin, V.; et al. The beta-Secretase-Derived C-Terminal Fragment of betaAPP, C99, But Not Abeta, Is a Key Contributor to Early Intraneuronal Lesions in Triple-Transgenic Mouse Hippocampus. *J. Neurosci.* **2012**, *32*, 16243–16255. [CrossRef] [PubMed]
24. Lauritzen, I.; Pardossi-Piquard, R.; Bourgeois, A.; Pagnotta, S.; Biferi, M.G.; Barkats, M.; Lacor, P.; Klein, W.; Bauer, C.; Checler, F. Intraneuronal aggregation of the beta-CTF fragment of APP (C99) induces Abeta-independent lysosomal-autophagic pathology. *Acta Neuropathol.* **2016**, *132*, 257–276. [CrossRef]
25. Vergara, C.; Houben, S.; Suain, V.; Yilmaz, Z.; De Decker, R.; Vanden Dries, V.; Boom, A.; Mansour, S.; Leroy, K.; Ando, K.; et al. Amyloid-beta pathology enhances pathological fibrillary tau seeding induced by Alzheimer PHF in vivo. *Acta Neuropathol.* **2019**, *137*, 397–412. [CrossRef]
26. He, Z.; Guo, J.L.; McBride, J.D.; Narasimhan, S.; Kim, H.; Changolkar, L.; Zhang, B.; Gathagan, R.J.; Yue, C.; Dengler, C.; et al. Amyloid-beta plaques enhance Alzheimer's brain tau-seeded pathologies by facilitating neuritic plaque tau aggregation. *Nat. Med.* **2018**, *24*, 29–38. [CrossRef]
27. Holbro, N.; Grunditz, A.; Oertner, T.G. Differential distribution of endoplasmic reticulum controls metabotropic signaling and plasticity at hippocampal synapses. *Proc. Natl. Acad. Sci. USA* **2009**, *106*, 15055–15060. [CrossRef]
28. Dailey, M.E.; Bridgman, P.C. Dynamics of the endoplasmic reticulum and other membranous organelles in growth cones of cultured neurons. *J. Neurosci.* **1989**, *9*, 1897–1909. [CrossRef]
29. Emptage, N.J.; Reid, C.A.; Fine, A. Calcium stores in hippocampal synaptic boutons mediate short-term plasticity, store-operated Ca2+ entry, and spontaneous transmitter release. *Neuron* **2001**, *29*, 197–208. [CrossRef]
30. Berridge, M.J.; Bootman, M.D.; Lipp, P. Calcium–a life and death signal. *Nature* **1998**, *395*, 645–648. [CrossRef]
31. Li, W.; Llopis, J.; Whitney, M.; Zlokarnik, G.; Tsien, R.Y. Cell-permeant caged InsP3 ester shows that Ca2+ spike frequency can optimize gene expression. *Nature* **1998**, *392*, 936–941. [CrossRef] [PubMed]
32. Bandtlow, C.E.; Schmidt, M.F.; Hassinger, T.D.; Schwab, M.E.; Kater, S.B. Role of intracellular calcium in NI-35-evoked collapse of neuronal growth cones. *Science* **1993**, *259*, 80–83. [CrossRef] [PubMed]
33. Popugaeva, E.; Bezprozvanny, I. Can the calcium hypothesis explain synaptic loss in Alzheimer's disease? *Neurodegener. Dis.* **2014**, *13*, 139–141. [CrossRef] [PubMed]
34. Bojarski, L.; Herms, J.; Kuznicki, J. Calcium dysregulation in Alzheimer's disease. *Neurochem. Int.* **2008**, *52*, 621–633. [CrossRef] [PubMed]
35. Tong, B.C.; Wu, A.J.; Li, M.; Cheung, K.H. Calcium signaling in Alzheimer's disease & therapies. *Biochim. Biophys. Acta Mol. Cell Res.* **2018**, *1865*, 1745–1760. [CrossRef]
36. Del Prete, D.; Checler, F.; Chami, M. Ryanodine receptors: Physiological function and deregulation in Alzheimer disease. *Mol. Neurodegener.* **2014**, *9*, 21. [CrossRef]
37. Cao, L.L.; Guan, P.P.; Liang, Y.Y.; Huang, X.S.; Wang, P. Calcium Ions Stimulate the Hyperphosphorylation of Tau by Activating Microsomal Prostaglandin E Synthase 1. *Front. Aging Neurosci.* **2019**, *11*, 108. [CrossRef]
38. Hayley, M.; Perspicace, S.; Schulthess, T.; Seelig, J. Calcium enhances the proteolytic activity of BACE1: An in vitro biophysical and biochemical characterization of the BACE1-calcium interaction. *Biochim. Biophys. Acta* **2009**, *1788*, 1933–1938. [CrossRef]
39. Ho, M.; Hoke, D.E.; Chua, Y.J.; Li, Q.X.; Culvenor, J.G.; Masters, C.; White, A.R.; Evin, G. Effect of Metal Chelators on gamma-Secretase Indicates That Calcium and Magnesium Ions Facilitate Cleavage of Alzheimer Amyloid Precursor Substrate. *Int. J. Alzheimer's Dis.* **2010**, *2011*, 950932. [CrossRef]
40. Miller, S.G.; Kennedy, M.B. Regulation of brain type II Ca2+/calmodulin-dependent protein kinase by autophosphorylation: A Ca2+-triggered molecular switch. *Cell* **1986**, *44*, 861–870. [CrossRef]

41. Oka, M.; Fujisaki, N.; Maruko-Otake, A.; Ohtake, Y.; Shimizu, S.; Saito, T.; Hisanaga, S.I.; Iijima, K.M.; Ando, K. Ca2+/calmodulin-dependent protein kinase II promotes neurodegeneration caused by tau phosphorylated at Ser262/356 in a transgenic Drosophila model of tauopathy. *J. Biochem.* **2017**, *162*, 335–342. [CrossRef] [PubMed]
42. Litersky, J.M.; Johnson, G.V.; Jakes, R.; Goedert, M.; Lee, M.; Seubert, P. Tau protein is phosphorylated by cyclic AMP-dependent protein kinase and calcium/calmodulin-dependent protein kinase II within its microtubule-binding domains at Ser-262 and Ser-356. *Biochem. J.* **1996**, *316 (Pt 2)*, 655–660. [CrossRef]
43. Chakroborty, S.; Stutzmann, G.E. Early calcium dysregulation in Alzheimer's disease: Setting the stage for synaptic dysfunction. *Sci. China Life Sci.* **2011**, *54*, 752–762. [CrossRef] [PubMed]
44. Mattson, M.P. ER calcium and Alzheimer's disease: In a state of flux. *Sci. Signal.* **2010**, *3*, pe10. [CrossRef] [PubMed]
45. LaFerla, F.M. Calcium dyshomeostasis and intracellular signalling in Alzheimer's disease. *Nat. Rev. Neurosci.* **2002**, *3*, 862–872. [CrossRef] [PubMed]
46. Supnet, C.; Bezprozvanny, I. The dysregulation of intracellular calcium in Alzheimer disease. *Cell Calcium* **2010**, *47*, 183–189. [CrossRef] [PubMed]
47. Bezprozvanny, I.; Mattson, M.P. Neuronal calcium mishandling and the pathogenesis of Alzheimer's disease. *Trends Neurosci.* **2008**, *31*, 454–463. [CrossRef] [PubMed]
48. Berridge, M.J. Calcium signalling and Alzheimer's disease. *Neurochem. Res.* **2011**, *36*, 1149–1156. [CrossRef]
49. Chakroborty, S.; Stutzmann, G.E. Calcium channelopathies and Alzheimer's disease: Insight into therapeutic success and failures. *Eur. J. Pharmacol.* **2014**, *739*, 83–95. [CrossRef]
50. Arispe, N.; Rojas, E.; Pollard, H.B. Alzheimer disease amyloid beta protein forms calcium channels in bilayer membranes: Blockade by tromethamine and aluminum. *Proc. Natl. Acad. Sci. USA* **1993**, *90*, 567–571. [CrossRef]
51. Alberdi, E.; Sanchez-Gomez, M.V.; Cavaliere, F.; Perez-Samartin, A.; Zugaza, J.L.; Trullas, R.; Domercq, M.; Matute, C. Amyloid beta oligomers induce Ca2+ dysregulation and neuronal death through activation of ionotropic glutamate receptors. *Cell Calcium* **2010**, *47*, 264–272. [CrossRef] [PubMed]
52. Texido, L.; Martin-Satue, M.; Alberdi, E.; Solsona, C.; Matute, C. Amyloid beta peptide oligomers directly activate NMDA receptors. *Cell Calcium* **2011**, *49*, 184–190. [CrossRef] [PubMed]
53. Thibault, O.; Pancani, T.; Landfield, P.W.; Norris, C.M. Reduction in neuronal L-type calcium channel activity in a double knock-in mouse model of Alzheimer's disease. *Biochim. Biophys. Acta* **2012**, *1822*, 546–549. [CrossRef] [PubMed]
54. Ma, Z.; Siebert, A.P.; Cheung, K.H.; Lee, R.J.; Johnson, B.; Cohen, A.S.; Vingtdeux, V.; Marambaud, P.; Foskett, J.K. Calcium homeostasis modulator 1 (CALHM1) is the pore-forming subunit of an ion channel that mediates extracellular Ca2+ regulation of neuronal excitability. *Proc. Natl. Acad. Sci. USA* **2012**, *109*, E1963–E1971. [CrossRef]
55. Zeiger, W.; Vetrivel, K.S.; Buggia-Prevot, V.; Nguyen, P.D.; Wagner, S.L.; Villereal, M.L.; Thinakaran, G. Ca2+ influx through store-operated Ca2+ channels reduces Alzheimer disease beta-amyloid peptide secretion. *J. Biol. Chem.* **2013**, *288*, 26955–26966. [CrossRef]
56. Yoo, A.S.; Cheng, I.; Chung, S.; Grenfell, T.Z.; Lee, H.; Pack-Chung, E.; Handler, M.; Shen, J.; Xia, W.; Tesco, G.; et al. Presenilin-mediated modulation of capacitative calcium entry. *Neuron* **2000**, *27*, 561–572. [CrossRef]
57. Chernyuk, D.; Zernov, N.; Kabirova, M.; Bezprozvanny, I.; Popugaeva, E. Antagonist of neuronal store-operated calcium entry exerts beneficial effects in neurons expressing PSEN1DeltaE9 mutant linked to familial Alzheimer disease. *Neuroscience* **2019**, *410*, 118–127. [CrossRef]
58. Zhang, H.; Sun, S.; Wu, L.; Pchitskaya, E.; Zakharova, O.; Fon Tacer, K.; Bezprozvanny, I. Store-Operated Calcium Channel Complex in Postsynaptic Spines: A New Therapeutic Target for Alzheimer's Disease Treatment. *J. Neurosci.* **2016**, *36*, 11837–11850. [CrossRef]
59. Zhang, H.; Wu, L.; Pchitskaya, E.; Zakharova, O.; Saito, T.; Saido, T.; Bezprozvanny, I. Neuronal Store-Operated Calcium Entry and Mushroom Spine Loss in Amyloid Precursor Protein Knock-In Mouse Model of Alzheimer's Disease. *J. Neurosci.* **2015**, *35*, 13275–13286. [CrossRef]
60. Popugaeva, E.; Pchitskaya, E.; Speshilova, A.; Alexandrov, S.; Zhang, H.; Vlasova, O.; Bezprozvanny, I. STIM2 protects hippocampal mushroom spines from amyloid synaptotoxicity. *Mol. Neurodegener.* **2015**, *10*, 37. [CrossRef]

61. Tang, J.; Oliveros, A.; Jang, M.H. Dysfunctional Mitochondrial Bioenergetics and Synaptic Degeneration in Alzheimer Disease. *Int. Neurourol. J.* **2019**, *23*, S5–S10. [CrossRef] [PubMed]
62. Garcia-Escudero, V.; Martin-Maestro, P.; Perry, G.; Avila, J. Deconstructing mitochondrial dysfunction in Alzheimer disease. *Oxid. Med. Cell Longev.* **2013**, *2013*, 162152. [CrossRef] [PubMed]
63. Esteras, N.; Abramov, A.Y. Mitochondrial Calcium Deregulation in the Mechanism of Beta-Amyloid and Tau Pathology. *Cells* **2020**, *9*, 2135. [CrossRef] [PubMed]
64. Perez, M.J.; Ponce, D.P.; Aranguiz, A.; Behrens, M.I.; Quintanilla, R.A. Mitochondrial permeability transition pore contributes to mitochondrial dysfunction in fibroblasts of patients with sporadic Alzheimer's disease. *Redox Biol.* **2018**, *19*, 290–300. [CrossRef] [PubMed]
65. Jadiya, P.; Kolmetzky, D.W.; Tomar, D.; Di Meco, A.; Lombardi, A.A.; Lambert, J.P.; Luongo, T.S.; Ludtmann, M.H.; Pratico, D.; Elrod, J.W. Impaired mitochondrial calcium efflux contributes to disease progression in models of Alzheimer's disease. *Nat. Commun.* **2019**, *10*, 3885. [CrossRef] [PubMed]
66. Wolfe, D.M.; Lee, J.H.; Kumar, A.; Lee, S.; Orenstein, S.J.; Nixon, R.A. Autophagy failure in Alzheimer's disease and the role of defective lysosomal acidification. *Eur. J. Neurosci.* **2013**, *37*, 1949–1961. [CrossRef] [PubMed]
67. Lee, J.H.; Yu, W.H.; Kumar, A.; Lee, S.; Mohan, P.S.; Peterhoff, C.M.; Wolfe, D.M.; Martinez-Vicente, M.; Massey, A.C.; Sovak, G.; et al. Lysosomal proteolysis and autophagy require presenilin 1 and are disrupted by Alzheimer-related PS1 mutations. *Cell* **2010**, *141*, 1146–1158. [CrossRef]
68. Lee, J.H.; McBrayer, M.K.; Wolfe, D.M.; Haslett, L.J.; Kumar, A.; Sato, Y.; Lie, P.P.; Mohan, P.; Coffey, E.E.; Kompella, U.; et al. Presenilin 1 Maintains Lysosomal Ca(2+) Homeostasis via TRPML1 by Regulating vATPase-Mediated Lysosome Acidification. *Cell Rep.* **2015**, *12*, 1430–1444. [CrossRef]
69. Tu, H.; Nelson, O.; Bezprozvanny, A.; Wang, Z.; Lee, S.F.; Hao, Y.H.; Serneels, L.; De Strooper, B.; Yu, G.; Bezprozvanny, I. Presenilins form ER Ca2+ leak channels, a function disrupted by familial Alzheimer's disease-linked mutations. *Cell* **2006**, *126*, 981–993. [CrossRef]
70. Nelson, O.; Tu, H.; Lei, T.; Bentahir, M.; de Strooper, B.; Bezprozvanny, I. Familial Alzheimer disease-linked mutations specifically disrupt Ca2+ leak function of presenilin 1. *J. Clin. Invest.* **2007**, *117*, 1230–1239. [CrossRef]
71. Brunello, L.; Zampese, E.; Florean, C.; Pozzan, T.; Pizzo, P.; Fasolato, C. Presenilin-2 dampens intracellular Ca2+ stores by increasing Ca2+ leakage and reducing Ca2+ uptake. *J. Cell Mol. Med.* **2009**, *13*, 3358–3369. [CrossRef] [PubMed]
72. Shilling, D.; Muller, M.; Takano, H.; Mak, D.O.; Abel, T.; Coulter, D.A.; Foskett, J.K. Suppression of InsP3 receptor-mediated Ca2+ signaling alleviates mutant presenilin-linked familial Alzheimer's disease pathogenesis. *J. Neurosci.* **2014**, *34*, 6910–6923. [CrossRef] [PubMed]
73. Shilling, D.; Mak, D.O.; Kang, D.E.; Foskett, J.K. Lack of evidence for presenilins as endoplasmic reticulum Ca2+ leak channels. *J. Biol. Chem.* **2012**, *287*, 10933–10944. [CrossRef] [PubMed]
74. Green, K.N.; Demuro, A.; Akbari, Y.; Hitt, B.D.; Smith, I.F.; Parker, I.; LaFerla, F.M. SERCA pump activity is physiologically regulated by presenilin and regulates amyloid beta production. *J. Cell Biol.* **2008**, *181*, 1107–1116. [CrossRef]
75. Bussiere, R.; Oules, B.; Mary, A.; Vaillant-Beuchot, L.; Martin, C.; El Manaa, W.; Vallee, D.; Duplan, E.; Paterlini-Brechot, P.; Alves Da Costa, C.; et al. Upregulation of the Sarco-Endoplasmic Reticulum Calcium ATPase 1 Truncated Isoform Plays a Pathogenic Role in Alzheimer's Disease. *Cells* **2019**, *8*, 1539. [CrossRef]
76. Nelson, O.; Supnet, C.; Liu, H.; Bezprozvanny, I. Familial Alzheimer's disease mutations in presenilins: Effects on endoplasmic reticulum calcium homeostasis and correlation with clinical phenotypes. *J. Alzheimer's Dis.* **2010**, *21*, 781–793. [CrossRef]
77. Nelson, O.; Supnet, C.; Tolia, A.; Horre, K.; De Strooper, B.; Bezprozvanny, I. Mutagenesis mapping of the presenilin 1 calcium leak conductance pore. *J. Biol. Chem.* **2011**, *286*, 22339–22347. [CrossRef]
78. Zampese, E.; Fasolato, C.; Kipanyula, M.J.; Bortolozzi, M.; Pozzan, T.; Pizzo, P. Presenilin 2 modulates endoplasmic reticulum (ER)-mitochondria interactions and Ca2+ cross-talk. *Proc. Natl. Acad. Sci. USA* **2011**, *108*, 2777–2782. [CrossRef]
79. Stutzmann, G.E.; Caccamo, A.; LaFerla, F.M.; Parker, I. Dysregulated IP3 signaling in cortical neurons of knock-in mice expressing an Alzheimer's-linked mutation in presenilin1 results in exaggerated Ca2+ signals and altered membrane excitability. *J. Neurosci.* **2004**, *24*, 508–513. [CrossRef]

80. Stutzmann, G.E.; Smith, I.; Caccamo, A.; Oddo, S.; Parker, I.; Laferla, F. Enhanced ryanodine-mediated calcium release in mutant PS1-expressing Alzheimer's mouse models. *Ann. N.Y. Acad. Sci.* **2007**, *1097*, 265–277. [CrossRef]
81. Cheung, K.H.; Shineman, D.; Muller, M.; Cardenas, C.; Mei, L.; Yang, J.; Tomita, T.; Iwatsubo, T.; Lee, V.M.; Foskett, J.K. Mechanism of Ca2+ disruption in Alzheimer's disease by presenilin regulation of InsP(3) receptor channel gating. *Neuron* **2008**, *58*, 871–883. [CrossRef] [PubMed]
82. Querfurth, H.W.; Jiang, J.; Geiger, J.D.; Selkoe, D.J. Caffeine stimulates amyloid beta-peptide release from beta-amyloid precursor protein-transfected HEK293 cells. *J. Neurochem.* **1997**, *69*, 1580–1591. [CrossRef] [PubMed]
83. Chan, S.L.; Mayne, M.; Holden, C.P.; Geiger, J.D.; Mattson, M.P. Presenilin-1 mutations increase levels of ryanodine receptors and calcium release in PC12 cells and cortical neurons. *J. Biol. Chem.* **2000**, *275*, 18195–18200. [CrossRef] [PubMed]
84. Smith, I.F.; Hitt, B.; Green, K.N.; Oddo, S.; LaFerla, F.M. Enhanced caffeine-induced Ca2+ release in the 3xTg-AD mouse model of Alzheimer's disease. *J. Neurochem.* **2005**, *94*, 1711–1718. [CrossRef]
85. Stutzmann, G.E.; Smith, I.; Caccamo, A.; Oddo, S.; Laferla, F.M.; Parker, I. Enhanced ryanodine receptor recruitment contributes to Ca2+ disruptions in young, adult, and aged Alzheimer's disease mice. *J. Neurosci.* **2006**, *26*, 5180–5189. [CrossRef]
86. Supnet, C.; Grant, J.; Kong, H.; Westaway, D.; Mayne, M. Amyloid-beta-(1-42) increases ryanodine receptor-3 expression and function in neurons of TgCRND8 mice. *J. Biol. Chem.* **2006**, *281*, 38440–38447. [CrossRef]
87. Chakroborty, S.; Goussakov, I.; Miller, M.B.; Stutzmann, G.E. Deviant ryanodine receptor-mediated calcium release resets synaptic homeostasis in presymptomatic 3xTg-AD mice. *J. Neurosci.* **2009**, *29*, 9458–9470. [CrossRef]
88. Paula-Lima, A.C.; Adasme, T.; SanMartin, C.; Sebollela, A.; Hetz, C.; Carrasco, M.A.; Ferreira, S.T.; Hidalgo, C. Amyloid beta-peptide oligomers stimulate RyR-mediated Ca2+ release inducing mitochondrial fragmentation in hippocampal neurons and prevent RyR-mediated dendritic spine remodeling produced by BDNF. *Antioxid. Redox Signal.* **2011**, *14*, 1209–1223. [CrossRef]
89. Ito, E.; Oka, K.; Etcheberrigaray, R.; Nelson, T.J.; McPhie, D.L.; Tofel-Grehl, B.; Gibson, G.E.; Alkon, D.L. Internal Ca2+ mobilization is altered in fibroblasts from patients with Alzheimer disease. *Proc. Natl. Acad. Sci. USA* **1994**, *91*, 534–538. [CrossRef]
90. Goussakov, I.; Miller, M.B.; Stutzmann, G.E. NMDA-mediated Ca(2+) influx drives aberrant ryanodine receptor activation in dendrites of young Alzheimer's disease mice. *J. Neurosci.* **2010**, *30*, 12128–12137. [CrossRef]
91. Jensen, L.E.; Bultynck, G.; Luyten, T.; Amijee, H.; Bootman, M.D.; Roderick, H.L. Alzheimer's disease-associated peptide Abeta42 mobilizes ER Ca(2+) via InsP3R-dependent and -independent mechanisms. *Front. Mol. Neurosci.* **2013**, *6*, 36. [CrossRef] [PubMed]
92. Oules, B.; Del Prete, D.; Greco, B.; Zhang, X.; Lauritzen, I.; Sevalle, J.; Moreno, S.; Paterlini-Brechot, P.; Trebak, M.; Checler, F.; et al. Ryanodine receptor blockade reduces amyloid-beta load and memory impairments in Tg2576 mouse model of Alzheimer disease. *J. Neurosci.* **2012**, 32, 11820–11834. [CrossRef] [PubMed]
93. Chakroborty, S.; Briggs, C.; Miller, M.B.; Goussakov, I.; Schneider, C.; Kim, J.; Wicks, J.; Richardson, J.C.; Conklin, V.; Cameransi, B.G.; et al. Stabilizing ER Ca2+ channel function as an early preventative strategy for Alzheimer's disease. *PLoS ONE* **2012**, *7*, e52056. [CrossRef] [PubMed]
94. Chakroborty, S.; Kim, J.; Schneider, C.; Jacobson, C.; Molgo, J.; Stutzmann, G.E. Early presynaptic and postsynaptic calcium signaling abnormalities mask underlying synaptic depression in presymptomatic Alzheimer's disease mice. *J. Neurosci.* **2012**, *32*, 8341–8353. [CrossRef] [PubMed]
95. Santos, S.F.; Pierrot, N.; Morel, N.; Gailly, P.; Sindic, C.; Octave, J.N. Expression of human amyloid precursor protein in rat cortical neurons inhibits calcium oscillations. *J. Neurosci.* **2009**, *29*, 4708–4718. [CrossRef] [PubMed]
96. Gazda, K.; Kuznicki, J.; Wegierski, T. Knockdown of amyloid precursor protein increases calcium levels in the endoplasmic reticulum. *Sci. Rep.* **2017**, *7*, 14512. [CrossRef]
97. Mahoney, R.; Ochoa Thomas, E.; Ramirez, P.; Miller, H.E.; Beckmann, A.; Zuniga, G.; Dobrowolski, R.; Frost, B. Pathogenic Tau Causes a Toxic Depletion of Nuclear Calcium. *Cell Rep.* **2020** *32*, 107900. [CrossRef]

98. Esteras, N.; Kundel, F.; Amodeo, G.F.; Pavlov, E.V.; Klenerman, D.; Abramov, A.Y. Insoluble tau aggregates induce neuronal death through modification of membrane ion conductance, activation of voltage-gated calcium channels and NADPH oxidase. *FEBS J.* **2020**. [CrossRef]
99. Britti, E.; Ros, J.; Esteras, N.; Abramov, A.Y. Tau inhibits mitochondrial calcium efflux and makes neurons vulnerable to calcium-induced cell death. *Cell Calcium* **2020**, *86*, 102150. [CrossRef]
100. Furuichi, T.; Furutama, D.; Hakamata, Y.; Nakai, J.; Takeshima, H.; Mikoshiba, K. Multiple types of ryanodine receptor/Ca2+ release channels are differentially expressed in rabbit brain. *J. Neurosci.* **1994**, *14*, 4794–4805. [CrossRef]
101. Lehnart, S.E.; Mongillo, M.; Bellinger, A.; Lindegger, N.; Chen, B.X.; Hsueh, W.; Reiken, S.; Wronska, A.; Drew, L.J.; Ward, C.W.; et al. Leaky Ca2+ release channel/ryanodine receptor 2 causes seizures and sudden cardiac death in mice. *J. Clin. Investig.* **2008**, *118*, 2230–2245. [CrossRef] [PubMed]
102. Meissner, G.; Darling, E.; Eveleth, J. Kinetics of rapid Ca2+ release by sarcoplasmic reticulum. Effects of Ca2+, Mg2+, and adenine nucleotides. *Biochemistry* **1986**, *25*, 236–244. [CrossRef] [PubMed]
103. Meissner, G. The structural basis of ryanodine receptor ion channel function. *J. Gen. Physiol.* **2017**, *149*, 1065–1089. [CrossRef] [PubMed]
104. Laver, D.R.; Honen, B.N. Luminal Mg2+, a key factor controlling RYR2-mediated Ca2+ release: Cytoplasmic and luminal regulation modeled in a tetrameric channel. *J. Gen. Physiol.* **2008**, *132*, 429–446. [CrossRef] [PubMed]
105. Tencerova, B.; Zahradnikova, A.; Gaburjakova, J.; Gaburjakova, M. Luminal Ca2+ controls activation of the cardiac ryanodine receptor by ATP. *J. Gen. Physiol.* **2012**, *140*, 93–108. [CrossRef] [PubMed]
106. Yan, Z.; Bai, X.; Yan, C.; Wu, J.; Li, Z.; Xie, T.; Peng, W.; Yin, C.; Li, X.; Scheres, S.H.W.; et al. Structure of the rabbit ryanodine receptor RyR1 at near-atomic resolution. *Nature* **2015**, *517*, 50–55. [CrossRef]
107. Peng, W.; Shen, H.; Wu, J.; Guo, W.; Pan, X.; Wang, R.; Chen, S.R.; Yan, N. Structural basis for the gating mechanism of the type 2 ryanodine receptor RyR2. *Science* **2016**, *354*. [CrossRef]
108. Denniss, A.; Dulhunty, A.F.; Beard, N.A. Ryanodine receptor Ca(2+) release channel post-translational modification: Central player in cardiac and skeletal muscle disease. *Int. J. Biochem. Cell Biol.* **2018**, *101*, 49–53. [CrossRef]
109. Lanner, J.T.; Georgiou, D.K.; Joshi, A.D.; Hamilton, S.L. Ryanodine receptors: Structure, expression, molecular details, and function in calcium release. *Cold Spring Harb. Perspect. Biol.* **2010**, *2*, a003996. [CrossRef]
110. Balshaw, D.M.; Yamaguchi, N.; Meissner, G. Modulation of intracellular calcium-release channels by calmodulin. *J. Membr. Biol.* **2002**, *185*, 1–8. [CrossRef]
111. MacMillan, D. FK506 binding proteins: Cellular regulators of intracellular Ca2+ signalling. *Eur. J. Pharmacol.* **2013**, *700*, 181–193. [CrossRef] [PubMed]
112. Zalk, R.; Lehnart, S.E.; Marks, A.R. Modulation of the ryanodine receptor and intracellular calcium. *Annu. Rev. Biochem.* **2007**, *76*, 367–385. [CrossRef] [PubMed]
113. Marx, S.O.; Reiken, S.; Hisamatsu, Y.; Jayaraman, T.; Burkhoff, D.; Rosemblit, N.; Marks, A.R. PKA phosphorylation dissociates FKBP12.6 from the calcium release channel (ryanodine receptor): Defective regulation in failing hearts. *Cell* **2000**, *101*, 365–376. [CrossRef]
114. Currie, S. Cardiac ryanodine receptor phosphorylation by CaM Kinase II: Keeping the balance right. *Front. Biosci.* **2009**, *14*, 5134–5156. [CrossRef]
115. Allen, P.B.; Ouimet, C.C.; Greengard, P. Spinophilin, a novel protein phosphatase 1 binding protein localized to dendritic spines. *Proc. Natl. Acad. Sci. USA* **1997**, *94*, 9956–9961. [CrossRef]
116. Chami, M.; Checler, F. Targeting Post-Translational Remodeling of Ryanodine Receptor: A New Track for Alzheimer's Disease Therapy? *Curr. Alzheimer Res.* **2020**, *17*, 313–323. [CrossRef]
117. Lee, S.Y.; Hwang, D.Y.; Kim, Y.K.; Lee, J.W.; Shin, I.C.; Oh, K.W.; Lee, M.K.; Lim, J.S.; Yoon, D.Y.; Hwang, S.J.; et al. PS2 mutation increases neuronal cell vulnerability to neurotoxicants through activation of caspase-3 by enhancing of ryanodine receptor-mediated calcium release. *FASEB J.* **2006**, *20*, 151–153.
118. Guo, Q.; Sopher, B.L.; Furukawa, K.; Pham, D.G.; Robinson, N.; Martin, G.M.; Mattson, M.P. Alzheimer's presenilin mutation sensitizes neural cells to apoptosis induced by trophic factor withdrawal and amyloid beta-peptide: Involvement of calcium and oxyradicals. *J. Neurosci.* **1997**, *17*, 4212–4222. [CrossRef]
119. Leissring, M.A.; Murphy, M.P.; Mead, T.R.; Akbari, Y.; Sugarman, M.C.; Jannatipour, M.; Anliker, B.; Muller, U.; Saftig, P.; De Strooper, B.; et al. A physiologic signaling role for the gamma -secretase-derived intracellular fragment of APP. *Proc. Natl. Acad. Sci. USA* **2002**, *99*, 4697–4702. [CrossRef]

120. Lopez, J.R.; Lyckman, A.; Oddo, S.; Laferla, F.M.; Querfurth, H.W.; Shtifman, A. Increased intraneuronal resting [Ca(2+)] in adult Alzheimer's disease mice. *J. Neurochem.* **2008**, *105*, 262–271. [CrossRef]
121. Rojas, G.; Cardenas, A.M.; Fernandez-Olivares, P.; Shimahara, T.; Segura-Aguilar, J.; Caviedes, R.; Caviedes, P. Effect of the knockdown of amyloid precursor protein on intracellular calcium increases in a neuronal cell line derived from the cerebral cortex of a trisomy 16 mouse. *Exp. Neurol.* **2008**, *209*, 234–242. [CrossRef] [PubMed]
122. Niu, Y.; Su, Z.; Zhao, C.; Song, B.; Zhang, X.; Zhao, N.; Shen, X.; Gong, Y. Effect of amyloid beta on capacitive calcium entry in neural 2a cells. *Brain Res. Bull.* **2009**, *78*, 152–157. [CrossRef] [PubMed]
123. Paula-Lima, A.C.; Hidalgo, C. Amyloid beta-peptide oligomers, ryanodine receptor-mediated Ca(2+) release, and Wnt-5a/Ca(2+) signaling: Opposing roles in neuronal mitochondrial dynamics? *Front. Cell Neurosci.* **2013**, *7*, 120. [CrossRef] [PubMed]
124. Shtifman, A.; Ward, C.W.; Laver, D.R.; Bannister, M.L.; Lopez, J.R.; Kitazawa, M.; LaFerla, F.M.; Ikemoto, N.; Querfurth, H.W. Amyloid-beta protein impairs Ca2+ release and contractility in skeletal muscle. *Neurobiol. Aging* **2010**, *31*, 2080–2090. [CrossRef] [PubMed]
125. Kelliher, M.; Fastbom, J.; Cowburn, R.F.; Bonkale, W.; Ohm, T.G.; Ravid, R.; Sorrentino, V.; O'Neill, C. Alterations in the ryanodine receptor calcium release channel correlate with Alzheimer's disease neurofibrillary and beta-amyloid pathologies. *Neuroscience* **1999**, *92*, 499–513. [CrossRef]
126. Wu, B.; Yamaguchi, H.; Lai, F.A.; Shen, J. Presenilins regulate calcium homeostasis and presynaptic function via ryanodine receptors in hippocampal neurons. *Proc. Natl. Acad. Sci. USA* **2013**, *110*, 15091–15096. [CrossRef]
127. Kipanyula, M.J.; Contreras, L.; Zampese, E.; Lazzari, C.; Wong, A.K.; Pizzo, P.; Fasolato, C.; Pozzan, T. Ca2+ dysregulation in neurons from transgenic mice expressing mutant presenilin 2. *Aging Cell* **2012**, *11*, 885–893. [CrossRef]
128. Cisse, M.; Duplan, E.; Lorivel, T.; Dunys, J.; Bauer, C.; Meckler, X.; Gerakis, Y.; Lauritzen, I.; Checler, F. The transcription factor XBP1s restores hippocampal synaptic plasticity and memory by control of the Kalirin-7 pathway in Alzheimer model. *Mol. Psychiatry* **2017**, *22*, 1562–1575. [CrossRef]
129. Gerakis, Y.; Dunys, J.; Bauer, C.; Checler, F. Abeta42 oligomers modulate beta-secretase through an XBP-1s-dependent pathway involving HRD1. *Sci. Rep.* **2016**, *6*, 37436. [CrossRef]
130. Casas-Tinto, S.; Zhang, Y.; Sanchez-Garcia, J.; Gomez-Velazquez, M.; Rincon-Limas, D.E.; Fernandez-Funez, P. The ER stress factor XBP1s prevents amyloid-beta neurotoxicity. *Hum. Mol. Genet.* **2011**, *20*, 2144–2160. [CrossRef]
131. Liu, J.; Supnet, C.; Sun, S.; Zhang, H.; Good, L.; Popugaeva, E.; Bezprozvanny, I. The role of ryanodine receptor type 3 in a mouse model of Alzheimer disease. *Channels* **2014**, *8*, 230–242. [CrossRef] [PubMed]
132. Mickelson, J.R.; Gallant, E.M.; Litterer, L.A.; Johnson, K.M.; Rempel, W.E.; Louis, C.F. Abnormal sarcoplasmic reticulum ryanodine receptor in malignant hyperthermia. *J. Biol. Chem.* **1988**, *263*, 9310–9315. [PubMed]
133. Kushnir, A.; Wajsberg, B.; Marks, A.R. Ryanodine receptor dysfunction in human disorders. *Biochim. Biophys. Acta Mol. Cell Res.* **2018**, *1865*, 1687–1697. [CrossRef] [PubMed]
134. Kushnir, A.; Betzenhauser, M.J.; Marks, A.R. Ryanodine receptor studies using genetically engineered mice. *FEBS Lett.* **2010**, *584*, 1956–1965. [CrossRef]
135. Takeshima, H.; Iino, M.; Takekura, H.; Nishi, M.; Kuno, J.; Minowa, O.; Takano, H.; Noda, T. Excitation-contraction uncoupling and muscular degeneration in mice lacking functional skeletal muscle ryanodine-receptor gene. *Nature* **1994**, *369*, 556–559. [CrossRef]
136. Takeshima, H.; Ikemoto, T.; Nishi, M.; Nishiyama, N.; Shimuta, M.; Sugitani, Y.; Kuno, J.; Saito, I.; Saito, H.; Endo, M.; et al. Generation and characterization of mutant mice lacking ryanodine receptor type 3. *J. Biol. Chem.* **1996**, *271*, 19649–19652. [CrossRef]
137. Matsuo, N.; Tanda, K.; Nakanishi, K.; Yamasaki, N.; Toyama, K.; Takao, K.; Takeshima, H.; Miyakawa, T. Comprehensive behavioral phenotyping of ryanodine receptor type 3 (RyR3) knockout mice: Decreased social contact duration in two social interaction tests. *Front. Behav. Neurosci.* **2009**, *3*, 3. [CrossRef]
138. Balschun, D.; Wolfer, D.P.; Bertocchini, F.; Barone, V.; Conti, A.; Zuschratter, W.; Missiaen, L.; Lipp, H.P.; Frey, J.U.; Sorrentino, V. Deletion of the ryanodine receptor type 3 (RyR3) impairs forms of synaptic plasticity and spatial learning. *EMBO J.* **1999**, *18*, 5264–5273. [CrossRef]

139. Futatsugi, A.; Kato, K.; Ogura, H.; Li, S.T.; Nagata, E.; Kuwajima, G.; Tanaka, K.; Itohara, S.; Mikoshiba, K. Facilitation of NMDAR-independent LTP and spatial learning in mutant mice lacking ryanodine receptor type 3. *Neuron* **1999**, *24*, 701–713. [CrossRef]
140. Shimuta, M.; Yoshikawa, M.; Fukaya, M.; Watanabe, M.; Takeshima, H.; Manabe, T. Postsynaptic modulation of AMPA receptor-mediated synaptic responses and LTP by the type 3 ryanodine receptor. *Mol. Cell Neurosci.* **2001**, *17*, 921–930. [CrossRef]
141. Gong, S.; Su, B.B.; Tovar, H.; Mao, C.; Gonzalez, V.; Liu, Y.; Lu, Y.; Wang, K.S.; Xu, C. Polymorphisms Within RYR3 Gene Are Associated With Risk and Age at Onset of Hypertension, Diabetes, and Alzheimer's Disease. *Am. J. Hypertens.* **2018**, *31*, 818–826. [CrossRef] [PubMed]
142. Sun, J.; Song, F.; Wang, J.; Han, G.; Bai, Z.; Xie, B.; Feng, X.; Jia, J.; Duan, Y.; Lei, H. Hidden risk genes with high-order intragenic epistasis in Alzheimer's disease. *J. Alzheimer's Dis.* **2014**, *41*, 1039–1056. [CrossRef] [PubMed]
143. Koran, M.E.; Hohman, T.J.; Thornton-Wells, T.A. Genetic interactions found between calcium channel genes modulate amyloid load measured by positron emission tomography. *Hum. Genet.* **2014**, *133*, 85–93. [CrossRef] [PubMed]
144. Wehrens, X.H.; Lehnart, S.E.; Reiken, S.R.; Deng, S.X.; Vest, J.A.; Cervantes, D.; Coromilas, J.; Landry, D.W.; Marks, A.R. Protection from cardiac arrhythmia through ryanodine receptor-stabilizing protein calstabin2. *Science* **2004**, *304*, 292–296. [CrossRef]
145. Andersson, D.C.; Betzenhauser, M.J.; Reiken, S.; Meli, A.C.; Umanskaya, A.; Xie, W.; Shiomi, T.; Zalk, R.; Lacampagne, A.; Marks, A.R. Ryanodine receptor oxidation causes intracellular calcium leak and muscle weakness in aging. *Cell Metab.* **2011**, *14*, 196–207. [CrossRef] [PubMed]
146. Bellinger, A.M.; Reiken, S.; Carlson, C.; Mongillo, M.; Liu, X.; Rothman, L.; Matecki, S.; Lacampagne, A.; Marks, A.R. Hypernitrosylated ryanodine receptor calcium release channels are leaky in dystrophic muscle. *Nat. Med.* **2009**, *15*, 325–330. [CrossRef]
147. Bellinger, A.M.; Reiken, S.; Dura, M.; Murphy, P.W.; Deng, S.X.; Landry, D.W.; Nieman, D.; Lehnart, S.E.; Samaru, M.; LaCampagne, A.; et al. Remodeling of ryanodine receptor complex causes "leaky" channels: A molecular mechanism for decreased exercise capacity. *Proc. Natl. Acad. Sci. USA* **2008**, *105*, 2198–2202. [CrossRef]
148. Fauconnier, J.; Meli, A.C.; Thireau, J.; Roberge, S.; Shan, J.; Sassi, Y.; Reiken, S.R.; Rauzier, J.M.; Marchand, A.; Chauvier, D.; et al. Ryanodine receptor leak mediated by caspase-8 activation leads to left ventricular injury after myocardial ischemia-reperfusion. *Proc. Natl. Acad. Sci. USA* **2011**, *108*, 13258–13263. [CrossRef]
149. Liu, X.; Betzenhauser, M.J.; Reiken, S.; Meli, A.C.; Xie, W.; Chen, B.X.; Arancio, O.; Marks, A.R. Role of leaky neuronal ryanodine receptors in stress-induced cognitive dysfunction. *Cell* **2012**, *150*, 1055–1067. [CrossRef]
150. Lacampagne, A.; Liu, X.; Reiken, S.; Bussiere, R.; Meli, A.C.; Lauritzen, I.; Teich, A.F.; Zalk, R.; Saint, N.; Arancio, O.; et al. Post-translational remodeling of ryanodine receptor induces calcium leak leading to Alzheimer's disease-like pathologies and cognitive deficits. *Acta Neuropathol.* **2017**, *134*, 749–767. [CrossRef]
151. Petrotchenko, E.V.; Yamaguchi, N.; Pasek, D.A.; Borchers, C.H.; Meissner, G. Mass spectrometric analysis and mutagenesis predict involvement of multiple cysteines in redox regulation of the skeletal muscle ryanodine receptor ion channel complex. *Res. Rep. Biol.* **2011**, *2011*, 13–21. [CrossRef] [PubMed]
152. Sun, J.; Yamaguchi, N.; Xu, L.; Eu, J.P.; Stamler, J.S.; Meissner, G. Regulation of the cardiac muscle ryanodine receptor by O(2) tension and S-nitrosoglutathione. *Biochemistry* **2008**, *47*, 13985–13990. [CrossRef] [PubMed]
153. Bussiere, R.; Lacampagne, A.; Reiken, S.; Liu, X.; Scheuerman, V.; Zalk, R.; Martin, C.; Checler, F.; Marks, A.R.; Chami, M. Amyloid beta production is regulated by beta2-adrenergic signaling-mediated post-translational modifications of the ryanodine receptor. *J. Biol. Chem.* **2017**, *292*, 10153–10168. [CrossRef]
154. Hidalgo, C.; Carrasco, M.A. Redox control of brain calcium in health and disease. *Antioxid. Redox Signal.* **2011**, *14*, 1203–1207. [CrossRef] [PubMed]
155. Von Bernhardi, R.; Eugenin, J. Alzheimer's disease: Redox dysregulation as a common denominator for diverse pathogenic mechanisms. *Antioxid. Redox Signal.* **2012**, *16*, 974–1031. [CrossRef]
156. Echeverria, V.; Ducatenzeiler, A.; Chen, C.H.; Cuello, A.C. Endogenous beta-amyloid peptide synthesis modulates cAMP response element-regulated gene expression in PC12 cells. *Neuroscience* **2005**, *135*, 1193–1202. [CrossRef] [PubMed]
157. Igbavboa, U.; Johnson-Anuna, L.N.; Rossello, X.; Butterick, T.A.; Sun, G.Y.; Wood, W.G. Amyloid beta-protein1-42 increases cAMP and apolipoprotein E levels which are inhibited by beta1 and

beta2-adrenergic receptor antagonists in mouse primary astrocytes. *Neuroscience* **2006**, *142*, 655–660. [CrossRef] [PubMed]

158. Prapong, T.; Uemura, E.; Hsu, W.H. G protein and cAMP-dependent protein kinase mediate amyloid beta-peptide inhibition of neuronal glucose uptake. *Exp. Neurol.* **2001**, *167*, 59–64. [CrossRef]
159. Palavicini, J.P.; Wang, H.; Bianchi, E.; Xu, S.; Rao, J.S.; Kang, D.E.; Lakshmana, M.K. RanBP9 aggravates synaptic damage in the mouse brain and is inversely correlated to spinophilin levels in Alzheimer's brain synaptosomes. *Cell Death Dis.* **2013**, *4*, e667. [CrossRef]
160. Marambaud, P.; Ancolio, K.; Alves da Costa, C.; Checler, F. Effect of protein kinase A inhibitors on the production of Abeta40 and Abeta42 by human cells expressing normal and Alzheimer's disease-linked mutated betaAPP and presenilin 1. *Br. J. Pharmacol.* **1999**, *126*, 1186–1190. [CrossRef]
161. Bekris, L.M.; Yu, C.E.; Bird, T.D.; Tsuang, D.W. Genetics of Alzheimer disease. *J. Geriatr. Psychiatry Neurol.* **2010**, *23*, 213–227. [CrossRef] [PubMed]
162. Branca, C.; Wisely, E.V.; Hartman, L.K.; Caccamo, A.; Oddo, S. Administration of a selective beta2 adrenergic receptor antagonist exacerbates neuropathology and cognitive deficits in a mouse model of Alzheimer's disease. *Neurobiol. Aging* **2014**, *35*, 2726–2735. [CrossRef] [PubMed]
163. Dobarro, M.; Gerenu, G.; Ramirez, M.J. Propranolol reduces cognitive deficits, amyloid and tau pathology in Alzheimer's transgenic mice. *Int. J. Neuropsychopharmacol.* **2013**, *16*, 2245–2257. [CrossRef] [PubMed]
164. Dang, V.; Medina, B.; Das, D.; Moghadam, S.; Martin, K.J.; Lin, B.; Naik, P.; Patel, D.; Nosheny, R.; Wesson Ashford, J.; et al. Formoterol, a long-acting beta2 adrenergic agonist, improves cognitive function and promotes dendritic complexity in a mouse model of Down syndrome. *Biol. Psychiatry* **2014**, *75*, 179–188. [CrossRef]
165. Peng, J.; Liang, G.; Inan, S.; Wu, Z.; Joseph, D.J.; Meng, Q.; Peng, Y.; Eckenhoff, M.F.; Wei, H. Dantrolene ameliorates cognitive decline and neuropathology in Alzheimer triple transgenic mice. *Neurosci. Lett.* **2012**, *516*, 274–279. [CrossRef]
166. Mikoshiba, K. IP3 receptor/Ca2+ channel: From discovery to new signaling concepts. *J. Neurochem.* **2007**, *102*, 1426–1446. [CrossRef]
167. Ross, C.A.; Meldolesi, J.; Milner, T.A.; Satoh, T.; Supattapone, S.; Snyder, S.H. Inositol 1,4,5-trisphosphate receptor localized to endoplasmic reticulum in cerebellar Purkinje neurons. *Nature* **1989**, *339*, 468–470. [CrossRef]
168. Furuichi, T.; Yoshikawa, S.; Miyawaki, A.; Wada, K.; Maeda, N.; Mikoshiba, K. Primary structure and functional expression of the inositol 1,4,5-trisphosphate-binding protein P400. *Nature* **1989**, *342*, 32–38. [CrossRef]
169. Mignery, G.A.; Sudhof, T.C.; Takei, K.; De Camilli, P. Putative receptor for inositol 1,4,5-trisphosphate similar to ryanodine receptor. *Nature* **1989**, *342*, 192–195. [CrossRef]
170. Foskett, J.K.; White, C.; Cheung, K.H.; Mak, D.O. Inositol trisphosphate receptor Ca2+ release channels. *Physiol. Rev.* **2007**, *87*, 593–658. [CrossRef]
171. Inoue, T.; Kato, K.; Kohda, K.; Mikoshiba, K. Type 1 inositol 1,4,5-trisphosphate receptor is required for induction of long-term depression in cerebellar Purkinje neurons. *J. Neurosci.* **1998**, *18*, 5366–5373. [CrossRef] [PubMed]
172. Baker, K.D.; Edwards, T.M.; Rickard, N.S. The role of intracellular calcium stores in synaptic plasticity and memory consolidation. *Neurosci. Biobehav. Rev.* **2013**, *37*, 1211–1239. [CrossRef] [PubMed]
173. Sugawara, T.; Hisatsune, C.; Le, T.D.; Hashikawa, T.; Hirono, M.; Hattori, M.; Nagao, S.; Mikoshiba, K. Type 1 inositol trisphosphate receptor regulates cerebellar circuits by maintaining the spine morphology of purkinje cells in adult mice. *J. Neurosci.* **2013**, *33*, 12186–12196. [CrossRef] [PubMed]
174. Egorova, P.A.; Bezprozvanny, I.B. Inositol 1,4,5-trisphosphate receptors and neurodegenerative disorders. *FEBS J.* **2018**, *285*, 3547–3565. [CrossRef]
175. Leissring, M.A.; Paul, B.A.; Parker, I.; Cotman, C.W.; LaFerla, F.M. Alzheimer's presenilin-1 mutation potentiates inositol 1,4,5-trisphosphate-mediated calcium signaling in Xenopus oocytes. *J. Neurochem.* **1999**, *72*, 1061–1068. [CrossRef]
176. Cedazo-Minguez, A.; Popescu, B.O.; Ankarcrona, M.; Nishimura, T.; Cowburn, R.F. The presenilin 1 deltaE9 mutation gives enhanced basal phospholipase C activity and a resultant increase in intracellular calcium concentrations. *J. Biol. Chem.* **2002**, *277*, 36646–36655. [CrossRef]

177. Bezprozvanny, I.; Supnet, C.; Sun, S.; Zhang, H.; De Strooper, B. Response to Shilling et al. (10.1074/jbc.M111.300491). *J. Biol. Chem.* **2012**, *287*, 20469. [CrossRef]
178. Mak, D.O.; Cheung, K.H.; Toglia, P.; Foskett, J.K.; Ullah, G. Analyzing and Quantifying the Gain-of-Function Enhancement of IP3 Receptor Gating by Familial Alzheimer's Disease-Causing Mutants in Presenilins. *PLoS Comput. Biol.* **2015**, *11*, e1004529. [CrossRef]
179. Toglia, P.; Ullah, G. The gain-of-function enhancement of IP3-receptor channel gating by familial Alzheimer's disease-linked presenilin mutants increases the open probability of mitochondrial permeability transition pore. *Cell Calcium* **2016**, *60*, 13–24. [CrossRef]
180. Wang, Z.J.; Zhao, F.; Wang, C.F.; Zhang, X.M.; Xiao, Y.; Zhou, F.; Wu, M.N.; Zhang, J.; Qi, J.S.; Yang, W. Xestospongin C, a Reversible IP3 Receptor Antagonist, Alleviates the Cognitive and Pathological Impairments in APP/PS1 Mice of Alzheimer's Disease. *J. Alzheimer's Dis.* **2019**, *72*, 1217–1231. [CrossRef]
181. Ronco, V.; Grolla, A.A.; Glasnov, T.N.; Canonico, P.L.; Verkhratsky, A.; Genazzani, A.A.; Lim, D. Differential deregulation of astrocytic calcium signalling by amyloid-beta, TNFalpha, IL-1beta and LPS. *Cell Calcium* **2014**, *55*, 219–229. [CrossRef] [PubMed]
182. Grolla, A.A.; Sim, J.A.; Lim, D.; Rodriguez, J.J.; Genazzani, A.A.; Verkhratsky, A. Amyloid-beta and Alzheimer's disease type pathology differentially affects the calcium signalling toolkit in astrocytes from different brain regions. *Cell Death Dis.* **2013**, *4*, e623. [CrossRef] [PubMed]
183. De Strooper, B.; Beullens, M.; Contreras, B.; Levesque, L.; Craessaerts, K.; Cordell, B.; Moechars, D.; Bollen, M.; Fraser, P.; George-Hyslop, P.S.; et al. Phosphorylation, subcellular localization, and membrane orientation of the Alzheimer's disease-associated presenilins. *J. Biol. Chem.* **1997**, *272*, 3590–3598. [CrossRef] [PubMed]
184. Sherrington, R.; Rogaev, E.I.; Liang, Y.; Rogaeva, E.A.; Levesque, G.; Ikeda, M.; Chi, H.; Lin, C.; Li, G.; Holman, K.; et al. Cloning of a gene bearing missense mutations in early-onset familial Alzheimer's disease. *Nature* **1995**, *375*, 754–760. [CrossRef]
185. Rogaev, E.I.; Sherrington, R.; Rogaeva, E.A.; Levesque, G.; Ikeda, M.; Liang, Y.; Chi, H.; Lin, C.; Holman, K.; Tsuda, T.; et al. Familial Alzheimer's disease in kindreds with missense mutations in a gene on chromosome 1 related to the Alzheimer's disease type 3 gene. *Nature* **1995**, *376*, 775–778. [CrossRef]
186. Levy-Lahad, E.; Wasco, W.; Poorkaj, P.; Romano, D.M.; Oshima, J.; Pettingell, W.H.; Yu, C.E.; Jondro, P.D.; Schmidt, S.D.; Wang, K.; et al. Candidate gene for the chromosome 1 familial Alzheimer's disease locus. *Science* **1995**, *269*, 973–977. [CrossRef]
187. Lu, P.; Bai, X.C.; Ma, D.; Xie, T.; Yan, C.; Sun, L.; Yang, G.; Zhao, Y.; Zhou, R.; Scheres, S.H.W.; et al. Three-dimensional structure of human gamma-secretase. *Nature* **2014**, *512*, 166–170. [CrossRef]
188. Bai, X.C.; Yan, C.; Yang, G.; Lu, P.; Ma, D.; Sun, L.; Zhou, R.; Scheres, S.H.W.; Shi, Y. An atomic structure of human gamma-secretase. *Nature* **2015**, *525*, 212–217. [CrossRef]
189. Yang, G.; Zhou, R.; Shi, Y. Cryo-EM structures of human gamma-secretase. *Curr. Opin. Struct. Biol.* **2017**, *46*, 55–64. [CrossRef]
190. Lee, M.K.; Slunt, H.H.; Martin, L.J.; Thinakaran, G.; Kim, G.; Gandy, S.E.; Seeger, M.; Koo, E.; Price, D.L.; Sisodia, S.S. Expression of presenilin 1 and 2 (PS1 and PS2) in human and murine tissues. *J. Neurosci.* **1996**, *16*, 7513–7525. [CrossRef]
191. Wong, P.C.; Zheng, H.; Chen, H.; Becher, M.W.; Sirinathsinghji, D.J.; Trumbauer, M.E.; Chen, H.Y.; Price, D.L.; Van der Ploeg, L.H.; Sisodia, S.S. Presenilin 1 is required for Notch1 and DII1 expression in the paraxial mesoderm. *Nature* **1997**, *387*, 288–292. [CrossRef] [PubMed]
192. Donoviel, D.B.; Hadjantonakis, A.K.; Ikeda, M.; Zheng, H.; Hyslop, P.S.; Bernstein, A. Mice lacking both presenilin genes exhibit early embryonic patterning defects. *Genes Dev.* **1999**, *13*, 2801–2810. [CrossRef] [PubMed]
193. Beglopoulos, V.; Sun, X.; Saura, C.A.; Lemere, C.A.; Kim, R.D.; Shen, J. Reduced beta-amyloid production and increased inflammatory responses in presenilin conditional knock-out mice. *J. Biol. Chem.* **2004**, *279*, 46907–46914. [CrossRef] [PubMed]
194. Zhang, C.; Wu, B.; Beglopoulos, V.; Wines-Samuelson, M.; Zhang, D.; Dragatsis, I.; Sudhof, T.C.; Shen, J. Presenilins are essential for regulating neurotransmitter release. *Nature* **2009**, *460*, 632–636. [CrossRef]
195. Wolfe, M.S.; Xia, W.; Ostaszewski, B.L.; Diehl, T.S.; Kimberly, W.T.; Selkoe, D.J. Two transmembrane aspartates in presenilin-1 required for presenilin endoproteolysis and gamma-secretase activity. *Nature* **1999**, *398*, 513–517. [CrossRef]

196. Borchelt, D.R.; Thinakaran, G.; Eckman, C.B.; Lee, M.K.; Davenport, F.; Ratovitsky, T.; Prada, C.M.; Kim, G.; Seekins, S.; Yager, D.; et al. Familial Alzheimer's disease-linked presenilin 1 variants elevate Abeta1-42/1-40 ratio in vitro and in vivo. *Neuron* **1996**, *17*, 1005–1013. [CrossRef]
197. Tomita, T.; Maruyama, K.; Saido, T.C.; Kume, H.; Shinozaki, K.; Tokuhiro, S.; Capell, A.; Walter, J.; Grunberg, J.; Haass, C.; et al. The presenilin 2 mutation (N141I) linked to familial Alzheimer disease (Volga German families) increases the secretion of amyloid beta protein ending at the 42nd (or 43rd) residue. *Proc. Natl. Acad. Sci. USA* **1997**, *94*, 2025–2030. [CrossRef]
198. Scheuner, D.; Eckman, C.; Jensen, M.; Song, X.; Citron, M.; Suzuki, N.; Bird, T.D.; Hardy, J.; Hutton, M.; Kukull, W.; et al. Secreted amyloid beta-protein similar to that in the senile plaques of Alzheimer's disease is increased in vivo by the presenilin 1 and 2 and APP mutations linked to familial Alzheimer's disease. *Nat. Med.* **1996**, *2*, 864–870. [CrossRef]
199. Mehra, R.; Kepp, K.P. Identification of Structural Calcium Binding Sites in Membrane-Bound Presenilin 1 and 2. *J. Phys. Chem. B* **2020**, *124*, 4697–4711. [CrossRef]
200. Thinakaran, G.; Borchelt, D.R.; Lee, M.K.; Slunt, H.H.; Spitzer, L.; Kim, G.; Ratovitsky, T.; Davenport, F.; Nordstedt, C.; Seeger, M.; et al. Endoproteolysis of presenilin 1 and accumulation of processed derivatives in vivo. *Neuron* **1996**, *17*, 181–190. [CrossRef]
201. Takeda, T.; Asahi, M.; Yamaguchi, O.; Hikoso, S.; Nakayama, H.; Kusakari, Y.; Kawai, M.; Hongo, K.; Higuchi, Y.; Kashiwase, K.; et al. Presenilin 2 regulates the systolic function of heart by modulating Ca2+ signaling. *FASEB J.* **2005**, *19*, 2069–2071. [CrossRef] [PubMed]
202. Pack-Chung, E.; Meyers, M.B.; Pettingell, W.P.; Moir, R.D.; Brownawell, A.M.; Cheng, I.; Tanzi, R.E.; Kim, T.W. Presenilin 2 interacts with sorcin, a modulator of the ryanodine receptor. *J. Biol. Chem.* **2000**, *275*, 14440–14445. [CrossRef] [PubMed]
203. Hayrapetyan, V.; Rybalchenko, V.; Rybalchenko, N.; Koulen, P. The N-terminus of presenilin-2 increases single channel activity of brain ryanodine receptors through direct protein-protein interaction. *Cell Calcium* **2008**, *44*, 507–518. [CrossRef] [PubMed]
204. Rybalchenko, V.; Hwang, S.Y.; Rybalchenko, N.; Koulen, P. The cytosolic N-terminus of presenilin-1 potentiates mouse ryanodine receptor single channel activity. *Int. J. Biochem. Cell Biol.* **2008**, *40*, 84–97. [CrossRef] [PubMed]
205. Greotti, E.; Capitanio, P.; Wong, A.; Pozzan, T.; Pizzo, P.; Pendin, D. Familial Alzheimer's disease-linked presenilin mutants and intracellular Ca(2+) handling: A single-organelle, FRET-based analysis. *Cell Calcium* **2019**, *79*, 44–56. [CrossRef] [PubMed]
206. Baba-Aissa, F.; Raeymaekers, L.; Wuytack, F.; Dode, L.; Casteels, R. Distribution and isoform diversity of the organellar Ca2+ pumps in the brain. *Mol. Chem. Neuropathol.* **1998**, *33*, 199–208. [CrossRef] [PubMed]
207. Britzolaki, A.; Saurine, J.; Klocke, B.; Pitychoutis, P.M. A Role for SERCA Pumps in the Neurobiology of Neuropsychiatric and Neurodegenerative Disorders. *Adv. Exp. Med. Biol.* **2020**, *1131*, 131–161. [CrossRef]
208. Jin, H.; Sanjo, N.; Uchihara, T.; Watabe, K.; St George-Hyslop, P.; Fraser, P.E.; Mizusawa, H. Presenilin-1 holoprotein is an interacting partner of sarco endoplasmic reticulum calcium-ATPase and confers resistance to endoplasmic reticulum stress. *J. Alzheimer's Dis.* **2010**, *20*, 261–273. [CrossRef]
209. Krajnak, K.; Dahl, R. A new target for Alzheimer's disease: A small molecule SERCA activator is neuroprotective in vitro and improves memory and cognition in APP/PS1 mice. *Bioorg. Med. Chem. Lett.* **2018**, *28*, 1591–1594. [CrossRef]
210. Zhao, L.; Ackerman, S.L. Endoplasmic reticulum stress in health and disease. *Curr. Opin. Cell Biol.* **2006**, *18*, 444–452. [CrossRef]
211. Hetz, C.; Papa, F.R. The Unfolded Protein Response and Cell Fate Control. *Mol. Cell* **2018**, *69*, 169–181. [CrossRef] [PubMed]
212. Hoozemans, J.J.; Veerhuis, R.; Van Haastert, E.S.; Rozemuller, J.M.; Baas, F.; Eikelenboom, P.; Scheper, W. The unfolded protein response is activated in Alzheimer's disease. *Acta Neuropathol.* **2005**, *110*, 165–172. [CrossRef] [PubMed]
213. Hoozemans, J.J.; van Haastert, E.S.; Nijholt, D.A.; Rozemuller, A.J.; Eikelenboom, P.; Scheper, W. The unfolded protein response is activated in pretangle neurons in Alzheimer's disease hippocampus. *Am. J. Pathol.* **2009**, *174*, 1241–1251. [CrossRef] [PubMed]
214. Chang, R.C.; Suen, K.C.; Ma, C.H.; Elyaman, W.; Ng, H.K.; Hugon, J. Involvement of double-stranded RNA-dependent protein kinase and phosphorylation of eukaryotic initiation factor-2alpha in neuronal degeneration. *J. Neurochem.* **2002**, *83*, 1215–1225. [CrossRef]

215. Page, G.; Rioux Bilan, A.; Ingrand, S.; Lafay-Chebassier, C.; Pain, S.; Perault Pochat, M.C.; Bouras, C.; Bayer, T.; Hugon, J. Activated double-stranded RNA-dependent protein kinase and neuronal death in models of Alzheimer's disease. *Neuroscience* **2006**, *139*, 1343–1354. [CrossRef]
216. Kim, H.S.; Choi, Y.; Shin, K.Y.; Joo, Y.; Lee, Y.K.; Jung, S.Y.; Suh, Y.H.; Kim, J.H. Swedish amyloid precursor protein mutation increases phosphorylation of eIF2alpha in vitro and in vivo. *J. Neurosci. Res.* **2007**, *85*, 1528–1537. [CrossRef]
217. Chami, M.; Gozuacik, D.; Lagorce, D.; Brini, M.; Falson, P.; Peaucellier, G.; Pinton, P.; Lecoeur, H.; Gougeon, M.L.; le Maire, M.; et al. SERCA1 truncated proteins unable to pump calcium reduce the endoplasmic reticulum calcium concentration and induce apoptosis. *J. Cell Biol.* **2001**, *153*, 1301–1314. [CrossRef]
218. Chami, M.; Oules, B.; Szabadkai, G.; Tacine, R.; Rizzuto, R.; Paterlini-Brechot, P. Role of SERCA1 truncated isoform in the proapoptotic calcium transfer from ER to mitochondria during ER stress. *Mol. Cell* **2008**, *32*, 641–651. [CrossRef]
219. Nishitsuji, K.; Tomiyama, T.; Ishibashi, K.; Ito, K.; Teraoka, R.; Lambert, M.P.; Klein, W.L.; Mori, H. The E693Delta mutation in amyloid precursor protein increases intracellular accumulation of amyloid beta oligomers and causes endoplasmic reticulum stress-induced apoptosis in cultured cells. *Am. J. Pathol.* **2009**, *174*, 957–969. [CrossRef]
220. O'Connor, T.; Sadleir, K.R.; Maus, E.; Velliquette, R.A.; Zhao, J.; Cole, S.L.; Eimer, W.A.; Hitt, B.; Bembinster, L.A.; Lammich, S.; et al. Phosphorylation of the translation initiation factor eIF2alpha increases BACE1 levels and promotes amyloidogenesis. *Neuron* **2008**, *60*, 988–1009. [CrossRef]
221. Devi, L.; Ohno, M. PERK mediates eIF2alpha phosphorylation responsible for BACE1 elevation, CREB dysfunction and neurodegeneration in a mouse model of Alzheimer's disease. *Neurobiol. Aging* **2014**, *35*, 2272–2281. [CrossRef] [PubMed]
222. Chami, L.; Checler, F. BACE1 is at the crossroad of a toxic vicious cycle involving cellular stress and beta-amyloid production in Alzheimer's disease. *Mol. Neurodegener.* **2012**, *7*, 52. [CrossRef] [PubMed]
223. Salminen, A.; Kauppinen, A.; Suuronen, T.; Kaarniranta, K.; Ojala, J. ER stress in Alzheimer's disease: A novel neuronal trigger for inflammation and Alzheimer's pathology. *J. Neuroinflamm.* **2009**, *6*, 41. [CrossRef] [PubMed]
224. Popugaeva, E.; Bezprozvanny, I. STIM proteins as regulators of neuronal store-operated calcium influx. *Neurodegener. Dis. Manag.* **2018**, *8*, 5–7. [CrossRef] [PubMed]
225. Secondo, A.; Bagetta, G.; Amantea, D. On the Role of Store-Operated Calcium Entry in Acute and Chronic Neurodegenerative Diseases. *Front. Mol. Neurosci.* **2018**, *11*, 87. [CrossRef]
226. Kraft, R. STIM and ORAI proteins in the nervous system. *Channels* **2015**, *9*, 245–252. [CrossRef]
227. Luik, R.M.; Wu, M.M.; Buchanan, J.; Lewis, R.S. The elementary unit of store-operated Ca2+ entry: Local activation of CRAC channels by STIM1 at ER-plasma membrane junctions. *J. Cell Biol.* **2006**, *174*, 815–825. [CrossRef]
228. Ambudkar, I.S.; Ong, H.L.; Liu, X.; Bandyopadhyay, B.C.; Cheng, K.T. TRPC1: The link between functionally distinct store-operated calcium channels. *Cell Calcium* **2007**, *42*, 213–223. [CrossRef]
229. Chen, X.; Sooch, G.; Demaree, I.S.; White, F.A.; Obukhov, A.G. Transient Receptor Potential Canonical (TRPC) Channels: Then and Now. *Cells* **2020**, *9*, 1983. [CrossRef]
230. Moccia, F.; Zuccolo, E.; Soda, T.; Tanzi, F.; Guerra, G.; Mapelli, L.; Lodola, F.; D'Angelo, E. Stim and Orai proteins in neuronal Ca(2+) signaling and excitability. *Front. Cell Neurosci.* **2015**, *9*, 153. [CrossRef]
231. Wegierski, T.; Kuznicki, J. Neuronal calcium signaling via store-operated channels in health and disease. *Cell Calcium* **2018**, *74*, 102–111. [CrossRef] [PubMed]
232. Heine, M.; Heck, J.; Ciuraszkiewicz, A.; Bikbaev, A. Dynamic compartmentalization of calcium channel signalling in neurons. *Neuropharmacology* **2020**, *169*, 107556. [CrossRef] [PubMed]
233. Sun, S.; Zhang, H.; Liu, J.; Popugaeva, E.; Xu, N.J.; Feske, S.; White, C.L., 3rd; Bezprozvanny, I. Reduced synaptic STIM2 expression and impaired store-operated calcium entry cause destabilization of mature spines in mutant presenilin mice. *Neuron* **2014**, *82*, 79–93. [CrossRef] [PubMed]
234. Tong, B.C.; Lee, C.S.; Cheng, W.H.; Lai, K.O.; Foskett, J.K.; Cheung, K.H. Familial Alzheimer's disease-associated presenilin 1 mutants promote gamma-secretase cleavage of STIM1 to impair store-operated Ca2+ entry. *Sci. Signal.* **2016** *9*, ra89. [CrossRef]

235. Ryazantseva, M.; Goncharova, A.; Skobeleva, K.; Erokhin, M.; Methner, A.; Georgiev, P.; Kaznacheyeva, E. Presenilin-1 Delta E9 Mutant Induces STIM1-Driven Store-Operated Calcium Channel Hyperactivation in Hippocampal Neurons. *Mol. Neurobiol.* **2018**, *55*, 4667–4680. [CrossRef]
236. Linde, C.I.; Baryshnikov, S.G.; Mazzocco-Spezzia, A.; Golovina, V.A. Dysregulation of Ca2+ signaling in astrocytes from mice lacking amyloid precursor protein. *Am. J. Physiol. Cell Physiol.* **2011**, *300*, C1502–C1512. [CrossRef]
237. Wang, J.; Lu, R.; Yang, J.; Li, H.; He, Z.; Jing, N.; Wang, X.; Wang, Y. TRPC6 specifically interacts with APP to inhibit its cleavage by gamma-secretase and reduce Abeta production. *Nat. Commun.* **2015**, *6*, 8876. [CrossRef]
238. Lessard, C.B.; Lussier, M.P.; Cayouette, S.; Bourque, G.; Boulay, G. The overexpression of presenilin2 and Alzheimer's-disease-linked presenilin2 variants influences TRPC6-enhanced Ca2+ entry into HEK293 cells. *Cell Signal.* **2005**, *17*, 437–445. [CrossRef]
239. Prikhodko, V.; Chernyuk, D.; Sysoev, Y.; Zernov, N.; Okovityi, S.; Popugaeva, E. Potential Drug Candidates to Treat TRPC6 Channel Deficiencies in the Pathophysiology of Alzheimer's Disease and Brain Ischemia. *Cells* **2020**, *9*, 2351. [CrossRef]
240. Giorgi, C.; Missiroli, S.; Patergnani, S.; Duszynski, J.; Wieckowski, M.R.; Pinton, P. Mitochondria-associated membranes: Composition, molecular mechanisms, and physiopathological implications. *Antioxid. Redox Signal.* **2015**, *22*, 995–1019. [CrossRef]
241. Area-Gomez, E.; de Groof, A.; Bonilla, E.; Montesinos, J.; Tanji, K.; Boldogh, I.; Pon, L.; Schon, E.A. A key role for MAM in mediating mitochondrial dysfunction in Alzheimer disease. *Cell Death Dis.* **2018**, *9*, 335. [CrossRef] [PubMed]

12

Biomarkers for Alzheimer's Disease Early Diagnosis

Eva Ausó, Violeta Gómez-Vicente and Gema Esquiva *

Department of Optics, Pharmacology and Anatomy, University of Alicante, 03690 Alicante, Spain; eva.auso@ua.es (E.A.); vgvicente@ua.es (V.G.-V.)
* Correspondence: gema.esquiva@ua.es

Abstract: Alzheimer's disease (AD) is the most common cause of dementia, affecting the central nervous system (CNS) through the accumulation of intraneuronal neurofibrillary tau tangles (NFTs) and β-amyloid plaques. By the time AD is clinically diagnosed, neuronal loss has already occurred in many brain and retinal regions. Therefore, the availability of early and reliable diagnosis markers of the disease would allow its detection and taking preventive measures to avoid neuronal loss. Current diagnostic tools in the brain, such as magnetic resonance imaging (MRI), positron emission tomography (PET) imaging, and cerebrospinal fluid (CSF) biomarkers (Aβ and tau) detection are invasive and expensive. Brain-secreted extracellular vesicles (BEVs) isolated from peripheral blood have emerged as novel strategies in the study of AD, with enormous potential as a diagnostic evaluation of therapeutics and treatment tools. In addition; similar mechanisms of neurodegeneration have been demonstrated in the brain and the eyes of AD patients. Since the eyes are more accessible than the brain, several eye tests that detect cellular and vascular changes in the retina have also been proposed as potential screening biomarkers. The aim of this study is to summarize and discuss several potential markers in the brain, eye, blood, and other accessible biofluids like saliva and urine, and correlate them with earlier diagnosis and prognosis to identify individuals with mild symptoms prior to dementia.

Keywords: Alzheimer's disease; biomarkers; early diagnosis; biofluids

1. Introduction

1.1. Pathophysiology of AD and Clinical Manifestations

The lesions of Alzheimer's disease (AD) include pathological changes in the brain such as the accumulation of proteins (amyloid-β (Aβ) peptide and Tau); the degeneration of neurons and synapses, most noticeably in the neocortex and the hippocampus, which leads to structural changes as well as to the loss of functional connectivity, and the alterations of reactive processes like neuroinflammation and plasticity, related to oxidative stress and mitochondrial dysfunction [1]. Some of these hallmarks can be detected in the prodromal stage of the disease, also referred to as mild cognitive impairment (MCI) due to AD, when the symptoms are not yet obvious.

Amyloid-β deposits are widely distributed in the brain and follow an anterograde sequence originating in five phases in which different brain regions are hierarchically involved [2–4]. The five phases go from phase 1, when the deposits are exclusively found in the isocortex, to phase 5, when the cerebellum and several brainstem nuclei, such as the pontine nuclei and the locus coeruleus, among others, are involved [2,4]. The progression of Tau pathology is also staggered from the transentorhinal and entorhinal cortex to the isocortex via the hippocampus, with a heterogeneous and area-specific neuronal loss [2–4]. It is well-established that the accumulation of Tau protein takes place specifically in neurons and occurs in their cell body as neurofibrillary tangles (NFTs), in their dendrites as neuropil threads (NT), and in their axons forming the senile plaque neuritic corona [3].

The Braak stages, based on phospho-Tau accumulation within connected brain regions, defines the progression of AD neuropathology. I–II refer to the entorhinal cortex, III–IV to the hippocampus/limbic system, and V–VI to the frontal and parietal lobes.

1.2. Diagnostic Tools

The progress in the diagnosis of AD has noticeably improved with the development in the last decades of noninvasive neuroimaging techniques that allow the visualization of structures in vivo. Some examples are novel magnetic resonance imaging (MRI), metabolic changes detected by positron emission tomography (PET), and amyloid imaging. These techniques permit the detection of pre-symptomatic diagnostic biomarkers in the brains of cognitively normal elderly individuals and also serve to monitor disease progression after the onset of symptoms [1]. Due to their reliability and high discriminative capacity in the pre-dementia state, volumetric approaches of the high-resolution subfield are useful, as well as diagnostic techniques in order to study the early changes in the most affected brain structures [2–4]. With all these tools, the typical lesions related to protein accumulation and the structural changes in certain brain areas are easier to detect and; therefore, constitute the basis of the diagnosis.

In addition, the advancement in the past few years of omics technologies (genomics, transcriptomics, proteomics, metabolomics, secretomics, etc.) has made possible the analysis of a wide range of AD hallmarks referring to both, sporadic and familial cases. These tools facilitate the analysis of human fluid samples of diverse nature such as blood, tears, urine, or saliva, whose collection in most cases does not require trained professionals and has the advantage of being noninvasive due to easy accessibility. The importance of identifying and developing reliable and sensitive tools for the early diagnosis of AD relies on the potential benefits for the patients, including timely access to medical treatments to slow down the progression of the disease and; therefore, preservation of longer cognitive capacity, or even the possibility to plan for the future.

2. Invasive Biomarkers

2.1. Changes in Specific Brain Areas as Early Biomarkers

The locus coeruleus (LC) is a neuromelanin-rich brainstem structure thought to modulate attention and memory and is the major source of noradrenaline in the brain. In the asymptomatic stage of AD, Tau NFTs are observed in the LC [5,6] prior to their presence in other cerebral areas such as the entorhinal cortex and the neocortex [7–10]. These Tau aggregates precede typical neuronal loss in the LC during AD progression [11]. Studies using unbiased stereology have revealed an average decrease in LC volume of 8.4% for each Braak stage increment, as well as neuronal loss mainly in the rostral/middle area of the LC, progressing from 30% in the prodromal stage to 55% when dementia is diagnosed [11]. Functionally, this neuronal loss has correlated with cognitive dysfunction [12] and reduced noradrenaline levels in the hippocampus and the cortex [13]. Additionally, a two-fold increase in Tau accumulation was also observed from Braak stage 0 to I [9]. Therefore, the detection using in vivo imaging of early structural tissue modifications such as the decrease in the LC volume or metabolic changes would support the diagnosis and could potentially slow down disease progression if the patient benefits from treatments in the appropriate time [14,15].

Although there is controversy regarding the accelerated rates of brain atrophy at the preclinical stage of the disease, it seems that the medial temporal lobe and, particularly, the hippocampus are brain structures early affected by NFTs and neurite loss. Studies using voxel-based morphometry and high-resolution MRI have revealed hippocampal atrophy in AD patients' brains at the preclinical stage, up to 10 years before the diagnosis of dementia [16], and even before MCI [17,18]. The magnitude of atrophy in the hippocampus and its subfields determines the progression to either MCI or AD [19–21]. Thus, studies using radial atrophy measurements have shown that CA1 and the subicular atrophy in cognitively healthy individuals is associated with an increased risk of developing MCI, while the gradual involvement of the CA1 and subiculum fields, along with atrophy spread to the rest of the hippocampus (CA2–3 subfields) in amnestic MCI, suggests the future diagnosis of AD [22,23]. Moreover, apolipoprotein E (ApoE) plays a significant role in AD pathogenesis by affecting amyloid and Tau pathology. The presence of the allele ε4 (APOEε4) [24] influences the reduction of the hippocampal volume and the accumulation of Aβ filaments in the brains of elderly people without cognitive impairment and normal levels of Aβ-peptides morphologically [25–27]. In this direction, MRI imaging has revealed a significant reduction in the hippocampal volume in amnestic MCI people carrying APOEε4, especially in those who progressed to AD [28]. Even cognitively normal APOEε4 carriers have shown hippocampal volume and cortical thickness reduction together with memory decline and accelerated brain atrophy rates before the onset of cognitive impairment [24,27].

Regarding neuronal connectivity dysfunction, a novel PET tracer that binds to synaptic vesicle glycoprotein 2A (SV2A) can be used to quantify synaptic density in vivo, predicting the stage of AD [29]. Several morphological studies have shown that synaptic loss appears early in the pathology [30,31], so the study of markers of neuronal death may derive in promising results for the early diagnosis of AD.

In conclusion, in vivo morphological studies of different brain areas (LC, hippocampus, etc.), along with genetic studies that detect alleles or mutations closely related to the pathology, point out their usefulness as biomarkers for the early detection of AD. Despite the high prognostic ability of these techniques in AD and MCI [32], sometimes, there are limitations that make it difficult to use them in the routine analysis [33]. For this reason, biomarkers in cerebrospinal fluid (CSF) are being extensively studied worldwide as potential candidates for the diagnosis of AD before the appearance of cognitive symptoms [34].

2.2. Cerebrospinal Fluid

There is no doubt the ideal fluid biomarker should have a series of characteristics—reliable, reproducible, and noninvasive in terms of collection, specific for a particular disease, simple, and inexpensive to measure, and easy to implement in large populations. In this regard, blood biomarkers meet several of these criteria and could be used in primary care to identify patients with risk of AD [35]. In contrast, CSF collection does not meet the criteria of being a noninvasive procedure, which certainly limits its use but given the close relationship between the brain and the CSF, this fluid could provide valuable information about the biochemical changes that occur in the brain at the preclinical stages of AD [36]. For instance, it is well established that decreased Aβ-42 and elevated total Tau and phospho-Tau in CSF are considered specific markers of AD [37,38], and that these biomarkers can predict cognitive decline over time [39]. The advantages and disadvantages of each category of fluid biomarkers (blood, CSF, and other matrices such as tears, saliva, and urine) are summarized in Table 1.

Table 1. Advantages and disadvantages for each category of biological fluids used to isolate Alzheimer's disease biomarkers.

	Advantages	Disadvantages
CSF	Close relationship with the brain High accuracy in the diagnostic process Ability to test a large number of candidate pathophysiological biomarkers High concentration of the biomarkers	Invasive Clinicians require training Positioned in later disease stages, after blood samples, as a confirmatory diagnostic modality Process less accepted by the population and at the risk of causing harm, anxiety, and fear to the patient

Table 1. *Cont.*

	Advantages	Disadvantages
Blood	Noninvasive, fast and convenient Inexpensive and reproducible Simple to measure (well-established as part of clinical routines globally) No prior training of the clinicians is required Can be performed in a large variety of settings (primary care, hospitals, patient's home ...) Easy to implement in large populations Ability to test a large number of candidate pathophysiological biomarkers First-step of the multi-stage diagnostic process (identification of patients at the earliest stages of the disease)	Less accurate Presence of very low concentrations of the biomarkers once they have crossed the blood-brain barrier and decreased time window for testing Less consistent results (susceptibility to interference with other components)
Other matrices (tears, saliva, and urine)	Extremely noninvasive Repeatable collections Easy, no risk of infection, can be self-collected by the patient Cheap Stress-free	Remarkable lack of validated studies Lack of results replicated in larger, multicenter and longitudinal studies

Nowadays, novel molecular markers are being evaluated in CSF through omics technologies, which allow measuring a large number of analytes at a time (Figure 1). For example, a mass spectroscopy-based analysis revealed that similar levels of ApoE and its isoforms (ApoE2, ApoE3, and ApoE4) were found in the CSF of AD patients and non-AD individuals, independent of their APOE genotype (APOEε2, APOEε3, or APOEε4). However, CSF total ApoE concentrations were positively associated with CSF total Tau and phospho-Tau levels [40,41].

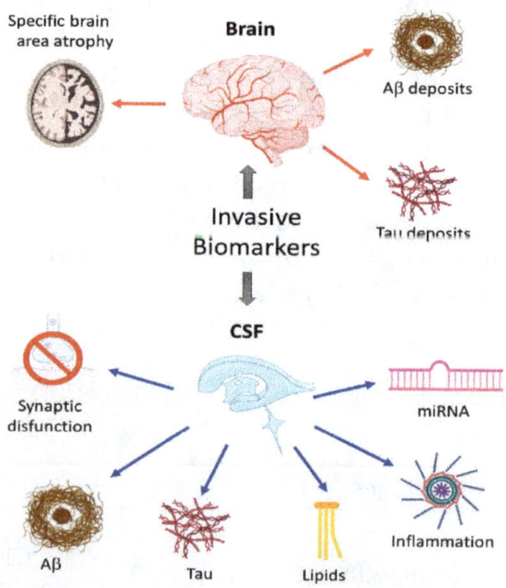

Figure 1. Schematic overview of invasive biomarkers. Different biomarkers have been used to detect early anatomical changes in the brains of people with mild cognitive impairment, including the atrophy of specific brain areas like the locus coeruleus or the hippocampus, and the presence of typical protein aggregates such as extracellular amyloid plaques or intracellular Tau-containing neurofibrillary tangles (upper panel). Additionally, biomarkers of Alzheimer's disease (AD)-related degenerative processes like synaptic dysfunction, neuroinflammation, oxidative stress, or neuronal loss can be measured in the cerebrospinal fluid of AD patients. The detection of miRNAs represents a novel and promising tool for the early AD diagnosis (lower panel).

Proteins involved in the pathological processing of the amyloid precursor protein (APP) could be biomarker candidates for early AD diagnosis and must be considered. Presenilin 1 (PSEN1) and β-secretase 1 (BACE1) are both enzymes involved in the cleavage of APP. In MCI patients, both PSEN1 and BACE1 levels and their activity were increased in CSF [42,43]. Moreover, elevated BACE1 expression has been associated with the APOEε4 genotype [43]. It is worth noting that BACE1 activity was only increased in MCI patients whose impairment was progressing to more advanced stages of dementia, and not occurring in stable MCI patients [44]. So, while BACE1 seems to be highlighted as a sensitive early biomarker to detect alterations in the amyloidogenic process in APOEε4 carriers [43], it does not seem to be a good candidate in APOEε4 non-carriers.

Other early aspects to highlight in AD are neuroinflammation and the synaptic dysfunction; thus, specific markers of these processes could also play a very important role and may correlate more directly with cognitive decline [45]. In this sense, many proteins involved in vesicular transport (secretogranin II (SCG2), chromogranin A (CHGA)), in synapses formation and stabilization (neurexins (NRXNs), neuronal pentraxin 1 (NPTX1), neurocan core protein (NCANP)), and in the immune system (lysozime C (LysC) and β_2-microglobulin (β_2M)) were significantly higher in the CSF of patients with MCI, especially in patients with MCI progressing to AD pathology than in AD and healthy control patients [46]. According to one study, higher levels of CHGA in the CSF of healthy elderly people predicted future decreases in Aβ-42 [47]. Other proteins that play a crucial role in inflammation are YKL-40 and visinin-like protein-1 (VILIP-1). Increased expression of these molecules has been seen in both MCI and AD patients, contrary to cognitively normal elderly subjects. While YKL-40 was increased from the prodromal stage until the severe stage of the disease, VILIP-1 was only increased in the prodromal stage [48]. Some studies have found an association between the upregulation of YKL-40 with an increased risk of progression from the normal conditions to MCI [49]. Another potential inflammatory marker is the interferon-γ-induced protein 10 (IP-10), whose level was increased in the CSF of asymptomatic elderly adults that also presented elevated levels of total-Tau and phospho-Tau [50]. Likewise, monocyte chemoattractant protein 1 (MCP-1), a low-molecular-weight cytokine involved in the inflammatory process, was found elevated in the CSF of MCI and AD patients [51]. The triggering receptor expressed on myeloid cells 2 (TREM2), expressed by microglial cells, among others, plays an important role in regulating immune responses in the brain and in the production of inflammatory cytokines [52]. Its haplodeficiency has been associated with increased axonal dystrophy and phospho-Tau accumulation around Aβ-plaques [53]. An increased level of CSF soluble TREM2 has been seen in carriers of an autosomal dominant AD mutation, at least five years before the onset of symptoms, although later to brain amyloidosis and Tau pathology [54]. All these findings reveal that a large number of proteins involved in the inflammatory response can be potential early biomarkers of AD.

One protein that plays an important role in memory enhancement is neurogranin. It is involved in post-synaptic signaling pathways, and its CSF levels differentiated patients with early symptomatic AD from controls with a comparable diagnostic utility to the other CSF biomarkers [55]. The potential of neurogranin as a biomarker of AD depended on the fragment measured [56].

Regarding neuronal damage, some proteins such as neurofilament light chain (NF-L), a protein involved in protecting neurites, and neuron-specific enolase (NSE), which plays a role in neuronal metabolism, have revealed increased CSF concentrations in MCI patients in comparison with cognitively elderly, and with patients at advanced AD stages [57,58]. In AD patients with advanced pathology, high CSF NF-L levels are associated with cognitive decline and morphological changes in the brain that indicate neuronal loss [57]. Schmidt et al. showed a correlation between high CSF NSE levels and Tau pathology [58]. These results agree with studies, where plasma protein levels were also studied and support the use of NF-L and NSE as early AD biomarkers [56].

Lipid alterations in CSF participate as well in the modulation of neuropathological events related to AD and can be an AD biomarker candidate. In patients with incipient dementia, a reduction of up to 40% of sulfatide levels was observed [59] The levels of some other lipids such as phosphocholine and sphingomyelin were increased in patients at the prodromal stage and correlated with amyloid and Tau pathology [60]. Another biomarker candidate is the fatty acid-binding protein (FABP3), which may play a role in neuronal synapse formation. In MCI and AD patients, the FABP3 level was higher than in cognitively healthy people [61], and it was related to early structural brain changes typical of AD patients (entorhinal cortex atrophy). Also, high FABP3 levels have been found in non-amnestic elderly APOEε4 carriers [62], showing their increase occurs at a very early stage of the disease [63].

Overall, all the findings mentioned above reflect changes in specific areas of the brain detected using novel imaging techniques (MRI, PET), the presence of two classical AD proteins (Aβ and Tau), and the progression of processes such as neuronal apoptosis, synaptic loss, and inflammation. Many of them are still under consideration as potential early biomarkers of AD, and larger longitudinal studies are required for validation of the results [56]. Unfortunately, most AD patients are asymptomatic during the preclinical stages, complicating the recruitment for these kinds of studies and emphasizing the importance of rapid diagnosis.

It is also relevant to investigate the presence of microRNAs (miRNAs), a big family of endogenous short non-coding RNAs that regulate the number of mature mRNAs at the post-transcriptional level [64]. About 70% of identified miRNAs are expressed in the brain, and some miRNAs species are present in exosomes, both good biomarker candidates in clinical diagnostics. Of the approximately 2000 human miRNAs identified to date, no more than 40 are abundantly expressed in the brain [65]. The core CSF biomarkers (Aβ-42, total-tau, and phospho-tau) are relatively stable in clinical AD, and although they are useful for diagnosis, they are not good enough as indicators of disease progression. Although CSF miRNAs are obtained in an invasive manner, which is far from ideal, they have the advantage of targeting important pathological AD genes. A single miRNA has the potential to interfere with the expression of a small family of genes. This is the case with miRNA-125b (upregulated in AD), which targets the synaptic protein synapsin-2 (SYN-2), the enzyme 15-lipoxygenase (15-LOX), and the cell cycle regulator CDKN2A. This opens up the door for the use of miRNAs as therapeutic agents in the future. Furthermore, the misregulation of specific miRNAs could contribute to AD etiopathogenesis [66] and partially explain the large number of brain mRNAs gradually and significantly downregulated in anatomical regions sensitive to AD progression (reviewed in Lukiv 2013)[65]. Other attractive points that favor the use of CSF miRNAs as diagnosis tools are their high stability in body fluids [67,68], the low concentration required for their detection by standard molecular biology techniques, such as quantitative RT-PCR, and the proven high predictive accuracy in the pathogenic process of AD. All of the above supports the huge potential miRNAs offer as diagnostic and prognostic biomarkers and, at the same time, as plausible therapeutic tools against AD [69].

In the hippocampus of AD patients, in comparison with healthy volunteers, upregulation of three out of the 13 brain-associated miRNAs studied was observed: miRNA-9, miRNA125b, and miRNA128 [66]. Very similar results were found in the CSF of AD patients. Using microarrays, qRT-PCR and novel highly sensitive LNA, EDC and DIG (LED)-Northern dot-blot (an improved northern blot-based protocol for small RNA detection that combines the use of digoxigenin (DIG)-labeled oligonucleotide probes containing locked nucleic acids (LNA) and 1-ethyl-3-(3-dimethylaminopropyl) carbodiimide (EDC) for cross-linking the RNA to the membrane), high amounts of proinflammatory miRNAs such as miRNA146a, miRNA-155, miRNA-9, and miRNA-125b have been detected in AD patients CSF compared with age-matched controls [65,70,71]. Briefly, miRNA-125b targets synaptic proteins, neurotrophic factors and cell regulator proteins, and miRNA146a targets immune system regulators and proteins involved in proinflammatory signaling, as well as in Aβ accumulation [65]. Both miRNA-125b and miRNA-146a can explain many of the pathogenic effects of AD, so they could be excellent candidates as AD biomarkers. In areas such as the frontal gyrus and the neocortex, the up- and downregulation of an elevated number of miRNAs has been seen, and even some of them showed different regulations according to the area studied [72]. miRNA-29a seems a promising biomarker because it targets BACE1, which promotes the formation of Aβ from APP. In the cortex of AD patients, decreased miRNA29a has been reported, while a two-fold increase in miR-29a levels was found in the

CSF of AD patients in comparison with cognitively healthy people [73,74]. The decrease in miR-29 brain expression in AD patients can be associated with an increase of BACE1, leading to the subsequent increase in Aβ levels [75]. Another miRNA that is upregulated in the neocortex, hippocampus, and CSF is miRNA-9 [65,70]. MiRNA-9 is mainly involved in neurogenesis and brain cell proliferation [76,77] and also targets BACE1, decreasing its expression [78]. In this sense, miRNA-29a and miRNA-9 could be indicators of pathology acting as biomarkers. We have only named a few microRNAs involved in AD, although it is worth noting that there are many more with promising results [79].

3. Noninvasive Biomarkers

3.1. *Blood Biomarkers*

Blood pressure has been pointed out as an early marker of AD. High blood pressure has been associated with senile plaques, neurofilament tangles, and hippocampal atrophy, and advanced age and hypertension have been linked to AD development [80]. In addition, selected low amounts of brain proteins/substances can cross the blood-brain barrier, reaching the bloodstream. Therefore, it is possible the detection in the blood of specific substances derived exclusively from the brain or systemic pathologies [81]. Despite blood is a more complex matrix for investigating neuronal processes, making the research of neurodegenerative biomarkers in blood challenging; its accessibility makes the study and validation interesting. To this effect, blood represents a noninvasive way of monitoring AD development and progression [82].

Compared with CSF, blood is easily collected and, therefore, represents the matrix of choice for the discovery of new accessible biomarkers. In addition, CSF and brain Aβ and Tau correlated with plasma Aβ and Tau in sporadic AD [83,84]. To this end, measurements in the bloodstream of proteins and peptide concentrations that originate in the brain are very promising. A decrease in the levels of Aβ-42, Aβ-40,and the Aβ-42/Aβ-40 ratio was found in the plasma of preclinical AD patients [85]. Other studies focused on Aβ-0 and showed higher levels in samples of AD patients [86]. Blood-based Tau levels have also been investigated in some studies and found to be elevated in the plasma of AD patients [87,88]. However, the relatively low levels of Aβ and Tau proteins in peripheral blood necessitate more sensitive detection techniques to consolidate as diagnostic biomarkers of AD.

Recent studies have revealed that serum neurofilament protein levels correlated with AD [89]. However, this fact was not specific of AD but was also reported in other neurodegenerative diseases [90]. Henceforth, Aβ, Tau, and neurofilaments are not strong enough biomarkers to predict sporadic AD [91], and it would be useful to account for additional molecules for a more accurate early diagnosis. It has been found that changes in the plasma concentration of brain-derived neurotrophic factor (BDNF) depend on the severity of AD [92]. Also, plasma clusterin levels are significantly increased in both, MCI and AD patients [93], and have been related to increased risk of progression from MCI to AD, but a slower cognitive decline in AD patients [94].

Extracellular RNA (exRNA) from human biofluids has been recently characterized. In neurological disorders, brain-derived exRNAs can reach the bloodstream in different ways. One possibility is the elimination of waste from the brain by the lymphatic system into the bloodstream [95]. A second one is that blood-brain barrier leakiness described in early AD facilitates the passage of all types of extracellular molecules [96]. Thus, the presence of exRNAs in the blood allows the study of gene expression in the central nervous system. In this context, it has been recently described that phosphoglycerate dehydrogenase (PHGDH) exhibits consistent upregulation in the AD brain transcriptome and is increased in presymptomatic AD plasma as compared to controls, suggesting the potential utility of plasma PHGDH exRNA as a presymptomatic indicator of AD [97].

Like in CSF, miRNAs are also considered to be one of the potential candidates for blood-based biomarkers. It has been reported that several miRNAs downregulate AD-related proteins, including BACE-1 and APP [98]. Four miRNAs (miR-31, miR-93, miR-143, and miR-146a) were significantly decreased in AD patients' serum, suggesting that these could be used as potential diagnostic and prognostic markers for dementia. Notably, miR-31, miR-146a, and miR-93 were related to inflammation, cell apoptosis, and fibrosis. Furthermore, miR-93 and miR-146a were significantly elevated in MCI compared to controls and miR-31, miR-93, and miR-146a can be used to discriminate AD from other types of dementia [99]. In addition, the level of miR-206, involved in cognitive decline and memory deficits, was increased in AD plasma, so it could also be a good AD biomarker candidate [100].

Circulating exRNAs are usually protected by exosomes and other extracellular carriers [101]. Extracellular vesicles (EVs), including exosomes, are small (50–150 nm) membrane microvesicles involved in cell-to-cell communication, which can go across a healthy blood-brain barrier. EVs contain not only exRNAs but also other biologically active cargo of molecules specific of their tissue of origin, such as metabolites and proteins, making EVs a good blood-based biomarker candidate, prognostic indicator, and therapeutic tool in AD. Isolation of brain-secreted EVs (BEVs) from the blood provides a minimally invasive way to sample components of brain tissue. Cerebrovascular-derived BEV studies are sparse in human AD patients, so more research would be needed in this field. Nonetheless, it has been reported that pathophysiological alterations in AD are, in fact, reflected in the number and composition of BEVs from neurons, neural precursor cells, and astrocytes [102,103].

As mentioned above, blood is a more complex matrix than CSF, and the high number of cells and soluble molecules contained in it can lead to interferences. Moreover, the low number of brain-derived biomarkers in blood requires highly sensitive techniques for their detection. Great variability in the results depending on the methodology used has been reported, and the fact that several studies show conflicting results represents a limitation for the use of blood biomarkers as an AD diagnostic tool [104]. For all these reasons, the use of blood biomarkers has not yet been validated [81], and the research of alternative fluids as urine, tears, and saliva, is challenging (Figure 2).

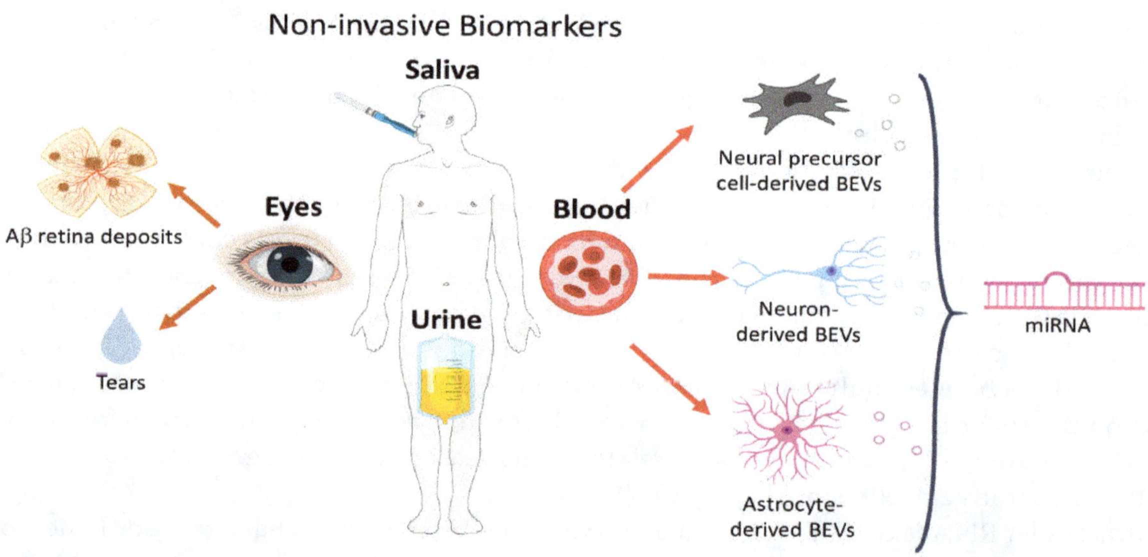

Figure 2. Schematic overview of noninvasive biomarkers: eyes, saliva, urine and blood. Besides fluid biomarkers (tears) that can be collected from the eyes, the promising advances in in vivo retinal imaging could provide an AD diagnosis tool in the near future. Blood-isolated brain secreted extracellular vesicles (BEVs) derive from three possible brain cell types: neural precursors, neurons and astrocytes. The content of this blood-isolated BEVs, mainly miRNAs, have been investigated as potential AD biomarker.

3.1.1. Neuron-Derived BEVs in Blood

Several studies reported significantly elevated Aβ-42 levels in plasma-isolated neuron-derived BEVs in AD dementia relative to cognitively normal individuals. EVs may mediate the transcellular spread of Aβ peptide by destabilizing calcium cell homeostasis and damaging mitochondrial function; thus making neurons more vulnerable to excitotoxicity [105]. Plasma Aβ-42 has the potential to be used both, as a novel earlier biomarkers of AD, as well as a marker of AD progression, having the same capacity as Aβ-42 in CSF for the diagnosis of AD [83]. Nonetheless, the EV concentration is higher in blood plasma than in CSF [105], making this a more sensitive biomarker.

Regarding Tau levels in the plasma, the association of neuron-derived BEVs with AD has yet to reach a consensus. Although three studies [83,106,107] found elevated phospho-Tau levels in AD dementia, these reached a plateau as early as 10 years before AD diagnosis, making it a worse marker of AD progression than Aβ-42 [107]. In addition, three other studies [108–110] showed no statistical difference in Tau fragments.

Protein cargo form plasma and serum isolated neuron-derived BEVs included synaptic proteins like neurogranin, synaptotagmin, synaptopodin, and synaptophysin, which was reduced in individuals with AD dementia [111]. However, the potential of being selective biomarkers of AD appears low because these synaptic proteins were also reduced in MCI and Parkinson's disease. Decreased levels of the growth-associated protein 43 (GAP43), synaptosomal-associated protein-25 (SNAP-25), and synapsin 1 were also observed in blood-isolated neuron-derived BEVs of AD patients [103]. Therefore, synaptic proteins cargo of neuron-derived BEVs demonstrates some biomarker potential in AD, although more studies are needed to confirm this.

Insulin pathway proteins are deregulated in AD as well. Specifically, higher phospho-Ser312-insulin receptor substrate-1 (IRS-1) and lower phospho-panTyr-IRS-1 levels were reported in blood isolated neuron-derived BEVS of AD patients [112,113]. So IRS-1 level, as well as being used to monitor insulin administration [114], could also be used as an AD biomarker.

Lysosomal proteins of neuron-derived BEVs from plasma were also found to discriminate AD dementia. Levels of cathepsin D, alysosome-associated membrane protein, and ubiquitinated proteins were significantly increased in AD patients, and levels of heat-shock protein-70 were diminished in preclinical and clinical AD, suggesting that neuronal lysosomal dysfunction is an early phenomenon in AD [115].

Finally, research from Winston et al. [106] demonstrated that the level of the repressor element 1-silencing transcription factor (REST) was significantly lower in AD patients and MCI compared to control subjects.

3.1.2. Neural Precursor Cell-Derived BEVs in Blood

Chondroitin sulfate proteoglycan (CSPG4) cells are a subtype of neuronal precursor cells that release neurotrophic factors implicated in neuronal growth and survival. Four assessed neurotrophic factors (hepatocyte growth factor, fibroblast growth factors 2 and 13, and type 1 insulin-like growth factor) were significantly lower in CSPG4 neuronal precursor cells-derived BEVs from preclinical AD patients, being able to use these neurotrophic factors as early biomarkers of AD. No significant further decrease was found during the course of the disease [116], though.

3.1.3. Astrocyte-Derived BEVs in Blood

Astrocyte-derived BEVs have also been reported to cargo Tau, Aβ-42, and APP pathway proteins. However, only levels of BACE1, sAPPβ, complement proteins, and glial-derived neurotrophic factor (GDNF) were significantly deregulated in AD. The levels of BACE1, sAPPβ, and complement proteins were higher [117], and the levels of GDNF were lower in AD patients compared to control individuals [118].

3.1.4. MicroRNA Cargo of Blood-Isolated EVs

The levels of miRNAs in peripheral blood can be affected by multiple factors and may also vary among different sample types. In this regard, exosomal miRNAs effectively avoid that problem because of their stable expression. Exosomes are a subtype of EV with a size of 40–100 nm that are released from most types of cells, including neurons [106]. Recent studies have shown that exosomes, in addition to functional proteins, carry mRNA and miRNAs [119], and abnormal expression of these exosomal miRNAs has been detected in AD [120].

More than 40 differentially expressed plasma- and serum-isolated EV-associated miRNAs have been described in AD and MCI relative to control individuals [121–127]. For example, exosomal miR-342-3p [123], miR-125a-5p, miR-125b-5p, and miR-451a, associated with fatty acid biosynthesis, hippo signaling, and protein processing in the endoplasmic reticulum were significantly lower in AD patients, and their level correlated with the extent of cognitive impairment [128]. Decreased levels of exosomal miRNA 23a-3p, ex-let-7i-5p, ex-miR-126-3p, and ex-miR-151a-3p, which target genes involved in cell death, among others, suggest that changes in the plasma level of AD individuals exhibit diagnostic value [129]. The exosomal miR-223, which regulates inflammation by interacting with different targets, was also significantly decreased in AD patients [125]. On the other hand, Barbagallo et al. found that exosomal miR-29a was significantly increased in AD patients [130] and Cheng et al. reported 14 significantly upregulated exosomal miRNAs [122]. It is also important to mention three of those exosomal miRNAs that have been reported in at least two different studies—the decrease of miR-193b and miR-342-3p [121,124], and both, the increase and decrease of miR3065-5p [122,123]. miR-193b is known to repress the expression of APP and PSEN1 mRNAs, so its reduction may promote amyloidosis, and miR 342-3p is suggested to affect Tau phosphorylation and aggregation.

These studies suggest that specific blood exosome miRNAs can be used as diagnostic biomarkers of AD and, additionally, are able to reflect the disease progression. It has also been reported that the combination of miR-135a, miR-193b, and miR-384, modulators of APP or BACE1 expression, are good for early AD diagnosis [124], demonstrating that a combined biomarker signature is better than a particular one for diagnosis. These studies have been carried out in already clinically diagnosed AD patients, so further studies will be necessary to evaluate the potential of these miRNAs as early biomarkers of AD. Table 2 summarizes all the information regarding AD-related miRNAs found in blood, as well as in CSF.

Table 2. AD-related main miRNA.

miRNAs	Regulation and Localization	References
miR-let-7d-5p, miR-let-7g-5p, miR-26b-5p, miR-191-5p	↓ Blood	[131]
miR-125a-5p	↓ Blood	[128]
miR-126-3p, miR-23a-3p, miR-151a-3p	↓ Blood	[129]
miR-135b	↓ Blood	[132]
miR-181a	↓ Blood	[133]
miR-194-5p	↓ Blood	[134]
miR-19b-3p, miR-29c-3p, miR-125b-3p	↓ Blood	[135]
miR-31, miR-93	↓ Blood	[99]
miR-3613-3p, miR-3916, miR-4772-3p, miR-185-5p, miR-20b-3p	↓ Blood	[123]
miR-501-3p	↓ Blood	[136]
miR-545-3p	↓ Blood	[137]
miR-181c	↓ Blood, ↓ Brain	[133,138]
miR-139-5p, miR-141-3p, miR-150-5p, miR-152-3p, miR-23b-3p, miR-24-3p, miR-338-3p, miR-342-3p, miR-125b-5p, miR-342-5p	↓ Blood, ↓ CSF	[123]
miR-1306-5p	↓ Blood, ↓ CSF	[122,139]
miR-143	↓ Blood, ↓ CSF	[99,133]
miR-15b	↓ Blood, ↓ CSF	[131,133]
miR-15b-3p	↓ Blood, ↓ CSF	[122,139]
miR-193b	↓ Blood, ↓ CSF	[121,124]
miR-223	↓ Blood, ↓ CSF	[125,140]
miR-451a	↓ Blood, ↓ CSF	[128,139]

Table 2. *Cont.*

miRNAs	Regulation and Localization	References
miR-106, miR-107, miR-181	↓ Brain	[69]
miR-106b	↓ Brain	[138]
miR-137, miR-139, miR-153, miR-183, miR-135, miR-124b	↓ Brain	[66]
miR-15a, miR-19b, miR-26b, miR-330	↓ Brain	[138]
miR-425	↓ Brain	[133]
miR-146b	↓ Brain, ↓ CSF	[133]
miR-210	↓ Brain, ↓ CSF	[133,141]
miR-10, miR-126, miR-127, miR-154, miR-194, miR-195, miR-199a, miR-214, miR-221, miR-338, miR-422b, miR-451, miR-455, miR-497, miR-99a, miR-27a-3p	↓ CSF	[133]
miR-16-2, miR-16-5p, miR-605-5p, mir-9-5p, miR-598, miR-136-3p	↓ CSF	[139]
miR-200b	↓ CSF	[142]
miR-214-3p, miR-299-5p	↓ CSF	[132,143]
miR-29b-3p	↓ CSF	[123]
miR-29c	↓ CSF	[134]
miR-29	↓ Blood, ↓ Brain, ↑Brain	[69,131,133]
miR-125b	↓ Blood, ↑ Brain, ↑ CSF	[65,66,123]
miR-146a	↓ Blood, ↑ Brain, ↑ CSF	[69,71,99]
miR-26a	↓ Brain (frontal cortex), ↑ Brain (hippocampus)	[133]
miR-3065-5p	↓ Blood, ↑ Brain	[122,123]
let-7i-5p	↓ Blood, ↑ CSF	[129,134]
miR-106a-5p, miR-20-5p, miR-425-5p, miR-18b-5p, miR-582-5p	↑ Blood	[122]
miR-106b-3p, miR-20b-5p, miR-146a-5p, miR-195-5p, niR-497-5p	↑ Blood	[135]
miR-455-3p, miR-4668-5p	↑ Blood	[144]
miR-5001-3p	↑ Blood	[123]
miR-519	↑ Blood	[140]
miR-548at-5p	↑ Blood	[123]
miR-590-5p	↑ Blood	[134]
miR-101-3p, miR-106b-5p, miR-143-3p, miR-335-5p, miR-361-5p,	↑ Blood, ↑ CSF	[122]
miR-138-5p	↑ Blood, ↑ CSF	[123]
miR-155	↑ Blood, ↑ CSF	[71,131]
miR-15a-5p	↑ Blood, ↑ CSF	[122,134]
miR-659-5p	↑ Blood, ↑ CSF	[123]
miR-100, miR-145, miR-148a, miR-27, miR-34a, miR-381, miR-422a, miR-423, miR-92	↑ Brain	[133]
miR-128	↑ Brain	[66]
miR-34	↑ Brain	[69]
miR-98	↑ Brain	[138]
miR-let-7b, miR-let7e	↑ CSF	[145]
miR-let-7f, miR-105, miR-138, miR-141, miR-151, miR-186, miR-191, miR-197, miR-204, miR-205, miR-216, miR-302b, miR-30a-3p, miR-30a-5p, miR-30b, miR-30d, miR-32, miR-345, miR-362, miR-371, miR-374, miR-375, miR-380-3p, miR-429, miR-448, miR-449, miR-494, miR-501, miR-517, miR-518, miR-520, miR-526	↑ CSF	[133]
miR-20a-5p	↑ CSF	[122]
miR-222	↑ CSF	[146]

Table 2. *Cont.*

miRNAs	Regulation and Localization	References
miR-331-5p, miR-485-5p, miR-132-5p	↑ CSF	[139]
miR-613	↑ CSF	[147]
miR-200b-5p	↑ Eyes	[148]
miR-93-5p	↑ ↓ Blood, ↑ CSF	[122,135]
miR-101	↑ Blood, ↓ Brain	[131,138]
miR-132, miR-212	↑ Blood, ↓ Brain	[126,133]
miR-200c	↑ Blood, ↓ Brain (frontal cortex), ↑ Brain (hippocampus)	[133,149]
miR-9	↑ Blood, ↓ Brain (frontal cortex, cortex), ↑ Brain (hippocampus), ↑ CSF	[66,71,131,133,138]
miR-30e-5p	↑ Blood, ↑ Brain, ↑ CSF,	[122,133]
miR-29a	↑ Blood, ↓ Brain, ↑ CSF	[73,74,130]
miR-206	↑ Blood, ↑ CSF, ↑ Eyes	[100,150]
miR-142-5p	↑ Blood, ↓ CSF	[133,134]
miR-384	↑ Blood, ↓ CSF	[124]
miR-135a	↑ Blood, ↓ CSF, ↑ CSF	[124,133,142]
miR-125a	↓ Brain, ↑ CSF	[66,133]
miR-29b	↓ Blood, ↓ Brain, ↑ CSF	[73,74,131]
miR-30c	↑ Brain (frontal cortex), ↓ Brain (hippocampus), ↑ CSF	[133]

3.2. Ocular Biomarkers

AD not only causes neurodegenerative changes in the brain but also produces structural and functional alterations in the retinal neural and non-neural ocular tissues [151]. Engagingly, specific biomarkers of AD have been reported as well in retinal degeneration and visual function impairment [152], sharing pathophysiological features with glaucoma and age-related macular degeneration (AMD) [153]. The similarity between ocular and cerebral tissues suggests that these ocular manifestations may be used as early biomarkers of AD.

Numerous studies have identified Aβ depositions in the lens and retina. Aβ-accumulates in the retina in an age-dependent manner in a mouse model of AD and correlates with amyloid plaques in the brain. Interestingly, the appearance of retinal amyloid plaques precedes that in the brain [154]. Elevated levels of Aβ1-42 and amyloid plaques were also reported in the retinas of confirmed AD patients [152]. This retinal Aβ can be detected noninvasively by using hyperspectral imaging microscopy or with modified endoscope applied to the corneal surface [155].

In the same way, Aβ has been identified in the lens of rodents, monkeys, and humans in several studies. The accumulation of the isoforms Aβ1-40 and Aβ1-42 has been demonstrated in the lenses of AD people *post mortem* at concentrations comparable with those in the brain [156]. In the same way, a clinical trial carried out on AD patients, and age-matched healthy volunteers confirmed the presence of Aβ in the lens of the first and its correlation in the brain using imaging techniques [157].

Moreover, changes such as thinning of the nerve cell layer, optic nerve atrophy, and the loss of retinal ganglion cells [156,158] were reported in AD, resulting in visual functional impairment and circadian disturbances [159]. Specifically, a study of melanopsin retinal ganglion cells (mRGCs), a photosensitive subtype of ganglion cells in charge of the circadian rhythms, has shown a significant decrease of this neuronal cell type in people with AD but not in healthy controls, with a prominent Aβ accumulation around mRGCs [160,161].

Other ocular tissues, such as the cornea, which is the outermost layer of the eye and, therefore, grants accessibility, could be used as potential biomarker for the diagnosis of AD. Dutescu et al. [162] found the cytoplasmic expression of APP in the epithelial cell layer of the cornea of transgenic mouse models of AD. More recently, Choi et al. corroborated the expression of APP, together with proteins involved in its processing such as BACE1, in human corneal fibroblasts, and the corneal epithelium [163].

For the development of a novel noninvasive screening and diagnostic tool, the ocular examination sector appears promising. In this context, tear fluid provides a viable source widely used for biomarker studies [164], including neurodegenerative diseases [165]. Tear samples are easy to collect and contain a lot of proteins, most notably lipocalin-1, lactotransferrin, and lysozyme C, involved in immune and inflammatory processes [166].

Against this backdrop, total protein concentration and composition modifications in tears and an abnormal flow rate and tear function have been described in AD patients [167], supporting the use of tears as a new noninvasive method to discriminate AD patients. Specifically, lipocalin-1, dermcidin, lysozyme C, and lacritin were shown to be potential biomarkers, with an 81% sensitivity and 77% specificity [168]. In addition, the elongation initiation factor 4E (eIF4E) was exclusively expressed in tear samples from AD patients. Total miRNA content was also higher in tears from AD individuals and miR-200b-5p was significantly elevated in AD tear fluid samples compared to controls [148]. Tears could be useful for first screening, and patients with a positive tear analysis test might be further evaluated to establish an early diagnosis. Assessments of pupillary responses and retinal vasculature have also been considered as biomarkers of AD, but are not yet conclusively validated for clinical diagnosis. Further research is needed in order to use ocular biomarkers as AD early diagnostic tools.

Regarding the use of ocular biomarkers, as well as other novel matrices, some limitations arise, like the amall volume of the samples or the standardization of the collection procedures.

3.3. *Salivary Biomarkers*

Due to the link between the decline of the salivary glands and AD [169,170], it seems likely that AD-specific proteins are expressed in the salivary glands. Salivary epithelial cells express APP and Aβ, and changes in the CSF may be reflected in the saliva [171,172]. Saliva is a novel matrix; therefore, there are still some conflicts between studies. One study has revealed no changes in Aβ-40 protein between AD patients and age-matched controls and high levels of Aβ-42 only in MCI patients (in severe AD stages, these levels returned to control values) [173]. A second study has shown that salivary levels of Aβ-40 and Aβ-42 peptides increase as the severity of AD grows, even as far as a three-fold increase in the case of Aβ-42 levels [174,175]. Moreover, studies where the genetic condition was considered, suggested that salivary Aβ-42 levels were associated with familial AD more than with sporadic AD [173,176]. Among the reasons for these different results may be the distinct Aβ peptide detection and saliva collection techniques, as well as the different disease stages of the patients. There is a clear need for more studies and larger sample size to conclude whether there is a relationship between salivary Aβ-42 and Aβ-40 levels and AD progression.

Another typical candidate protein for analysis in the saliva is Tau, which is expressed and secreted by the acinar epithelial cells of the salivary glands [177]. No changes have been seen in total Tau levels between healthy elderly, MCI, and AD patients [178]. In contrast, the phospho-Tau/total-Tau ratio looks promising in this regard. A high phospho-Tau/total-Tau ratio was found in AD patients compared with non-amnestic people [179]. Though no conclusive results were found that pointed in a particular direction, the few results available suggest that studies should be directed at investigating different sites of Tau protein phosphorylation as possible candidates for biomarkers of the pathology [180].

Interestingly, the study of one of the most important antimicrobial peptides in saliva, lactoferrin, seems to have a high accuracy in AD diagnosis. Lactoferrin participates in modulating the immune response and inflammation process due to its high defense action. It has been seen that low lactoferrin levels in saliva of healthy people mean a clear risk factor to develop amnestic MCI and AD dementia [181].

Another proposed candidate in the saliva is the acetylcholinesterase enzyme (AChE), which plays a role in removing the accumulation of acetylcholine (ACh) in Aβ-plaques and NFTs. Although there are still few studies, no evidence has been found to suggest that AChE activity is different between AD patients and control individuals of the same cognitive age not taking anticholinergics [182,183].

All these results support the need for longitudinal studies with a larger number of subjects to find conclusive results regarding the potential use of the expression of certain molecules in saliva as biomarkers in AD.

3.4. Urine Biomarkers

Oxidative stress plays an important role in AD, and the study of guide molecules of oxidative brain damage might be promising early hallmarks of AD in urine. Some metabolites such as the isoprostane 8,12-iso-iPF(2alpha)-VI, a free amino acid generated by lipid peroxidation whose levels in urine were higher at advanced AD stages, might predict the progression of the pathology from MCI to AD dementia [184,185].

Other metabolite candidates that reflect oxidative DNA damage can be oxidized nucleosides such as pseudouridine, 1-methyladenosine, 3-methyluridine, N2, N2-dimethylguanosine, 8-hydroxy-2′-deoxyguanosine, and 2-deoxyguanosine, whose levels were higher in AD patients than in healthy elderly [186].

Other promising markers are some proteins found in urine. Given that the AD-associated neuronal thread protein (AD7c-NTP) was isolated from brain tissue and was increased in the CSF of AD people, correlating with the severity of dementia [187], it has been suggested as a potential biomarker of AD. Recently, a high specificity of this protein has been demonstrated to predict Aβ-plaques in MCI patients when present in the urine [188]. These findings are supported by a meta-analysis proposing the use of urinary AD7c-NTP for the early diagnosis of probable AD [189]. In a longitudinal study carried out in 2018, high levels of albumin, a protein characteristic of chronic kidney disease, were detected in AD patients in comparison with age-matched healthy individuals [190]. According to Yao et al. [191], and in the same direction, the urine of patients with AD showed significantly decreased levels of osteopontin and increased levels of gelsolin and insulin-like growth factor-binding protein 7 in comparison with healthy elderly. All of them are proteins involved in several pathological processes of AD [192–194], and they may serve as potential novel urinary biomarkers.

Although it is evident the need for longitudinal studies with bigger samples to get conclusive results verifying the diagnostic value of these peripheral markers, the scientific community is hopeful that the biomarkers in these noninvasive new matrices will be able to demonstrate diagnostic value.

4. Concluding Remarks and Future Perspectives

In addition to the established Aβ-42, total-Tau, phospho-Tau, and CSF biomarkers, several candidate more accessible fluid biomarkers have shown potential for clinical use in AD to support diagnosis and prognosis.

Blood has been the most widely studied fluid biomarker, being neuron-derived BEVs the most investigated biomarker among blood-isolated EVs. The majority of the studies reported elevated Aβ-42 levels in blood-isolated neuron derived BEVs in AD and MCI patients early in the course of the disease, and also with disease progression. With regard to synaptic proteins assessed in neuron-derived BEVs, growth-associated protein 43 (GAP43) also showed some potential as a marker of AD progression. Henceforth, BEVs have emerged as a novel potential blood-based biomarker of AD. It would also be interesting to study BEVs from other components of the brain, such as the cerebrovasculature, that are affected in the early stages of AD and that would allow us to obtain more sensitive blood-based biomarkers.

Tear fluid also provides a viable source widely used for biomarker studies and lipocalin-1, dermcidin, lysozyme C, lacritin, eIF4E, and the microRNA-200b-5p were shown to be potential biomarkers. The relationship between salivary Aβ-42, Aβ-40, and lactoferrin levels and the progression of AD point out to also be biomarker candidates of AD and MCI in saliva. Lastly, several metabolites and proteins like AD7c-NTP, osteopontin, gelsolin, or insulin-like growth factor-binding protein 7 in urine are involved in several pathological processes in AD.

Inflammatory and oxidative stress markers are very common hallmarks of neurodegenerative diseases such as amyotrophic lateral sclerosis, Parkinson, Huntington, and AD. It has been suggested that these alterations reflect inflammatory mechanisms within the central nervous system that parallel the neurodegenerative process [56]. In this review, we have mentioned several neuroinflammation candidate biomarkers such as TREM2, MCP-1, and YKL-40, which have been extensively investigated in AD patients. Particularly, there is strong evidence regarding CSF YKL-40 levels, not only as a potential biomarker for AD diagnosis, but also as a predictor of disease progression from the asymptomatic stage to prodromal, and eventually dementia stages [51]. However, the idea that these inflammation-related proteins could differentiate AD from other dementias is controversial since neurodegeneration and neuroinflammation go hand in hand and inflammation on its own cannot be considered a marker of a specific pathology. There is a clear lack of reliable inflammatory biomarkers that can be used in the context of accurate diagnosis.

Despite recent studies strongly indicating the potential of fluid biomarkers as early diagnosis of AD, these biomarkers are not yet validated for clinical use and further research is needed before these can be regulatory qualified and applied clinically. Future work should establish normative ranges for the levels of these biomarkers to indicate a pathology that may find clinical applications. If we provided early diagnosis and treatment before the underlying pathology manifests clinically, AD patients' quality of life could notably improve and could be an approach to prevent its irreversible consequences.

Author Contributions: E.A. and G.E. carried out the literature review, conceptualized and prepared the initial draft. G.E. provided critical inputs. V.G.-V. edited and contributed in the final manuscript. All authors have read and agreed to the final version of the manuscript.

Acknowledgments: Figures created with BioRender.com.

References

1. Dubois, B.; Feldman, H.H.; Jacova, C.; DeKosky, S.T.; Barberger-Gateau, P.; Cummings, J.; Delacourte, A.; Galasko, D.; Gauthier, S.; Jicha, G.; et al. Research criteria for the diagnosis of Alzheimer's disease: Revising the NINCDS-ADRDA criteria. *Lancet Neurol.* **2007**, *6*, 734–746. [CrossRef]
2. Mueller, S.G.; Schuff, N.; Yaffe, K.; Madison, C.; Miller, B.; Weiner, M.W. Hippocampal atrophy patterns in mild cognitive impairment and alzheimer's disease. *Hum. Brain Mapp.* **2010**, *31*, 1339–1347. [CrossRef] [PubMed]
3. La Joie, R.; Perrotin, A.; De La Sayette, V.; Egret, S.; Doeuvre, L.; Belliard, S.; Eustache, F.; Desgranges, B.; Chételat, G. Hippocampal subfield volumetry in mild cognitive impairment, Alzheimer's disease and semantic dementia. *NeuroImage Clin.* **2013**, *3*, 155–162. [CrossRef] [PubMed]
4. Pluta, J.; Yushkevich, P.; Das, S.; Wolk, D. In vivo Analysis of Hippocampal Subfield Atrophy in Mild Cognitive Impairment via Semi-Automatic Segmentation of T2-Weighted MRI. *J. Alzheimer's Dis.* **2012**, *31*, 85–99. [CrossRef]
5. Arendt, T.; Brückner, M.K.; Morawski, M.; Jäger, C.; Gertz, H.J. Early neurone loss in Alzheimer's disease: Cortical or subcortical? *Acta Neuropathol. Commun.* **2015**, *3*, 10. [CrossRef]
6. Braak, H.; Del Tredici, K. Where, when, and in what form does sporadic Alzheimer's disease begin? *Curr. Opin. Neurol.* **2012**, *25*, 708–714. [CrossRef]
7. Andrés-Benito, P.; Fernández-Dueñas, V.; Carmona, M.; Escobar, L.A.; Torrejón-Escribano, B.; Aso, E.; Ciruela, F.; Ferrer, I. Locus coeruleus at asymptomatic early and middle Braak stages of neurofibrillary tangle pathology. *Neuropathol. Appl. Neurobiol.* **2017**, *43*, 373–392. [CrossRef]
8. Braak, H.; Thal, D.R.; Ghebremedhin, E.; Del Tredici, K. Stages of the pathologic process in alzheimer disease: Age categories from 1 to 100 years. *J. Neuropathol. Exp. Neurol.* **2011**, *70*, 960–969. [CrossRef]

9. Ehrenberg, A.J.; Nguy, A.K.; Theofilas, P.; Dunlop, S.; Suemoto, C.K.; Di Lorenzo Alho, A.T.; Leite, R.P.; Diehl Rodriguez, R.; Mejia, M.B.; Rüb, U.; et al. Quantifying the accretion of hyperphosphorylated tau in the locus coeruleus and dorsal raphe nucleus: The pathological building blocks of early Alzheimer's disease. *Neuropathol. Appl. Neurobiol.* **2017**, *43*, 393–408. [CrossRef]
10. Stratmann, K.; Heinsen, H.; Korf, H.-W.; Del Turco, D.; Ghebremedhin, E.; Seidel, K.; Bouzrou, M.; Grinberg, L.T.; Bohl, J.; Wharton, S.B.; et al. Precortical Phase of Alzheimer's Disease (AD)-Related Tau Cytoskeletal Pathology. *Brain Pathol.* **2016**, *26*, 371–386. [CrossRef]
11. Theofilas, P.; Ehrenberg, A.J.; Dunlop, S.; Di Lorenzo Alho, A.T.; Nguy, A.; Leite, R.E.P.; Rodriguez, R.D.; Mejia, M.B.; Suemoto, C.K.; Ferretti-Rebustini, R.E.D.L.; et al. Locus coeruleus volume and cell population changes during Alzheimer's disease progression: A stereological study in human postmortem brains with potential implication for early-stage biomarker discovery. *Alzheimer's Dement.* **2017**, *13*, 236–246. [CrossRef] [PubMed]
12. Kelly, S.C.; He, B.; Perez, S.E.; Ginsberg, S.D.; Mufson, E.J.; Counts, S.E. Locus coeruleus cellular and molecular pathology during the progression of Alzheimer's disease. *Acta Neuropathol. Commun.* **2017**, *5*, 8. [CrossRef] [PubMed]
13. Lyness, S.A.; Zarow, C.; Chui, H.C. Neuron loss in key cholinergic and aminergic nuclei in Alzheimer disease: A meta-analysis. *Neurobiol. Aging* **2003**, *24*, 1–23. [CrossRef]
14. Betts, M.J.; Cardenas-Blanco, A.; Kanowski, M.; Jessen, F.; Düzel, E. In vivo MRI assessment of the human locus coeruleus along its rostrocaudal extent in young and older adults. *Neuroimage* **2017**, *163*, 150–159. [CrossRef]
15. Priovoulos, N.; Jacobs, H.I.L.; Ivanov, D.; Uludağ, K.; Verhey, F.R.J.; Poser, B.A. High-resolution in vivo imaging of human locus coeruleus by magnetization transfer MRI at 3T and 7T. *Neuroimage* **2018**, *168*, 427–436. [CrossRef]
16. Tondelli, M.; Wilcock, G.K.; Nichelli, P.; de Jager, C.A.; Jenkinson, M.; Zamboni, G. Structural MRI changes detectable up to ten years before clinical Alzheimer's disease. *Neurobiol. Aging* **2012**, *33*, 825.e25–825.e36. [CrossRef]
17. Bernard, C.; Helmer, C.; Dilharreguy, B.; Amieva, H.; Auriacombe, S.; Dartigues, J.F.; Allard, M.; Catheline, G. Time course of brain volume changes in the preclinical phase of Alzheimer's disease. *Alzheimer's Dement.* **2014**, *10*, 143–151.e1. [CrossRef]
18. Smith, C.D.; Chebrolu, H.; Wekstein, D.R.; Schmitt, F.A.; Jicha, G.A.; Cooper, G.; Markesbery, W.R. Brain structural alterations before mild cognitive impairment. *Neurology* **2007**, *68*, 1268–1273. [CrossRef]
19. Apostolova, L.G.; Dutton, R.A.; Dinov, I.D.; Hayashi, K.M.; Toga, A.W.; Cummings, J.L.; Thompson, P.M. Conversion of mild cognitive impairment to alzheimer disease predicted by hippocampal atrophy maps. *Arch. Neurol.* **2006**, *63*, 693–699. [CrossRef]
20. Jack, C.R.; Petersen, R.C.; Xu, Y.C.; O'Brien, P.C.; Smith, G.E.; Ivnik, R.J.; Boeve, B.F.; Waring, S.C.; Tangalos, E.G.; Kokmen, E. Prediction of AD with MRI-based hippocampal volume in mild cognitive impairment. *Neurology* **1999**, *52*, 1397–1403. [CrossRef]
21. Korf, E.S.C.; Wahlund, L.O.; Visser, P.J.; Scheltens, P. Medial temporal lobe atrophy on MRI predicts dementia in patients with mild cognitive impairment. *Neurology* **2004**, *63*, 94–100. [CrossRef]
22. Apostolova, L.G.; Mosconi, L.; Thompson, P.M.; Green, A.E.; Hwang, K.S.; Ramirez, A.; Mistur, R.; Tsui, W.H.; de Leon, M.J. Subregional hippocampal atrophy predicts Alzheimer's dementia in the cognitively normal. *Neurobiol. Aging* **2010**, *31*, 1077–1088. [CrossRef] [PubMed]
23. Csernansky, J.G.; Wang, L.; Swank, J.; Miller, J.P.; Gado, M.; McKeel, D.; Miller, M.I.; Morris, J.C. Preclinical detection of Alzheimer's disease: Hippocampal shape and volume predict dementia onset in the elderly. *Neuroimage* **2005**, *25*, 783–792. [CrossRef] [PubMed]
24. Chen, K.; Reiman, E.M.; Alexander, G.E.; Caselli, R.J.; Gerkin, R.; Bandy, D.; Domb, A.; Osborne, D.; Fox, N.; Crum, W.R.; et al. Correlations between apolipoprotein E ε4 gene dose and whole brain atrophy rates. *Am. J. Psychiatry* **2007**, *164*, 916–921. [CrossRef] [PubMed]
25. Lim, Y.Y.; Mormino, E.C. APOE genotype and early β-amyloid accumulation in older adults without dementia. *Neurology* **2017**, *89*, 1028–1034. [CrossRef] [PubMed]
26. Castellano, J.M.; Kim, J.; Stewart, F.R.; Jiang, H.; DeMattos, R.B.; Patterson, B.W.; Fagan, A.M.; Morris, J.C.; Mawuenyega, K.G.; Cruchaga, C.; et al. Human apoE Isoforms Differentially Regulate Brain Amyloid-Peptide Clearance. *Sci. Transl. Med.* **2011**, *3*, 89ra57. [CrossRef]

27. Reiman, E.M.; Uecker, A.; Caselli, R.J.; Lewis, S.; Bandy, D.; De Leon, M.J.; De Santi, S.; Convit, A.; Osborne, D.; Weaver, A.; et al. Hippocampal volumes in cognitively normal persons at genetic risk for Alzheimer's disease. *Ann. Neurol.* **1998**, *44*, 288–291. [CrossRef]
28. Fang, Y.; Du, N.; Xing, L.; Duo, Y.; Zheng, L. Evaluation of hippocampal volume and serum brain-derived neurotrophic factor as potential diagnostic markers of conversion from amnestic mild cognitive impairment to Alzheimer disease A STROBE-compliant article. *Medicine (United States)* **2019**, *98*. [CrossRef]
29. Finnema, S.J.; Nabulsi, N.B.; Eid, T.; Detyniecki, K.; Lin, S.F.; Chen, M.K.; Dhaher, R.; Matuskey, D.; Baum, E.; Holden, D.; et al. Imaging synaptic density in the living human brain. *Sci. Transl. Med.* **2016**, *8*, 1–10. [CrossRef]
30. Terry, R.D.; Masliah, E.; Salmon, D.P.; Butters, N.; DeTeresa, R.; Hill, R.; Hansen, L.A.; Katzman, R. Physical basis of cognitive alterations in alzheimer's disease: Synapse loss is the major correlate of cognitive impairment. *Ann. Neurol.* **1991**, *30*, 572–580. [CrossRef]
31. Lista, S.; Hampel, H. Synaptic degeneration and neurogranin in the pathophysiology of Alzheimer's disease. *Expert Rev. Neurother.* **2017**, *17*, 47–57. [CrossRef] [PubMed]
32. Chandra, A.; Valkimadi, P.E.; Pagano, G.; Cousins, O.; Dervenoulas, G.; Politis, M. Applications of amyloid, tau, and neuroinflammation PET imaging to Alzheimer's disease and mild cognitive impairment. *Hum. Brain Mapp.* **2019**, *40*, 5424–5442. [CrossRef] [PubMed]
33. Johnson, K.A.; Fox, N.C.; Sperling, R.A.; Klunk, W.E. Brain Imaging in Alzheimer Disease. *Cold Spring Harb. Perspect. Med.* **2012**, *2*, a006213. [CrossRef] [PubMed]
34. Ferreira, D.; Perestelo-Pérez, L.; Westman, E.; Wahlund, L.O.; Sarrisa, A.; Serrano-Aguilar, P. Meta-review of CSF core biomarkers in Alzheimer's disease: The state-of-the-art after the new revised diagnostic criteria. *Front. Aging Neurosci.* **2014**, *6*, 1–24. [CrossRef]
35. Hampel, H.; O'Bryant, S.E.; Molinuevo, J.L.; Zetterberg, H.; Masters, C.L.; Lista, S.; Kiddle, S.J.; Batrla, R.; Blennow, K. Blood-based biomarkers for Alzheimer disease: Mapping the road to the clinic. *Nat. Rev. Neurol.* **2018**, *14*, 639–652. [CrossRef]
36. Fishman, R. Cerebrospinal fluid in diseases of the nervous system. *WB Saunders Co.* **1992**, 183–252.
37. Dubois, B.; Feldman, H.H.; Jacova, C.; Hampel, H.; Molinuevo, J.L.; Blennow, K.; Dekosky, S.T.; Gauthier, S.; Selkoe, D.; Bateman, R.; et al. Advancing research diagnostic criteria for Alzheimer's disease: The IWG-2 criteria. *Lancet Neurol.* **2014**, *13*, 614–629. [CrossRef]
38. McKhann, G.M.; Knopman, D.S.; Chertkow, H.; Hyman, B.T.; Jack, C.R.; Kawas, C.H.; Klunk, W.E.; Koroshetz, W.J.; Manly, J.J.; Mayeux, R.; et al. The diagnosis of dementia due to Alzheimer's disease: Recommendations from the National Institute on Aging-Alzheimer's Association workgroups on diagnostic guidelines for Alzheimer's disease. *Alzheimer's Dement.* **2011**, *7*, 263–269. [CrossRef]
39. Kester, M.I.; Van Der Vlies, A.E.; Blankenstein, M.A.; Pijnenburg, Y.A.L.; Van Elk, E.J.; Scheltens, P.; Van Der Flier, W.M. CSF biomarkers predict rate of cognitive decline in Alzheimer disease. *Neurology* **2009**, *73*, 1353–1358. [CrossRef]
40. Martínez-Morillo, E.; Hansson, O.; Atagi, Y.; Bu, G.; Minthon, L.; Diamandis, E.P.; Nielsen, H.M. Total apolipoprotein E levels and specific isoform composition in cerebrospinal fluid and plasma from Alzheimer's disease patients and controls. *Acta Neuropathol.* **2014**, *127*, 633–643. [CrossRef]
41. Strittmatter, W.J.; Saunders, A.M.; Goedert, M.; Weisgraber, K.H.; Dong, L.M.; Jakes, R.; Huang, D.Y.; Pericak-Vance, M.; Schmechel, D.; Roses, A.D. Isoform-specific interactions of apolipoprotein E with microtubule-associated protein tau: Implications for Alzheimer disease. *Proc. Natl. Acad. Sci. USA* **1994**, *91*, 11183–11186. [CrossRef] [PubMed]
42. García-Ayllón, M.-S.; Campanari, M.-L.; Brinkmalm, G.; Rábano, A.; Alom, J.; Saura, C.A.; Andreasen, N.; Blennow, K.; Sáez-Valero, J. CSF Presenilin-1 complexes are increased in Alzheimer's disease. *Acta Neuropathol. Commun.* **2013**, *1*, 46. [CrossRef] [PubMed]
43. Ewers, M.; Zhong, Z.; Bürger, K.; Wallin, A.; Blennow, K.; Teipel, S.J.; Shen, Y.; Hampel, H. Increased CSF-BACE 1 activity is associated with ApoE-ε4 genotype in subjects with mild cognitive impairment and Alzheimer's disease. *Brain* **2008**, *131*, 1252–1258. [CrossRef] [PubMed]
44. Zetterberg, H.; Andreasson, U.; Hansson, O.; Wu, G.; Sankaranarayanan, S.; Andersson, M.E.; Buchhave, P.; Londos, E.; Umek, R.M.; Minthon, L.; et al. Elevated cerebrospinal fluid BACE1 activity in incipient alzheimer disease. *Arch. Neurol.* **2008**, *65*, 1102–1107. [CrossRef]

45. Calsolaro, V.; Edison, P. Neuroinflammation in Alzheimer's disease: Current evidence and future directions. *Alzheimer's Dement.* **2016**, *12*, 719–732. [CrossRef]
46. Duits, F.H.; Brinkmalm, G.; Teunissen, C.E.; Brinkmalm, A.; Scheltens, P.; Van Der Flier, W.M.; Zetterberg, H.; Blennow, K. Synaptic proteins in CSF as potential novel biomarkers for prognosis in prodromal Alzheimer's disease. *Alzheimer's Res. Ther.* **2018**, *10*, 1–9. [CrossRef]
47. Mattsson, N.; Insel, P.; Nosheny, R.; Zetterberg, H.; Trojanowski, J.Q.; Shaw, L.M.; Tosun, D.; Weiner, M. CSF protein biomarkers predicting longitudinal reduction of CSF β-amyloid42 in cognitively healthy elders. *Transl. Psychiatry* **2013**, *3*. [CrossRef]
48. Kester, M.I.; Teunissen, C.E.; Sutphen, C.; Herries, E.M.; Ladenson, J.H.; Xiong, C.; Scheltens, P.; Van Der Flier, W.M.; Morris, J.C.; Holtzman, D.M.; et al. Cerebrospinal fluid VILIP-1 and YKL-40, candidate biomarkers to diagnose, predict and monitor Alzheimer's disease in a memory clinic cohort. *Alzheimer's Res. Ther.* **2015**, *7*, 1–9. [CrossRef]
49. Craig-Schapiro, R.; Perrin, R.J.; Roe, C.M.; Xiong, C.; Carter, D.; Cairns, N.J.; Mintun, M.A.; Peskind, E.R.; Li, G.; Galasko, D.R.; et al. YKL-40: A Novel Prognostic Fluid Biomarker for Preclinical Alzheimer's Disease. *Biol. Psychiatry* **2010**, *68*, 903–912. [CrossRef]
50. Bettcher, B.M.; Johnson, S.C.; Fitch, R.; Casaletto, K.B.; Heffernan, K.S.; Asthana, S.; Zetterberg, H.; Blennow, K.; Carlsson, C.M.; Neuhaus, J.; et al. Cerebrospinal Fluid and Plasma Levels of Inflammation Differentially Relate to CNS Markers of Alzheimer's Disease Pathology and Neuronal Damage. *J. Alzheimer's Dis.* **2018**, *62*, 385–397. [CrossRef]
51. Dhiman, K.; Blennow, K.; Zetterberg, H.; Martins, R.N.; Gupta, V.B. *Cerebrospinal Fluid Biomarkers for Understanding Multiple Aspects of Alzheimer's Disease Pathogenesis*; Springer International Publishing: New York, NY, USA, 2019; Volume 76, ISBN 0001801903040.
52. Takahashi, K.; Rochford, C.D.P.; Neumann, H. Clearance of apoptotic neurons without inflammation by microglial triggering receptor expressed on myeloid cells-2. *J. Exp. Med.* **2005**, *201*, 647–657. [CrossRef] [PubMed]
53. Yuan, P.; Condello, C.; Keene, C.D.; Wang, Y.; Bird, T.D.; Paul, S.M.; Luo, W.; Colonna, M.; Baddeley, D.; Grutzendler, J. TREM2 Haplodeficiency in Mice and Humans Impairs the Microglia Barrier Function Leading to Decreased Amyloid Compaction and Severe Axonal Dystrophy. *Neuron* **2016**, *90*, 724–739. [CrossRef] [PubMed]
54. Suárez-Calvet, M.; Kleinberger, G.; Araque Caballero, M.Á.; Brendel, M.; Rominger, A.; Alcolea, D.; Fortea, J.; Lleó, A.; Blesa, R.; Gispert, J.D.; et al. sTREM 2 cerebrospinal fluid levels are a potential biomarker for microglia activity in early-stage Alzheimer's disease and associate with neuronal injury markers. *EMBO Mol. Med.* **2016**, *8*, 466–476. [CrossRef]
55. Tarawneh, R.; D'Angelo, G.; Crimmins, D.; Herries, E.; Griest, T.; Fagan, A.M.; Zipfel, G.J.; Ladenson, J.H.; Morris, J.C.; Holtzman, D.M. Diagnostic and Prognostic Utility of the Synaptic Marker Neurogranin in Alzheimer Disease. *JAMA Neurol.* **2016**, *73*, 561. [CrossRef]
56. Molinuevo, J.L.; Ayton, S.; Batrla, R.; Bednar, M.M.; Bittner, T.; Cummings, J.; Fagan, A.M.; Hampel, H.; Mielke, M.M.; Mikulskis, A.; et al. *Current State of Alzheimer's Fluid Biomarkers*; Springer: Berlin/Heidelberg, Germany, 2018; Volume 136, ISBN 0040101819.
57. Zetterberg, H.; Skillbäck, T.; Mattsson, N.; Trojanowski, J.Q.; Portelius, E.; Shaw, L.M.; Weiner, M.W.; Blennow, K. Association of Cerebrospinal Fluid Neurofilament Light Concentration With Alzheimer Disease Progression. *JAMA Neurol.* **2016**, *73*, 60. [CrossRef]
58. Schmidt, F.M.; Mergl, R.; Stach, B.; Jahn, I.; Gertz, H.J.; Schönknecht, P. Elevated levels of cerebrospinal fluid neuron-specific enolase (NSE) in Alzheimer's disease. *Neurosci. Lett.* **2014**, *570*, 81–85. [CrossRef]
59. Mulder, C.; Wahlund, L.O.; Teerlink, T.; Blomberg, M.; Veerhuis, R.; Van Kamp, G.J.; Scheltens, P.; Scheffer, P.G. Decreased lysophosphatidylcholine/phosphatidylcholine ratio in cerebrospinal fluid in Alzheimer's disease. *J. Neural Transm.* **2003**, *110*, 949–955. [CrossRef]
60. Mielke, M.M.; Haughey, N.J.; Bandaru, V.V.R.; Zetterberg, H.; Blennow, K.; Andreasson, U.; Johnson, S.C.; Gleason, C.E.; Blazel, H.M.; Puglielli, L.; et al. Cerebrospinal fluid sphingolipids, β-amyloid, and tau in adults at risk for Alzheimer's disease. *Neurobiol. Aging* **2014**, *35*, 2486–2494. [CrossRef]
61. Hu, W.T.; Chen-Plotkin, A.; Arnold, S.E.; Grossman, M.; Clark, C.M.; Shaw, L.M.; Pickering, E.; Kuhn, M.; Chen, Y.; Mccluskey, L.; et al. Novel CSF biomarkers for Alzheimer's disease and mild cognitive impairment. *Acta Neuropathol.* **2010**, *119*, 669–678. [CrossRef] [PubMed]

62. Desikan, R.S.; Thompson, W.K.; Holland, D.; Hess, C.P.; Brewer, J.B.; Zetterberg, H.; Blennow, K.; Andreassen, O.A.; McEvoy, L.K.; Hyman, B.T.; et al. Heart fatty acid binding protein and Aβ-associated Alzheimer's neurodegeneration. *Mol. Neurodegener.* **2013**, *8*, 1. [CrossRef] [PubMed]
63. Chiasserini, D.; Parnetti, L.; Andreasson, U.; Zetterberg, H.; Giannandrea, D.; Calabresi, P.; Blennow, K. CSF levels of heart fatty acid binding protein are altered during early phases of Alzheimer's disease. *J. Alzheimer's Dis.* **2010**, *22*, 1281–1288. [CrossRef] [PubMed]
64. Provost, P. Interpretation and applicability of microrna datato the context of Alzheimer's and age-related diseases. *Aging (Albany. NY)* **2010**, *2*, 166–169. [CrossRef] [PubMed]
65. Lukiw, W.J.; Andreeva, T.V.; Grigorenko, A.P.; Rogaev, E.I. Studying micro RNA function and dysfunction in Alzheimer's disease. *Front. Genet.* **2013**, *3*, 1–13. [CrossRef] [PubMed]
66. Lukiw, W.J. Micro-RNA speciation in fetal, adult and Alzheimer's disease hippocampus. *Neuroreport* **2007**, *18*, 297–300. [CrossRef]
67. Cortez, M.A.; Calin, G.A. MicroRNA identification in plasma and serum: A new tool to diagnose and monitor diseases. *Expert Opin. Biol. Ther.* **2009**, *9*, 703–711. [CrossRef]
68. Gallego, J.A.; Gordon, M.L.; Claycomb, K.; Bhatt, M.; Lencz, T.; Malhotra, A.K. In Vivo MicroRNA Detection and Quantitation in Cerebrospinal Fluid. *J. Mol. Neurosci.* **2012**, *47*, 243–248. [CrossRef]
69. Femminella, G.D.; Ferrara, N.; Rengo, G. The emerging role of microRNAs in Alzheimer's disease. *Front. Physiol.* **2015**, *6*, 1–5. [CrossRef]
70. Alexandrov, P.N.; Dua, P.; Hill, J.M.; Bhattacharjee, S.; Zhao, Y.; Lukiw, W.J. MicroRNA (miRNA) speciation in Alzheimer's disease (AD) cerebrospinal fluid (CSF) and extracellular fluid (ECF). *Int. J. Biochem. Mol. Biol.* **2012**, *3*, 365–373.
71. Lukiw, W.J.; Alexandrov, P.N.; Zhao, Y.; Hill, J.M.; Bhattacharjee, S. Spreading of Alzheimer's disease inflammatory signaling through soluble micro-RNA. *Neuroreport* **2012**, *23*, 621–626. [CrossRef] [PubMed]
72. Basavaraju, M.; De Lencastre, A. Alzheimer's disease: Presence and role of microRNAs. *Biomol. Concepts* **2016**, *7*, 241–252. [CrossRef] [PubMed]
73. Shioya, M.; Obayashi, S.; Tabunoki, H.; Arima, K.; Saito, Y.; Ishida, T.; Satoh, J. Aberrant microRNA expression in the brains of neurodegenerative diseases: MiR-29a decreased in Alzheimer disease brains targets neurone navigator 3. *Neuropathol. Appl. Neurobiol.* **2010**, *36*, 320–330. [CrossRef] [PubMed]
74. Müller, M.; Jäkel, L.; Bruinsma, I.B.; Claassen, J.A.; Kuiperij, H.B.; Verbeek, M.M. MicroRNA-29a Is a Candidate Biomarker for Alzheimer's Disease in Cell-Free Cerebrospinal Fluid. *Mol. Neurobiol.* **2016**, *53*, 2894–2899. [CrossRef]
75. Qiu, L.; Tan, E.K.; Zeng, L. microRNAs and Neurodegenerative Diseases. In *Advances in Experimental Medicine and Biology*; Academic Press: Cambridge, MA, USA, 2015; Chapter 6; pp. 85–105. ISBN 978-3-319-22671-2.
76. Zhang, F.; Gradinaru, V.; Adamantidis, A.R.; Durand, R.; Airan, R.D.; de Lecea, L.; Deisseroth, K. Optogenetic interrogation of neural circuits: Technology for probing mammalian brain structures. *Nat. Protoc.* **2010**, *5*, 439–456. [CrossRef]
77. Shibata, M.; Nakao, H.; Kiyonari, H.; Abe, T.; Aizawa, S. MicroRNA-9 regulates neurogenesis in mouse telencephalon by targeting multiple transcription factors. *J. Neurosci.* **2011**, *31*, 3407–3422. [CrossRef]
78. Vassar, R.; Kovacs, D.M.; Yan, R.; Wong, P.C. The β-secretase enzyme BACE in health and Alzheimer's disease: Regulation, cell biology, function, and therapeutic potential. *J. Neurosci.* **2009**, *29*, 12787–12794. [CrossRef]
79. Zhao, Y.; Zhang, Y.; Zhang, L.; Dong, Y.; Ji, H.; Shen, L. The potential markers of circulating micrornas and long non-coding RNAs in Alzheimer's disease. *Aging Dis.* **2019**, *10*, 1293–1301. [CrossRef]
80. Skoog, I.; Gustafson, D. Update on hypertension and Alzheimer's disease. *Neurol. Res.* **2006**, *28*, 605–611. [CrossRef]
81. Sancesario, G.; Bernardini, S. AD biomarker discovery in CSF and in alternative matrices. *Clin. Biochem.* **2019**, *72*, 52–57. [CrossRef]
82. Nakamura, A.; Kaneko, N.; Villemagne, V.L.; Kato, T.; Doecke, J.; Doré, V.; Fowler, C.; Li, Q.X.; Martins, R.; Rowe, C.; et al. High performance plasma amyloid-β biomarkers for Alzheimer's disease. *Nature* **2018**, *554*, 249–254. [CrossRef] [PubMed]

83. Jia, L.; Qiu, Q.; Zhang, H.; Chu, L.; Du, Y.; Zhang, J.; Zhou, C.; Liang, F.; Shi, S.; Wang, S.; et al. Concordance between the assessment of Aβ42, T-tau, and P-T181-tau in peripheral blood neuronal-derived exosomes and cerebrospinal fluid. *Alzheimer's Dement.* **2019**, *15*, 1071–1080. [CrossRef] [PubMed]
84. Lim, C.Z.J.; Zhang, Y.; Chen, Y.; Zhao, H.; Stephenson, M.C.; Ho, N.R.Y.; Chen, Y.; Chung, J.; Reilhac, A.; Loh, T.P.; et al. Subtyping of circulating exosome-bound amyloid β reflects brain plaque deposition. *Nat. Commun.* **2019**, *10*, 1–11. [CrossRef] [PubMed]
85. Janelidze, S.; Stomrud, E.; Palmqvist, S.; Zetterberg, H.; Van Westen, D.; Jeromin, A.; Song, L.; Hanlon, D.; Tan Hehir, C.A.; Baker, D.; et al. Plasma β-amyloid in Alzheimer's disease and vascular disease. *Sci. Rep.* **2016**, *6*, 1–11. [CrossRef]
86. Xia, W.; Yang, T.; Shankar, G.; Smith, I.M.; Shen, Y.; Walsh, D.M.; Selkoe, D.J. A specific enzyme-linked immunosorbent assay for measuring β-amyloid protein oligomers in human plasma and brain tissue of patients with Alzheimer Disease. *Arch. Neurol.* **2009**, *66*, 190–199. [CrossRef]
87. Mattsson, N.; Zetterberg, H.; Janelidze, S.; Insel, P.S.; Andreasson, U.; Stomrud, E.; Palmqvist, S.; Baker, D.; Tan Hehir, C.A.; Jeromin, A.; et al. Plasma tau in Alzheimer disease. *Neurology* **2016**, *87*, 1827–1835. [CrossRef]
88. Tatebe, H.; Kasai, T.; Ohmichi, T.; Kishi, Y.; Kakeya, T.; Waragai, M.; Kondo, M.; Allsop, D.; Tokuda, T. Quantification of plasma phosphorylated tau to use as a biomarker for brain Alzheimer pathology: Pilot case-control studies including patients with Alzheimer's disease and down syndrome. *Mol. Neurodegener.* **2017**, *12*, 1–11. [CrossRef]
89. Preische, O.; Schultz, S.A.; Apel, A.; Kuhle, J.; Kaeser, S.A.; Barro, C.; Gräber, S.; Kuder-Buletta, E.; LaFougere, C.; Laske, C.; et al. Serum neurofilament dynamics predicts neurodegeneration and clinical progression in presymptomatic Alzheimer's disease. *Nat. Med.* **2019**, *25*, 277–283. [CrossRef]
90. Hrubešová, K.; Fousková, M.; Habartová, L.; Fišar, Z.; Jirák, R.; Raboch, J.; Setnička, V. Search for biomarkers of Alzheimer's disease: Recent insights, current challenges and future prospects. *Clin. Biochem.* **2019**, *72*, 39–51. [CrossRef]
91. Kapogiannis, D.; Mustapic, M.; Shardell, M.D.; Berkowitz, S.T.; Diehl, T.C.; Spangler, R.D.; Tran, J.; Lazaropoulos, M.P.; Chawla, S.; Gulyani, S.; et al. Association of Extracellular Vesicle Biomarkers with Alzheimer Disease in the Baltimore Longitudinal Study of Aging. *JAMA Neurol.* **2019**, *76*, 1340–1351. [CrossRef]
92. Pláteník, J.; Fišar, Z.; Buchal, R.; Jirák, R.; Kitzlerová, E.; Zvěřová, M.; Raboch, J. GSK3β, CREB, and BDNF in peripheral blood of patients with alzheimer's disease and depression. *Prog. Neuro-Psychopharmacol. Biol. Psychiatry* **2014**, *50*, 83–93. [CrossRef] [PubMed]
93. Gupta, V.B.; Doecke, J.D.; Hone, E.; Pedrini, S.; Laws, S.M.; Thambisetty, M.; Bush, A.I.; Rowe, C.C.; Villemagne, V.L.; Ames, D.; et al. Plasma apolipoprotein J as a potential biomarker for Alzheimer's disease: Australian Imaging, Biomarkers and Lifestyle study of aging. *Alzheimer's Dement. Diagn. Assess. Dis. Monit.* **2016**, *3*, 18–26. [CrossRef] [PubMed]
94. Jongbloed, W.; Van Dijk, K.D.; Mulder, S.D.; Van De Berg, W.D.J.; Blankenstein, M.A.; Van Der Flier, W.; Veerhuis, R. Clusterin Levels in Plasma Predict Cognitive Decline and Progression to Alzheimer's Disease. *J. Alzheimer's Dis.* **2015**, *46*, 1103–1110. [CrossRef] [PubMed]
95. Da Mesquita, S.; Louveau, A.; Vaccari, A.; Smirnov, I.; Cornelison, R.C.; Kingsmore, K.M.; Contarino, C.; Onengut-Gumuscu, S.; Farber, E.; Raper, D.; et al. Functional aspects of meningeal lymphatics in ageing and Alzheimer's disease. *Nature* **2018**, *560*, 185–191. [CrossRef]
96. van de Haar, H.J.; Burgmans, S.; Jansen, J.F.A.; van Osch, M.J.P.; van Buchem, M.A.; Muller, M.; Hofman, P.A.M.; Verhey, F.R.J.; Backes, W.H. Blood-Brain Barrier Leakage in Patients with Early Alzheimer Disease. *Radiology* **2016**, *281*, 527–535. [CrossRef]
97. Yan, Z.; Zhou, Z.; Wu, Q.; Chen, Z.B.; Koo, E.H.; Zhong, S. Presymptomatic Increase of an Extracellular RNA in Blood Plasma Associates with the Development of Alzheimer's Disease. *Curr. Biol.* **2020**, *30*, 1–12. [CrossRef] [PubMed]
98. Chopra, N.; Wang, R.; Maloney, B.; Nho, K.; Beck, J.S.; Pourshafie, N.; Niculescu, A.; Saykin, A.J.; Rinaldi, C.; Counts, S.E.; et al. MicroRNA-298 reduces levels of human amyloid-β precursor protein (APP), β-site APP-converting enzyme 1 (BACE1) and specific tau protein moieties. *Mol. Psychiatry* **2020**, *1*. [CrossRef] [PubMed]

99. Dong, H.; Li, J.; Huang, L.; Chen, X.; Li, D.; Wang, T.; Hu, C.; Xu, J.; Zhang, C.; Zen, K.; et al. Serum MicroRNA profiles serve as novel biomarkers for the diagnosis of alzheimer's disease. *Dis. Markers* **2015**, *2015*. [CrossRef]
100. Kenny, A.; McArdle, H.; Calero, M.; Rabano, A.; Madden, S.F.; Adamson, K.; Forster, R.; Spain, E.; Prehn, J.H.M.; Henshall, D.C.; et al. Elevated plasma microRNA-206 levels predict cognitive decline and progression to dementia from mild cognitive impairment. *Biomolecules* **2019**, *9*, 734. [CrossRef]
101. Murillo, O.D.; Thistlethwaite, W.; Rozowsky, J.; Subramanian, S.L.; Lucero, R.; Shah, N.; Jackson, A.R.; Srinivasan, S.; Chung, A.; Laurent, C.D.; et al. exRNA Atlas Analysis Reveals Distinct Extracellular RNA Cargo Types and Their Carriers Present across Human Biofluids. *Cell* **2019**, *177*, 463–477.e15. [CrossRef]
102. Musunuri, S.; Khoonsari, P.E.; Mikus, M.; Wetterhall, M.; Häggmark-Mänberg, A.; Lannfelt, L.; Erlandsson, A.; Bergquist, J.; Ingelsson, M.; Shevchenko, G.; et al. Increased Levels of Extracellular Microvesicle Markers and Decreased Levels of Endocytic/Exocytic Proteins in the Alzheimer's Disease Brain. *J. Alzheimer's Dis.* **2016**, *54*, 1671–1686. [CrossRef] [PubMed]
103. Badhwar, A.; Haqqani, A.S. Biomarker potential of brain-secreted extracellular vesicles in blood in Alzheimer's disease. *Alzheimer's Dement. Diagn. Assess. Dis. Monit.* **2020**, *12*, 1–14. [CrossRef] [PubMed]
104. Lewczuk, P.; Ermann, N.; Andreasson, U.; Schultheis, C.; Podhorna, J.; Spitzer, P.; Maler, J.M.; Kornhuber, J.; Blennow, K.; Zetterberg, H. Plasma neurofilament light as a potential biomarker of neurodegeneration in Alzheimer's disease. *Alzheimer's Res. Ther.* **2018**, *10*, 1–10. [CrossRef] [PubMed]
105. Eitan, E.; Hutchison, E.R.; Marosi, K.; Comotto, J.; Mustapic, M.; Nigam, S.M.; Suire, C.; Maharana, C.; Jicha, G.A.; Liu, D.; et al. Extracellular vesicle-associated aβ mediates trans-neuronal bioenergetic and ca2+-handling deficits in alzheimer's disease models. *NPJ Aging Mech. Dis.* **2016**, *2*, 16019. [CrossRef] [PubMed]
106. Winston, C.N.; Goetzl, E.J.; Akers, J.C.; Carter, B.S.; Rockenstein, E.M.; Galasko, D.; Masliah, E.; Rissman, R.A. Prediction of conversion from mild cognitive impairment to dementia with neuronally derived blood exosome protein profile. *Alzheimer's Dement. Diagn. Assess. Dis. Monit.* **2016**, *3*, 63–72. [CrossRef] [PubMed]
107. Fiandaca, M.S.; Kapogiannis, D.; Mapstone, M.; Boxer, A.; Eitan, E.; Schwartz, J.B.; Abner, E.L.; Petersen, R.C.; Federoff, H.J.; Miller, B.L.; et al. Identification of preclinical Alzheimer's disease by a profile of pathogenic proteins in neurally derived blood exosomes: A case-control study. *Alzheimer's Dement.* **2015**, *11*, 600–607.e1. [CrossRef] [PubMed]
108. Shi, M.; Kovac, A.; Korff, A.; Cook, T.J.; Ginghina, C.; Bullock, K.M.; Yang, L.; Stewart, T.; Zheng, D.; Aro, P.; et al. CNS tau efflux via exosomes is likely increased in Parkinson's disease but not in Alzheimer's disease. *Alzheimer's Dement.* **2016**, *12*, 1125–1131. [CrossRef]
109. Winston, C.N.; Goetzl, E.J.; Baker, L.D.; Vitiello, M.V.; Rissman, R.A. Growth Hormone-Releasing Hormone Modulation of Neuronal Exosome Biomarkers in Mild Cognitive Impairment. *J. Alzheimer's Dis.* **2018**, *66*, 971–981. [CrossRef]
110. Guix, F.X.; Corbett, G.T.; Cha, D.J.; Mustapic, M.; Liu, W.; Mengel, D.; Chen, Z.; Aikawa, E.; Young-Pearse, T.; Kapogiannis, D.; et al. Detection of aggregation-competent tau in neuron-derived extracellular vesicles. *Int. J. Mol. Sci.* **2018**, *19*, 663. [CrossRef]
111. Goetzl, E.J.; Kapogiannis, D.; Schwartz, J.B.; Lobach, I.V.; Goetzl, L.; Abner, E.L.; Jicha, G.A.; Karydas, A.M.; Boxer, A.; Miller, B.L. Decreased synaptic proteins in neuronal exosomes of frontotemporal dementia and Alzheimer's disease. *FASEB J.* **2016**, *30*, 4141–4148. [CrossRef]
112. Mullins, R.J.; Mustapic, M.; Goetz, E.J.; Kapogiannis, D. Exosomal biomarkers of brain insulin resistance associated with regional atrophy in Alzheimer's disease. *Hum. Brain Mapp.* **2017**, *38*, 1933–1940. [CrossRef] [PubMed]
113. Kapogiannis, D.; Boxer, A.; Schwartz, J.B.; Abner, E.L.; Biragyn, A.; Masharani, U.; Frassetto, L.; Petersen, R.C.; Miller, B.L.; Goetzl, E.J. Dysfunctionally phosphorylated type 1 insulin receptor substrate in neural-derived blood exosomes of preclinical Alzheimer's disease. *FASEB J.* **2015**, *29*, 589–596. [CrossRef] [PubMed]
114. Mustapic, M.; Tran, J.; Craft, S.; Kapogiannis, D. Extracellular Vesicle Biomarkers Track Cognitive Changes Following Intranasal Insulin in Alzheimer's Disease. *J. Alzheimer's Dis.* **2019**, *69*, 489–498. [CrossRef] [PubMed]

115. Goetzl, E.J.; Boxer, A.; Schwartz, J.B.; Abner, E.L.; Petersen, R.C.; Miller, B.L.; Kapogiannis, D. Altered lysosomal proteins in neural-derived plasma exosomes in preclinical Alzheimer disease. *Neurology* **2015**, *85*, 40–47. [CrossRef]
116. Goetzl, E.J.; Nogueras-Ortiz, C.; Mustapic, M.; Mullins, R.J.; Abner, E.L.; Schwartz, J.B.; Kapogiannis, D. Deficient neurotrophic factors of CSPG4-type neural cell exosomes in Alzheimer disease. *FASEB J.* **2019**, *33*, 231–238. [CrossRef]
117. Goetzl, E.J.; Schwartz, J.B.; Abner, E.L.; Jicha, G.A.; Kapogiannis, D. High complement levels in astrocyte-derived exosomes of Alzheimer disease. *Ann. Neurol.* **2018**, *83*, 544–552. [CrossRef]
118. Goetzl, E.J.; Mustapic, M.; Kapogiannis, D.; Eitan, E.; Lobach, I.V.; Goetzl, L.; Schwartz, J.B.; Miller, B.L. Cargo proteins of plasma astrocyte-derived exosomes in Alzheimer's disease. *FASEB J.* **2016**, *30*, 3853–3859. [CrossRef]
119. Pant, S.; Hilton, H.; Burczynski, M.E. The multifaceted exosome: Biogenesis, role in normal and aberrant cellular function, and frontiers for pharmacological and biomarker opportunities. *Biochem. Pharmacol.* **2012**, *83*, 1484–1494. [CrossRef]
120. Burgos, K.; Malenica, I.; Metpally, R.; Courtright, A.; Rakela, B.; Beach, T.; Shill, H.; Adler, C.; Sabbagh, M.; Villa, S.; et al. Profiles of extracellular miRNA in cerebrospinal fluid and serum from patients with Alzheimer's and Parkinson's diseases correlate with disease status and features of pathology. *PLoS ONE* **2014**, *9*. [CrossRef]
121. Liu, C.G.; Song, J.; Zhang, Y.Q.; Wang, P.C. MicroRNA-193b is a regulator of amyloid precursor protein in the blood and cerebrospinal fluid derived exosomal microRNA-193b is a biomarker of Alzheimer's disease. *Mol. Med. Rep.* **2014**, *10*, 2395–2400. [CrossRef]
122. Cheng, L.; Doecke, J.D.; Sharples, R.A.; Villemagne, V.L.; Fowler, C.J.; Rembach, A.; Martins, R.N.; Rowe, C.C.; Macaulay, S.L.; Masters, C.L.; et al. Prognostic serum miRNA biomarkers associated with Alzheimer's disease shows concordance with neuropsychological and neuroimaging assessment. *Mol. Psychiatry* **2015**, *20*, 1188–1196. [CrossRef] [PubMed]
123. Lugli, G.; Cohen, A.M.; Bennett, D.A.; Shah, R.C.; Fields, C.J.; Hernandez, A.G.; Smalheiser, N.R. Plasma exosomal miRNAs in persons with and without Alzheimer disease: Altered expression and prospects for biomarkers. *PLoS ONE* **2015**, *10*, 1–18. [CrossRef]
124. Yang, T.T.; Liu, C.G.; Gao, S.C.; Zhang, Y.; Wang, P.C. The Serum Exosome Derived MicroRNA−135a, −193b, and −384 Were Potential Alzheimer's Disease Biomarkers. *Biomed. Environ. Sci.* **2018**, *31*, 87–96. [CrossRef] [PubMed]
125. Wei, H.; Xu, Y.; Xu, W.; Zhou, Q.; Chen, Q.; Yang, M.; Feng, F.; Liu, Y.; Zhu, X.; Yu, M.; et al. *Serum Exosomal miR-223 Serves as a Potential Diagnostic and Prognostic Biomarker for Dementia*; Elsevier: Amsterdam, The Netherlands, 2018; Volume 379, ISBN 8651188773631.
126. Cha, D.J.; Mengel, D.; Mustapic, M.; Liu, W.; Selkoe, D.J.; Kapogiannis, D.; Galasko, D.; Rissman, R.A.; Bennett, D.A.; Walsh, D.M. miR-212 and miR-132 Are Downregulated in Neurally Derived Plasma Exosomes of Alzheimer's Patients. *Front. Neurosci.* **2019**, *13*, 1–14. [CrossRef] [PubMed]
127. Galimberti, D.; Villa, C.; Fenoglio, C.; Serpente, M.; Ghezzi, L.; Cioffi, S.M.G.; Arighi, A.; Fumagalli, G.; Scarpini, E. Circulating miRNAs as potential biomarkers in alzheimer's disease. *J. Alzheimer's Dis.* **2014**, *42*, 1261–1267. [CrossRef]
128. Rani, A.; O'Shea, A.; Ianov, L.; Cohen, R.A.; Woods, A.J.; Foster, T.C. miRNA in circulating microvesicles as biomarkers for age-related cognitive decline. *Front. Aging Neurosci.* **2017**, *9*, 1–10. [CrossRef]
129. Gámez-Valero, A.; Campdelacreu, J.; Vilas, D.; Ispierto, L.; Reñé, R.; Álvarez, R.; Armengol, M.P.; Borràs, F.E.; Beyer, K. Exploratory study on microRNA profiles from plasma-derived extracellular vesicles in Alzheimer's disease and dementia with Lewy bodies. *Transl. Neurodegener.* **2019**, *8*, 1–17. [CrossRef]
130. Barbagallo, C.; Mostile, G.; Baglieri, G.; Giunta, F.; Luca, A.; Raciti, L.; Zappia, M.; Purrello, M.; Ragusa, M.; Nicoletti, A. Specific Signatures of Serum miRNAs as Potential Biomarkers to Discriminate Clinically Similar Neurodegenerative and Vascular-Related Diseases. *Cell. Mol. Neurobiol.* **2020**, *40*, 531–546. [CrossRef]
131. Chen, J.; Qi, Y.; Liu, C.-F.; Lu, J.-M.; Shi, J.; Shi, Y. MicroRNA expression data analysis to identify key miRNAs associated with Alzheimer's disease. *J. Gene Med.* **2018**, *20*, e3014. [CrossRef]

132. Zhang, Y.; Lv, X.; Liu, C.; Gao, S.; Ping, H.; Wang, J.; Wang, P. MiR-214-3p attenuates cognition defects via the inhibition of autophagy in SAMP8 mouse model of sporadic Alzheimer's disease. *Neurotoxicology* **2016**, *56*, 139–149. [CrossRef] [PubMed]
133. Cogswell, J.P.; Ward, J.; Taylor, I.A.; Waters, M.; Shi, Y.; Cannon, B.; Kelnar, K.; Kemppainen, J.; Brown, D.; Chen, C.; et al. Identification of miRNA Changes in Alzheimer's Disease Brain and CSF Yields Putative Biomarkers and Insights into Disease Pathways. *J. Alzheimer's Dis.* **2008**, *14*, 27–41. [CrossRef] [PubMed]
134. Sørensen, S.S.; Nygaard, A.B.; Christensen, T. miRNA expression profiles in cerebrospinal fluid and blood of patients with Alzheimer's disease and other types of dementia—An exploratory study. *Transl. Neurodegener.* **2016**, *5*, 1–12. [CrossRef] [PubMed]
135. Wu, Y.; Xu, J.; Xu, J.; Cheng, J.; Jiao, D.; Zhou, C.; Dai, Y.; Chen, Q. Lower serum levels of miR-29c-3p and miR-19b-3p as biomarkers for Alzheimer's disease. *Tohoku J. Exp. Med.* **2017**, *242*, 129–136. [CrossRef] [PubMed]
136. Hara, N.; Kikuchi, M.; Miyashita, A.; Hatsuta, H.; Saito, Y.; Kasuga, K.; Murayama, S.; Ikeuchi, T.; Kuwano, R. Serum microRNA miR-501-3p as a potential biomarker related to the progression of Alzheimer's disease. *Acta Neuropathol. Commun.* **2017**, *5*, 10. [CrossRef] [PubMed]
137. Cosín-Tomás, M.; Antonell, A.; Lladó, A.; Alcolea, D.; Fortea, J.; Ezquerra, M.; Lleó, A.; Martí, M.J.; Pallàs, M.; Sanchez-Valle, R.; et al. Plasma miR-34a-5p and miR-545-3p as Early Biomarkers of Alzheimer's Disease: Potential and Limitations. *Mol. Neurobiol.* **2017**, *54*, 5550–5562. [CrossRef] [PubMed]
138. Hébert, S.S.; Horré, K.; Nicolaï, L.; Papadopoulou, A.S.; Mandemakers, W.; Silahtaroglu, A.N.; Kauppinen, S.; Delacourte, A.; De Strooper, B. Loss of microRNA cluster miR-29a/b-1 in sporadic Alzheimer's disease correlates with increased BACE1/β-secretase expression. *Proc. Natl. Acad. Sci. USA* **2008**, *105*, 6415–6420. [CrossRef]
139. Wang, L.; Zhang, L. Circulating Exosomal miRNA as Diagnostic Biomarkers of Neurodegenerative Diseases. *Front. Mol. Neurosci.* **2020**, *13*, 1–11. [CrossRef]
140. Jia, L.-H.; Liu, Y.-N. Downregulated serum miR-223 servers as biomarker in Alzheimer's disease. *Cell Biochem. Funct.* **2016**, *34*, 233–237. [CrossRef]
141. Zhu, Y.; Li, C.; Sun, A.; Wang, Y.; Zhou, S. Quantification of microRNA-210 in the cerebrospinal fluid and serum: Implications for Alzheimer's disease. *Exp. Ther. Med.* **2015**, *9*, 1013–1017. [CrossRef]
142. Liu, C.G.; Wang, J.L.; Li, L.; Xue, L.X.; Zhang, Y.Q.; Wang, P.C. MicroRNA-135a and -200b, potential Biomarkers for Alzheimer's disease, regulate β secretase and amyloid precursor protein. *Brain Res.* **2014**, *1583*, 55–64. [CrossRef] [PubMed]
143. Zhang, Y.; Liu, C.; Wang, J.; Li, Q.; Ping, H.; Gao, S.; Wang, P. MIR-299-5p regulates apoptosis through autophagy in neurons and ameliorates cognitive capacity in APPswe/PS1dE9 mice. *Sci. Rep.* **2016**, *6*, 1–14. [CrossRef] [PubMed]
144. Kumar, S.; Reddy, P.H. MicroRNA-455-3p as a Potential Biomarker for Alzheimer's Disease: An Update. *Front. Aging Neurosci.* **2018**, *10*, 41. [CrossRef]
145. Derkow, K.; Rössling, R.; Schipke, C.; Krüger, C.; Bauer, J.; Fähling, M.; Stroux, A.; Schott, E.; Ruprecht, K.; Peters, O.; et al. Distinct expression of the neurotoxic microRNA family let-7 in the cerebrospinal fluid of patients with Alzheimer's disease. *PLoS ONE* **2018**, *13*, 1–18. [CrossRef] [PubMed]
146. Dangla-Valls, A.; Molinuevo, J.L.; Altirriba, J.; Sánchez-Valle, R.; Alcolea, D.; Fortea, J.; Rami, L.; Balasa, M.; Muñoz-García, C.; Ezquerra, M.; et al. CSF microRNA Profiling in Alzheimer's Disease: A Screening and Validation Study. *Mol. Neurobiol.* **2017**, *54*, 6647–6654. [CrossRef]
147. Li, W.; Li, X.; Xin, X.; Kan, P.C.; Yan, Y. MicroRNA-613 regulates the expression of brain-derived neurotrophic factor in Alzheimer's disease. *Biosci. Trends* **2016**, *10*, 372–377. [CrossRef]
148. Kenny, A.; Jiménez-Mateos, E.M.; Zea-Sevilla, M.A.; Rábano, A.; Gili-Manzanaro, P.; Prehn, J.H.M.; Henshall, D.C.; Ávila, J.; Engel, T.; Hernández, F. Proteins and microRNAs are differentially expressed in tear fluid from patients with Alzheimer's disease. *Sci. Rep.* **2019**, *9*, 1–14. [CrossRef]
149. Wu, Q.; Ye, X.; Xiong, Y.; Zhu, H.; Miao, J.; Zhang, W.; Wan, J. The Protective Role of microRNA-200c in Alzheimer's Disease Pathologies Is Induced by Beta Amyloid-Triggered Endoplasmic Reticulum Stress. *Front. Mol. Neurosci.* **2016**, *9*, 140. [CrossRef]
150. Tian, N.; Cao, Z.; Zhang, Y. MiR-206 decreases brain-derived neurotrophic factor levels in a transgenic mouse model of Alzheimer's disease. *Neurosci. Bull.* **2014**, *30*, 191–197. [CrossRef]

151. Crooke, A.; Huete-toral, F.; Martı, A.; Colligris, B.; Pintor, J. Ocular disorders and the utility of animal models in the discovery of melatoninergic drugs with therapeutic potential. *Expert Opin. Drug Discov.* **2012**, *7*, 989–1001. [CrossRef]
152. van Wijngaarden, P.; Hadoux, X.; Alwan, M.; Keel, S.; Dirani, M. Emerging ocular biomarkers of Alzheimer disease. *Clin. Exp. Ophthalmol.* **2017**, *45*, 54–61. [CrossRef] [PubMed]
153. Singh, A.K.; Verma, S. Use of ocular biomarkers as a potential tool for early diagnosis of Alzheimer's disease. *Indian J. Ophthalmol.* **2020**, *68*, 555–561. [CrossRef] [PubMed]
154. Ning, A.; Cui, J.; To, E.; Ashe, K.H.; Matsubara, J. Amyloid-β deposits lead to retinal degeneration in a mouse model of Alzheimer disease. *Investig. Ophthalmol. Vis. Sci.* **2008**, *49*, 5136–5143. [CrossRef] [PubMed]
155. More, S.S.; Vince, R. Hyperspectral imaging signatures detect amyloidopathy in alzheimers mouse retina well before onset of cognitive decline. *ACS Chem. Neurosci.* **2015**, *6*, 306–315. [CrossRef]
156. Goldstein, L.E.; Muffat, J.A.; Cherny, R.A.; Moir, R.D.; Ericsson, M.H.; Huang, X.; Mavros, C.; Coccia, J.A.; Faget, K.Y.; Fitch, K.A.; et al. Cytosolic β-amyloid deposition and supranuclear cataracts in lenses from people with Alzheimer's disease. *Lancet* **2003**, *361*, 1258–1265. [CrossRef]
157. Kerbage, C.; Sadowsky, C.H.; Tariot, P.N.; Agronin, M.; Alva, G.; Turner, F.D.; Nilan, D.; Cameron, A.; Cagle, G.D.; Hartung, P.D. Detection of Amyloid β Signature in the Lens and Its Correlation in the Brain to Aid in the Diagnosis of Alzheimer's Disease. *Am. J. Alzheimers Dis. Other Demen.* **2015**, *30*, 738–745. [CrossRef]
158. Koronyo-Hamaoui, M.; Koronyo, Y.; Ljubimov, A.V.; Miller, C.A.; Ko, M.K.; Black, K.L.; Schwartz, M.; Farkas, D.L. Identification of amyloid plaques in retinas from Alzheimer's patients and noninvasive in vivo optical imaging of retinal plaques in a mouse model. *Neuroimage* **2011**, *54*, S204–S217. [CrossRef]
159. Armstrong, R.A.; Syed, A.B. Alzheimer's disease and the eye. *Ophthalmic Physiol. Opt.* **2008**, *16*, S2–S8. [CrossRef]
160. La Morgia, C.; Ross-Cisneros, F.N.; Koronyo, Y.; Hannibal, J.; Gallassi, R.; Cantalupo, G.; Sambati, L.; Pan, B.X.; Tozer, K.R.; Barboni, P.; et al. Melanopsin retinal ganglion cell loss in Alzheimer disease. *Ann. Neurol.* **2016**, *79*, 90–109. [CrossRef]
161. Esquiva, G.; Hannibal, J. Melanopsin-expressing retinal ganglion cells in aging and disease. *Histol. Histopathol.* **2019**, *34*, 1299–1311.
162. Dutescu, R.M.; Li, Q.X.; Crowston, J.; Masters, C.L.; Baird, P.N.; Culvenor, J.G. Amyloid precursor protein processing and retinal pathology in mouse models of Alzheimer's disease. *Graefe's Arch. Clin. Exp. Ophthalmol.* **2009**, *247*, 1213–1221. [CrossRef] [PubMed]
163. Choi, S.I.; Lee, B.; Woo, J.H.; Jeong, J.B.; Jun, I.; Kim, E.K. APP processing and metabolism in corneal fibroblasts and epithelium as a potential biomarker for Alzheimer's disease. *Exp. Eye Res.* **2019**, *182*, 167–174. [CrossRef]
164. Csosz, É.; Boross, P.; Csutak, A.; Berta, A.; Tóth, F.; Póliska, S.; Török, Z.; Tozsér, J. Quantitative analysis of proteins in the tear fluid of patients with diabetic retinopathy. *J. Proteom.* **2012**, *75*, 2196–2204. [CrossRef] [PubMed]
165. Çomoğlu, S.S.; Güven, H.; Acar, M.; Öztürk, G.; Koçer, B. Tear levels of tumor necrosis factor-alpha in patients with Parkinson's disease. *Neurosci. Lett.* **2013**, *553*, 63–67. [CrossRef] [PubMed]
166. Zhou, L.; Zhao, S.Z.; Koh, S.K.; Chen, L.; Vaz, C.; Tanavde, V.; Li, X.R.; Beuerman, R.W. In-depth analysis of the human tear proteome. *J. Proteom.* **2012**, *75*, 3877–3885. [CrossRef] [PubMed]
167. Örnek, N.; Dag, E.; Örnek, K. Corneal sensitivity and tear function in neurodegenerative diseases. *Curr. Eye Res.* **2015**, *40*, 423–428. [CrossRef] [PubMed]
168. Kalló, G.; Emri, M.; Varga, Z.; Ujhelyi, B.; Tozsér, J.; Csutak, A.; Csosz, É. Changes in the chemical barrier composition of tears in Alzheimer's disease reveal potential tear diagnostic biomarkers. *PLoS ONE* **2016**, *11*, 1–14. [CrossRef] [PubMed]
169. Ship, J.A.; Puckett, S.A. Longitudinal Study on Oral Health in Subjects with Alzheimer's Disease. *J. Am. Geriatr. Soc.* **1994**, *42*, 57–63. [CrossRef]
170. Ship, J.A.; DeCarli, C.; Friedland, R.P.; Baum, B.J. Diminished submandibular salivary flow in dementia of the Alzheimer Type. *J. Gerontol.* **1990**, *45*, 61–66. [CrossRef]
171. Reuster, T.; Rilke, O.; Oehler, J. High correlation between salivary MHPG and CSF MHPG. *Psychopharmacology (Berl)* **2002**, *162*, 415–418. [CrossRef]

172. Formichi, P.; Battisti, C.; Radi, E.; Federico, A. Cerebrospinal fluid tau, Aß, and phosphorylated tau protein for the diagnosis of Alzheimer's disease. *J. Cell. Physiol.* **2006**, *208*, 39–46. [CrossRef] [PubMed]
173. Bermejo-Pareja, F.; Antequera, D.; Vargas, T.; Molina, J.A.; Carro, E. Saliva levels of Abeta1-42 as potential biomarker of Alzheimer's disease: A pilot study. *BMC Neurol.* **2010**, *10*, 108. [CrossRef] [PubMed]
174. Kim, C.-B.; Choi, Y.Y.; Song, W.K.; Song, K.-B. Antibody-based magnetic nanoparticle immunoassay for quantification of Alzheimer's disease pathogenic factor. *J. Biomed. Opt.* **2013**, *19*, 051205. [CrossRef] [PubMed]
175. Sabbagh, M.N.; Shi, J.; Lee, M.; Arnold, L.; Al-Hasan, Y.; Heim, J.; McGeer, P. Salivary beta amyloid protein levels are detectable and differentiate patients with Alzheimer's disease dementia from normal controls: Preliminary findings. *BMC Neurol.* **2018**, *18*, 155. [CrossRef] [PubMed]
176. Lee, M.; Guo, J.P.; Kennedy, K.; Mcgeer, E.G.; McGeer, P.L. A method for diagnosing Alzheimer's disease based on salivary amyloid-β protein 42 levels. *J. Alzheimer's Dis.* **2017**, *55*, 1175–1182. [CrossRef] [PubMed]
177. Conrad, C.; Vianna, C.; Freeman, M.; Davies, P. A polymorphic gene nested within an intron of the tau gene: Implications for Alzheimer's disease. *Proc. Natl. Acad. Sci. USA* **2002**, *99*, 7751–7756. [CrossRef]
178. Ashton, N.J.; Ide, M.; Schöll, M.; Blennow, K.; Lovestone, S.; Hye, A.; Zetterberg, H. No association of salivary total tau concentration with Alzheimer's disease. *Neurobiol. Aging* **2018**, *70*, 125–127. [CrossRef]
179. Shi, M.; Sui, Y.-T.; Peskind, E.R.; Li, G.; Hwang, H.; Devic, I.; Ginghina, C.; Edgar, J.S.; Pan, C.; Goodlett, D.R.; et al. Salivary Tau Species are Potential Biomarkers of Alzheimer's Disease. *J. Alzheimer's Dis.* **2011**, *27*, 299–305. [CrossRef]
180. Pekeles, H.; Qureshi, H.Y.; Paudel, H.K.; Schipper, H.M.; Gornistky, M.; Chertkow, H. Development and validation of a salivary tau biomarker in Alzheimer's disease. *Alzheimer's Dement. Diagn. Assess. Dis. Monit.* **2019**, *11*, 53–60. [CrossRef]
181. Carro, E.; Bartolomé, F.; Bermejo-Pareja, F.; Villarejo-Galende, A.; Molina, J.A.; Ortiz, P.; Calero, M.; Rabano, A.; Cantero, J.L.; Orive, G. Early diagnosis of mild cognitive impairment and Alzheimer's disease based on salivary lactoferrin. *Alzheimer's Dement. Diagn. Assess. Dis. Monit.* **2017**, *8*, 131–138. [CrossRef]
182. Boston, P.F.; Gopalkaje, K.; Manning, L.; Middleton, L.; Loxley, M. Developing a simple laboratory test for Alzheimer's disease: Measuring acetylcholinesterase in saliva—A pilot study. *Int. J. Geriatr. Psychiatry* **2008**, *23*, 439–440. [CrossRef] [PubMed]
183. Bakhtiari, S.; Moghadam, N.B.; Ehsani, M.; Mortazavi, H.; Sabour, S.; Bakhshi, M. Can salivary acetylcholinesterase be a diagnostic biomarker for Alzheimer? *J. Clin. Diagn. Res.* **2017**, *11*, ZC58–ZC60. [CrossRef] [PubMed]
184. García-Blanco, A.; Peña-Bautista, C.; Oger, C.; Vigor, C.; Galano, J.-M.; Durand, T.; Martín-Ibáñez, N.; Baquero, M.; Vento, M.; Cháfer-Pericás, C. Reliable determination of new lipid peroxidation compounds as potential early Alzheimer Disease biomarkers. *Talanta* **2018**, *184*, 193–201. [CrossRef] [PubMed]
185. Praticò, D.; Clark, C.M.; Liun, F.; Lee, V.Y.M.; Trojanowski, J.Q. Increase of brain oxidative stress in mild cognitive impairment: A possible predictor of Alzheimer disease. *Arch. Neurol.* **2002**, *59*, 972–976. [CrossRef] [PubMed]
186. Hee Lee, S.; Kim, I.; Chul Chung, B. Increased urinary level of oxidized nucleosides in patients with mild-to-moderate Alzheimer's disease. *Clin. Biochem.* **2007**, *40*, 936–938. [CrossRef]
187. De La Monte, S.M.; Ghanbari, K.; Frey, W.H.; Beheshti, I.; Averback, P.; Hauser, S.L.; Ghanbari, H.A.; Wands, J.R. Characterization of the AD7C-NTP cDNA expression in Alzheimer's disease and measurement of a 41-kD protein in cerebrospinal fluid. *J. Clin. Investig.* **1997**, *100*, 3093–3104. [CrossRef]
188. Zhang, N.; Zhang, L.; Li, Y.; Gordon, M.L.; Cai, L.; Wang, Y.; Xing, M.; Cheng, Y. Urine AD7c-NTP predicts amyloid deposition and symptom of agitation in patients with Alzheimer's disease and mild cognitive impairment. *J. Alzheimer's Dis.* **2017**, *60*, 87–95. [CrossRef]
189. Zhang, J.; Zhang, C.H.; Li, R.J.; Lin, X.L.; Chen, Y.D.; Gao, H.Q.; Shi, S.L. Accuracy of urinary AD7c-NTP for diagnosing alzheimer's disease: A systematic review and meta-analysis. *J. Alzheimer's Dis.* **2014**, *40*, 153–159. [CrossRef]
190. Takae, K.; Hata, J.; Ohara, T.; Yoshida, D.; Shibata, M.; Mukai, N.; Hirakawa, Y.; Kishimoto, H.; Tsuruya, K.; Kitazono, T.; et al. Albuminuria increases the risks for both Alzheimer disease and vascular dementia in community-dwelling Japanese elderly: The hisayama study. *J. Am. Heart Assoc.* **2018**, *7*. [CrossRef]

191. Yao, F.; Hong, X.; Li, S.; Zhang, Y.; Zhao, Q.; Du, W.; Wang, Y.; Ni, J. Urine-Based Biomarkers for Alzheimer's Disease Identified Through Coupling Computational and Experimental Methods. *J. Alzheimers Dis.* **2018**, *65*, 421–431. [CrossRef]
192. Agbemenyah, H.Y.; Agis-Balboa, R.C.; Burkhardt, S.; Delalle, I.; Fischer, A. Insulin growth factor binding protein 7 is a novel target to treat dementia. *Neurobiol. Dis.* **2014**, *62*, 135–143. [CrossRef] [PubMed]
193. Rentsendorj, A.; Sheyn, J.; Fuchs, D.; Daley, D.; Salumbides, B.C.; Schubloom, H.E.; Hart, N.J.; Li, S.; Hayden, E.Y.; Teplow, D.B.; et al. A novel role for osteopontin in macrophage-mediated amyloid-β clearance in Alzheimer's models. *Brain Behav. Immun.* **2018**, *67*, 163–180. [CrossRef] [PubMed]
194. Yang, W.; Chauhan, A.; Mehta, S.; Mehta, P.; Gu, F.; Chauhan, V. Trichostatin A increases the levels of plasma gelsolin and amyloid beta-protein in a transgenic mouse model of Alzheimer's disease. *Life Sci.* **2014**, *99*, 31–36. [CrossRef] [PubMed]

13

Imaging and Molecular Mechanisms of Alzheimer's Disease

Grazia Daniela Femminella [1], Tony Thayanandan [2], Valeria Calsolaro [1], Klara Komici [3], Giuseppe Rengo [4,5], Graziamaria Corbi [3] and Nicola Ferrara [4,5,*]

1 Neurology Imaging Unit, Imperial College London, London W12 0NN, UK; g.femminella@imperial.ac.uk (G.D.F.); v.calsolaro@imperial.ac.uk (V.C.)
2 Imperial Memory Unit, Charing Cross Hospital, Imperial College London, London W6 8RF, UK; tony.thayanandan@nhs.net
3 Department of Medicine and Health Sciences, University of Molise, 86100 Campobasso, Italy; klara.komici@unimol.it (K.K.); graziamaria.corbi@unimol.it (G.C.)
4 Department of Translational Medical Sciences, Federico II University of Naples, 80131 Naples, Italy; giuseppe.rengo@unina.it
5 Istituti Clinici Scientifici Maugeri SPA—Società Benefit, IRCCS, 82037 Telese Terme, Italy
* Correspondence: nicola.ferrara@unina.it

Abstract: Alzheimer's disease is the most common form of dementia and is a significant burden for affected patients, carers, and health systems. Great advances have been made in understanding its pathophysiology, to a point that we are moving from a purely clinical diagnosis to a biological one based on the use of biomarkers. Among those, imaging biomarkers are invaluable in Alzheimer's, as they provide an in vivo window to the pathological processes occurring in Alzheimer's brain. While some imaging techniques are still under evaluation in the research setting, some have reached widespread clinical use. In this review, we provide an overview of the most commonly used imaging biomarkers in Alzheimer's disease, from molecular PET imaging to structural MRI, emphasising the concept that multimodal imaging would likely prove to be the optimal tool in the future of Alzheimer's research and clinical practice.

Keywords: Alzheimer's disease; positron emission tomography (PET); magnetic resonance imaging (MRI)

1. Introduction

Alzheimer's disease (AD) is a neurodegenerative disease that is responsible for 60–80% of all cases of dementia worldwide. Recent epidemiological data indicate that approximately 5.7 million Americans of all ages are living with AD in 2018 and 10.5 million people were suffering with dementia in Europe in 2015. The prevalence of dementia in Europe ranges from 4.7% to 6.8% [1]. Estimated projections suggest that by 2025, the number of people over 65 with AD will reach 7.1 million in the U.S., which is almost a 29 percent increase from the 2018 prevalence, and by 2050 the population affected will grow to 13.8 million, posing a great burden on health systems [2]. Clinically, AD is typically characterised by impairment in short-term memory to such an extent as to interfere with activities of daily living, while later symptoms include impairment in the other cognitive domains, such as language, orientation, judgment, executive functions, behavioural changes, and, ultimately, motor difficulties.

The first criteria proposed for AD diagnosis were developed in 1984 and focused only on clinical symptoms. However, the exceptional amount of research conducted since has helped clarify that the phase of dementia in AD is preceded by a long preclinical phase of several decades that evolves through a continuum, with the prodromal stage of mild cognitive impairment (MCI), and ultimately leads to dementia [3]. In this long preclinical phase, an early diagnosis can be made with the help of biomarkers. Based on this evidence, the National Institute on Aging (NIA) and the Alzheimer's Association in 2011 published new guidelines incorporating biomarker tests in addition to clinical symptoms, moving from a symptom-based definition to a biology-based definition of AD [4].

The biology of AD is characterised by two major protein abnormalities in the brain of affected individuals: the extracellular accumulation of amyloid β (Aβ) plaques and intraneuronal deposits of neurofibrillary tangles (NFTs). Insoluble Aβ plaques are formed of aggregated Aβ peptides that derive from the abnormal cleavage of the amyloid precursor protein (APP) into hydrophobic Aβ peptides. Aβ is thought to be the trigger or the driver of the disease process, mainly based on evidence from familial AD cases, leading to the amyloid hypothesis of AD [5]. NFTs are composed of hyperphosphorylated tau protein aggregates which accumulate in the neuron cytoplasm, leading to destabilisation of microtubules and axonal transport [6]. Both proteinopathies can trigger oxidative stress, microvascular dysfunction, and blood–brain barrier (BBB) disruption, and can induce the activation of an inflammatory response within the brain, ultimately resulting in neuronal damage and consequent neurodegeneration [3].

All these pathological changes that manifest at earlier or later phases of the AD continuum can now be explored with the use of biomarkers, some of which are still only used in a research framework and are awaiting clinical validation. Overall, the main biomarkers in AD can be broadly divided into cerebrospinal (CSF) and imaging biomarkers. Research is ongoing in the field of blood biomarkers, but large clinical studies are needed to assess their diagnostic potential [7]. In this review, we will focus on imaging biomarkers, both those currently available in clinical practice and those that are only part of the research framework [8]. Over CSF biomarkers that constitute an indirect measure of the ongoing pathological processes, imaging ones have the advantage of providing information on the in vivo pathological processes, giving a "window" to the changes happening in the brain at the different stages of the disease, and are less invasive and troublesome for the patients. We will focus on neurodegenerative imaging biomarkers (MRI and glucose metabolism), amyloid and tau imaging, and the newest in vivo biomarkers for neuroinflammation and BBB dysfunction.

2. Imaging of Neurodegeneration

2.1. Structural Magnetic Resonance Imaging (MRI)

Atrophy seems to be an unavoidable, inevitable progressive component of neurodegeneration. Brain tissue loss correlates well with cognitive deficits, both cross-sectionally and longitudinally in AD [9]. Structural brain changes are accurately consistent with upstream Braak stages of neurofibrillary tangle deposition [10,11] and downstream neuropsychological deficits [12]. Rates of change in several structural measures, including whole-brain [13], entorhinal cortex [14], hippocampus [15], and temporal lobe volumes [16], correlate closely with changes in cognitive performance, validating atrophy in these regions as markers of AD. For atrophy markers to be useful clinically, the subtleties should be known at the different stages of the disease, and their relationship with other imaging and biological markers should be understood. Atrophy measures change with disease progression over AD disease severity. Structural markers are more sensitive to change than are markers of Aβ deposition, both in MCI and in the moderate dementia stage of AD [17]. However, studies have shown that in the earliest forms of MCI, amyloid burden shows more abnormalities that are structural changes [18,19]. Atrophy is accompanied by microstructural changes, such as axonal loss and metabolite changes, all of which are measured with techniques other than MRI.

Structural MRI is still one of the most widely used neuroimaging techniques in the diagnosis of AD. T1-weighted scans are the most commonly used due to their ability to provide good contrast between grey and white matter and to detect subtle changes in grey matter. MRI gives the best spatial resolution of any clinical neuroimaging technique, so measures from an MRI include grey matter volume, cortical thickness, and volumetric measures of the hippocampus [20]. Measurements of grey matter are usually done visually, but recently there has been increased use of automated methods to calculate volume and cortical thickness [21,22] and subcortical segmentation of the hippocampus [23,24]. However, with these recent advances in more methodological techniques, visual reading is still the method most often used clinically to read an MRI. This shows the lack of a standardised protocol or method for the diagnosis of AD but is of high interest for researchers [24,25]. Clinicians also use structural MRI to determine whether cognitive impairment is due to reasons other than AD such as tumours or subdural hematomas [26].

Structural MRI studies have shown reduced hippocampal volume in individuals with amnestic MCI, and its reduction is thought to be one of the most predictive and sensitive measures of AD [27]; however, studies have shown other neuropsychiatric disorders such as schizophrenia [28] and depression [29] demonstrate a reduction in hippocampal volume as well. Figure 1, panel A, shows a coronal structural MRI session where hippocampal atrophy is shown (left larger than right). Therefore, the implementation of MRI-based biomarkers for clinical use requires validation across both clinical and analytical techniques. The diagnostic and prognostic accuracy of neuroimaging markers are dependent on both how the biomarker is measured (visual or quantitative) and which one is measured (MRI, Amyloid PET, fluorodeoxyglucose (FDG)-PET, etc.) [30]. Variation in methods and scanners can introduce noise and bias into the data which can impact the diagnostic accuracy.

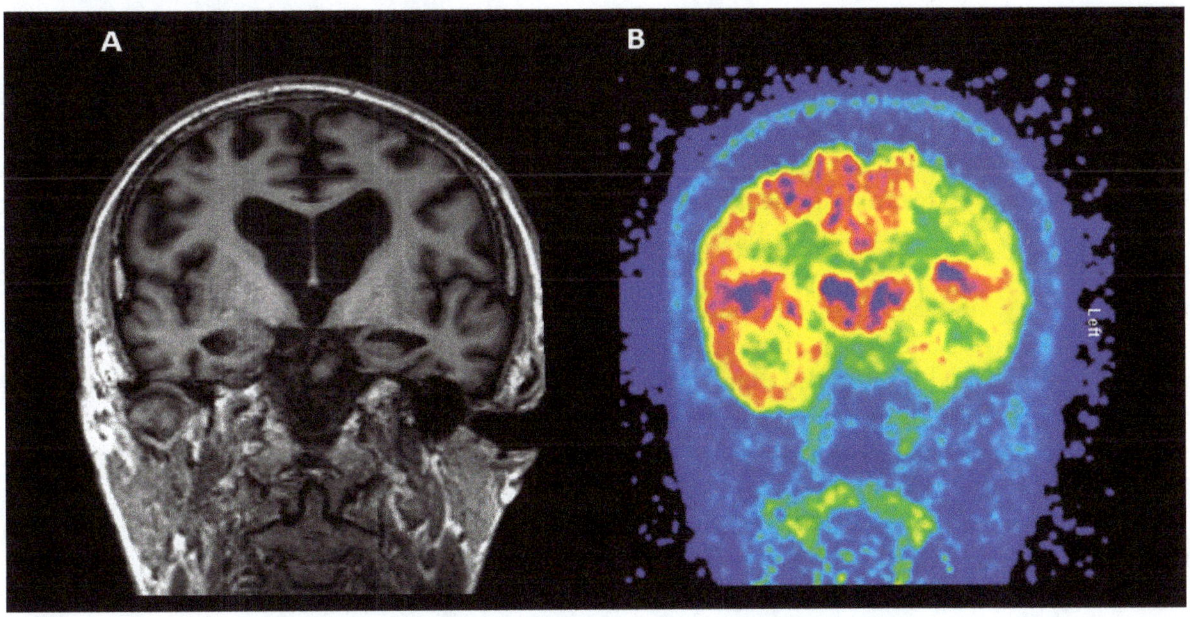

Figure 1. Imaging biomarkers of neurodegeneration. Coronal structural MRI section (panel **A**) and 18F-fluorodeoxyglucose (FDG) PET (panel **B**) from a patient with Alzheimer's disease (AD).

2.2. *Fluorodeoxyglucose (FDG) PET*

Glucose is the main source of energy used by the brain, which consumes around 25% of the amount circulating the whole body. The cerebral glucose metabolism is regulated by transport through the BBB, led by glucose transporters (GLUTs); GLUT1 is the main transporter on the BBB, while GLUT3 is the main transporter on neuron membranes, with a higher efficacy than GLUT1 [31]. GLUT1 is also present on astrocytes, which can uptake glucose in response to neuronal secretion of glutamate and produce lactate, another source of energy for neuronal activity [32]. The glucose consumption rate in the brain can be displayed in vivo using the PET tracer 18F-FDG, which reaches the neurons and enters the glycolytic process until the formation of FDG-6-phosphate, which will then stay trapped in the cells, at the same rate as the glucose [31]. The glucose consumption is not only an indicator of synaptic activity, whose loss is one of the main features of AD [33], but also reflects the excitatory glutamate release and recycling between astrocytes and neurons [34]. A reduction in the glucose metabolism is recognised as a biomarker of neurodegeneration, appearing years before the cognitive symptoms [33,35]. A pattern of reduced [18F]FDG uptake in posterior cingulate, hippocampi, and medial temporal structures is typical in AD and MCI, with subsequent spreading to the whole cortex as the disease progresses [33] (see Figure 1, panel B), while cerebellum, visual and primary motor cortices, and basal ganglia nuclei are less affected [36]. A different pattern of hypometabolism can be seen in other variants of AD, like posterior cortical atrophy and primary progressive aphasia [37]. It is interesting to note that the glucose hypometabolism is correlated with cognitive impairment and its severity, while the results of studies evaluating the same correlation between amyloid load and severity of cognitive impairment are less homogeneous [38,39]. The reduction in glucose metabolism in regions like the precuneus and posterior cingulate has been demonstrated to be associated with the severity of cognitive impairment [38]. A large study evaluated the baseline cerebral metabolic rate for glucose (CMRgl) in 298 subjects from the ADNI cohort (142 aMCI, 74 pAD, and 82 controls), correlating it with cognitive impairment severity; both the disease groups showed a reduction in the CMRgl in posterior cingulate, precuneus, and frontal and parietotemporal cortices compared with the cognitively intact subjects [40]. The CMRgl rate in the left frontal and temporal cortices was significantly correlated with low Mini-Mental State Examination (MMSE) scores when evaluating only the AD population [40]. In a different study, the pattern of regional hypometabolism appeared to be associated with specific cognitive domains, with visuospatial ability impairment correlated to a reduced metabolism in the posterior regions and impairment in language abilities with a left hemisphere reduction [38]. Interestingly, the impact of cognitive reserve in AD has also been studied with FDG-PET: Ewers et al. evaluated an ADNI cohort of cognitively normal subjects, classified as preclinical AD or healthy control based on the biomarkers profile, and they found that a higher level of education was associated with reduced FDG-PET in the amyloid-positive group [41]. This finding is in line with the literature, supporting the theory that high cognitive reserve can compensate the biological impairment, and highly educated subjects can show a degenerative profile worse than expected for the symptoms [41].

The accuracy of FDG-PET compared to serial clinical evaluation relative to post mortem pathological diagnosis was evaluated in a cohort of 44 subjects grouped as AD and not AD [42]. This study demonstrated that, in the diagnostic process, the FDG-PET is superior to clinical evaluation, which reached the same diagnostic power only later on in the follow-up [42].

Several studies demonstrated that FDG-PET is also a good predictor of disease progression from MCI to AD, according to a few longitudinal studies [43,44]. A longitudinal study aiming to establish the sensitivity and specificity of FDG-PET in patients evaluated and followed up for dementia proved an FDG-PET sensitivity of 93% in detecting progressive dementia and a specificity of 76%; it was also able to distinguish patients with AD from patients with other degenerative diseases with a sensitivity of 94% and a specificity of 73% for AD and 78% for other diseases [45]. It is also worth noticing that a negative scan at baseline indicates an unlikely progression across 3 years [45]. The use of FDG-PET in the clinical setting for the diagnostic process of MCI is more debated, with some studies showing hypometabolism in the cortex and others being inconclusive in the identification of MCIs [31]. In 2015, a Cochrane meta-analysis of 14 studies, for a total of 421 subjects, aimed to evaluate the effectiveness of FDG-PET in identifying MCI subjects converting to dementia at the follow-up [46]. According to the authors, the result of the meta-analysis did not support the use of FDG-PET in routine clinical use in MCI subjects. A limitation of this meta-analysis was the poor methodological quality of some of the studies, leading to risk of bias; therefore, more uniform protocols would be required to get to a satisfactory conclusion [46]. However, the use of FDG-PET is of high value in the diagnostic process, especially in the most difficult cases [37]. Few retrospective studies have actually demonstrated the usefulness of the FDG-PET in clarifying the diagnosis and increasing the cholinesterase inhibitor prescription; moreover, in atypical or uncertain cases, a repeated follow-up FDG-PET improved the diagnostic power and management [37]. FDG-PET is a widely used imaging technique, both in research and clinical settings, with a high predictive value and diagnostic power for Alzheimer's disease and different types of dementia. Together with the other biomarkers, such as cortical atrophy and amyloid and tau deposition, it is a fundamental tool for early diagnosis, selection criteria, and follow-up evaluation in clinical trials.

3. Amyloid Imaging

Accumulation of Aβ fibrils in the form of amyloid plaques is a neuropathological hallmark for autopsy-based diagnosis confirmation of dementia caused by AD [47]. Aβ deposition is thought to precede cognitive symptoms in AD and is therefore a potential preclinical marker of disease [48]. There have been different approaches to noninvasively visualise amyloid deposition in human brains with amyloid PET radiotracers. Typically, amyloid imaging agents bind to insoluble fibrillary forms of Aβ 40 and Aβ 42 deposits, which are major components of compact neuritic plaques and vascular deposits.

Clinical criteria for the suitable use of amyloid imaging in patients demonstrate the need to integrate scanning with detailed clinical and cognitive evaluations. These criteria state that amyloid imaging should only be used under certain circumstances such as in patients with persistent or progressive unexplained cognitive impairment or unclear clinical presentations [49]. Amyloid imaging, as stated by the clinical criteria, should not be used to determine severity of dementia or in patients with probable AD and of typical age, with a family history of dementia, and/or with the presence of the APOE4 allele [50,51]. 11C-Pittsburgh Compound B (PiB) was the first amyloid imaging PET agent used in human subjects in 2002 [52]. However, the PiB compound is labeled with 11C, with a short half-life of only 20 min, limiting its use. To overcome this problem, 18F-labeled Aβ tracers, with a longer half-life of 110 min, are used to show reliable assessment of brain amyloid in a single 15-minute scan. There are only three approved Aβ tracers for clinical use: 18F-Florbetapir [53], 18F-Florbetaben, and 18F-Flutemetamol.

18F-Florbetapir was the first tracer approved for the detection of in vivo amyloid and the first 18F-labelled tracer approved by the FDA since Fludeoxyglucose (FDG); subsequently, this has become the most widely used amyloid tracer. Multicentre studies showed that a high Aβ burden on 18F-Florbetapir PET was associated with poor memory performance in healthy participants [54]. It has also been shown that approximately 50% of MCI patients had a high Aβ burden on 18F-Florbetapir PET [55]. In phase III studies, 18F-Florbetapir demonstrated high sensitivity and specificity (92% and 100%, respectively) in detecting Aβ pathology with no tracer retention in control subjects [56,57]. 18F-Florbetaben reveals a high affinity for fibrillary Aβ in brain homogenates, selectively labelled Aβ plaques, and cerebral amyloid angiopathy in tissue sections from patients with AD [58]. 18F-Florbetaben PET can also detect Aβ pathology in a wide spectrum of neurodegenerative conditions such as frontotemporal lobar degeneration (FTLD). Cortical retention of 18F-Florbetaben was higher in patients with AD than in healthy controls or patients with frontotemporal dementia [59]. 18F-Flutemetamol, in phase I and II studies, was able to differentiate between patients with AD and healthy controls [60,61]. The prediction of progression to AD in patients with MCI was improved when combined with measures of brain atrophy [62]. The tracers discussed above have high affinity and selectivity for fibrillar Aβ in plaques and other Aβ-containing lesions [63,64]. When Aβ PET scans are visually read, cortical tracer retention is usually higher in patients with AD than in healthy controls, particularly in the frontal, cingulate, parietal, and lateral temporal cortices. Both visual and quantitative assessments of amyloid scans from different stages of disease progression reveal a consistent pattern of tracer retention that coincides with amyloid deposition found post mortem in patients with sporadic AD [65]. Longitudinal studies have shown that minute increases in Aβ deposition can be measured using PET; however, these changes can only be seen in those who have either have high or low burdens [66]. Acceptable Aβ loads in normal individuals have also been observed, and approximately 7% of these individuals have an increase of Aβ within 2.5 years above the threshold for "normal" levels [67].

The pivotal use of Aβ imaging is facilitating differential diagnosis in patients who present with atypical symptoms of dementia [68]. Clinical presentations of FTLD can be difficult to differentiate from early onset AD. FTLD does not have Aβ pathology, and these patients, for the most part, show no cortical retention of 11C-PiB—another amyloid tracer [69–71]. Therefore, using amyloid PET can help differentiate between FTLD and AD. The patterns of Aβ deposition can also help differential diagnosis. Patients with cognitively stable Parkinson's disease (PD) have no cortical Aβ deposition; however, Parkinson's disease dementia (PDD) shows signs of Aβ deposition [72,73].

4. Tau Imaging

Tau imaging is the latest innovation in the early detection of neurodegenerative proteinopathies. In the past few years, a number of first-generation tau-selective PET tracers have been developed. 18F-flortaucipir, 18F-THK5351, 18F-THK5317, and 11C-PBB3 have all been extensively used in research studies but have yet to be used clinically. Through imaging studies, tau tracer retention shows an affinity to not only known distributions of aggregated tau but also to mirror patterns of neuronal injury detected by FDG-PET [74,75]. FDG uptake and 18F-THK5317 retention show a negative correlation, primarily in frontal areas [76]. FDG also shows a mediating role in the association between tau pathology and cognitive decline in AD [77].

Tau imaging could be very useful to predict progression of AD due to the relationship between tau deposition, cognitive impairment, and neuronal injury. Tau imaging has the ability to assess the regional distribution and density of tau deposits in the brain which could also help with disease staging. While Aβ imaging studies indicate that total Aβ deposition in the brain is more important than regional differences in predicting cognitive decline, tau imaging data suggest that the topographical distribution of tau in the brain is more important than the total level of tau in the brain [78,79]. A combination of tau and Aβ imaging could be highly beneficial in predicting cognitive decline and neurodegeneration. Studies have demonstrated that high levels of cortical tau deposition in those with Aβ pathology showed increased cognitive impairment in several domains [80,81].

Most, if not all, applications of tau and amyloid imaging are used for the same purpose: accurate and early detection of AD pathology, disease staging, predicting disease progression, and use in disease-specific clinical treatment trials. However, several groups have suggested that tau imaging is better for disease staging and predicting progression than amyloid imaging [82,83]. These groups have compared patients with AD and non-AD tauopathies and have found significant differences in tracer retention between healthy controls, patients with AD, and patients presenting with atypical AD [84,85]. Interestingly, clinical presentations of patients with atypical AD significantly matched their tau deposits as assessed by 18F-flortaucipoir but not their Aβ burdens as assessed by 11C-PiB [86].

However, studies show that high levels of tau found in specific regions of interest (mesial and temporal lobes) are not found alongside a high level of Aβ. Conversely, high levels of tau are highly associated with high Aβ levels in the neocortex. This suggests that detectable levels of cortical Aβ deposits precede levels of cortical tau deposition. Post mortem studies have shown tau deposits in the mesial temporal cortex in elderly individuals, both healthy and with dementia [87]. These findings suggest that hippocampal tauopathy is age related, and not dependent on but magnified by Aβ pathology [74]; this is now known as primary age-related tauopathy (PART) [88].

The in vivo relationship between 18F-flortaucipir and grey matter intensity shows a negative correlation as measured by MRI in healthy controls. Moreover, a study by Wang et al. [89] showed that amyloid plaques affected the association between 18F-flortaucipir retention and cerebral atrophy. Amyloid-positive patients showed a significant association between tau imaging and volume loss, which suggests tau deposition and neuronal loss.

The best use of tau imaging would be a combination of amyloid imaging and selective tau imaging to explain whether Aβ accelerates or causes the spread of tau outside the mesial temporal cortex. This could also help elucidate whether this spreading into cortical areas corresponds clinically to the development of MCI [74,90].

Much like amyloid imaging, tau imaging can be used for differential diagnosis for neurodegenerative Aβ-related conditions such as Dementia Lewy Body (DLB) and other tauopathies such as progressive supranuclear palsy [91]. Also, approximately 40% of FTLD cases are caused by hyperphosphorylated tau, labelled FTLD-tau. As stated previously, Aβ deposition is not a pathological feature of FTLD; therefore, the tau imaging can help with correct diagnosis, especially for specific forms of the disease [92].

A low hippocampal signal has been observed in some tau tracers which is compounded by the unreliable and irregular tracer binding to the choroid plexus, which just lies above the hippocampus. Researchers have suggested that the tracers bind to the aggregated tau in the choroid plexus [93] despite the lack of in vitro autoradiographic studies showing a consistent failure of tracer binding [94]. Another theory suggests that the tracers actually bind to other β-sheet aggregated proteins, such as iron or transthyretin [95,96]. At the moment, no tau tracers have been validated for clinical use [97], and some researchers highlight the inconsistencies between the in vitro and in vivo binding profiles of the tracers [98].

Something that is even more alarming is the doubt over tau selectivity from some PET tracers. Studies show a there is "off-target" binding resulting from tracer binding to alternative targets. Selegiline, a selective and irreversible inhibitor of monoamine oxidase B, also known as MAO-B, can cause signal reductions in cortical and basal ganglia in 18F-THK5351 imaging. In fact, a single 5 mg dose of selegiline can cause signal reductions of up to 50%. This suggests that a certain percentage of tau binding seen in 18F-THK5351 is caused by MAO-B binding [99]. Newer second-generation tracers, such as 18F-RO69558948, have shown less off-target binding [100] with two other tracers (18F-MK6240 and 18F-PI2620) showing no off-target binding [101,102].

5. Imaging of Neuroinflammation

Neuroinflammation refers to the innate inflammatory response of the central nervous system (CNS) to any neuronal insult, such as infections, vascular lesions, trauma, and the presence of abnormal protein aggregates [103]. Data from studies conducted in the last decades indicate that in neurodegenerative diseases, and particularly in AD, neuroinflammation is not only an epiphenomenon secondary to Aβ and tau abnormalities, but it is an essential part of the disease pathophysiology. Results from genome-wide association studies indicate that many of the newly identified genetic risk variants associated with AD involve genes that play an important role in immune function [104]. The cellular players of inflammatory response in the brain are primarily microglia and astrocytes. Microglia activation and reactive astrocytosis can be evaluated in vivo by the use of PET imaging. Thus, in vivo detection of neuroinflammation could represent a useful tool to further clarify the role of immune response in AD pathology and to assess the effectiveness of novel treatments targeting neuroinflammation [105].

5.1. Imaging Microglia

Microglia are mononuclear resident phagocytes ubiquitously distributed in the brain, where they account for 10%–15% of non-neuronal cells [106]. Microglia are of myeloid lineage, originating from progenitors formed in the yolk sac, and their differentiation occurs in the CNS [107]. Under physiological conditions, microglial cells scan the brain parenchyma continuously in order to maintain the homeostasis and, in doing so, present in a ramified morphology. In this resting state they also provide supportive factors to tissue integrity and secrete trophic factors that help maintain neuronal plasticity [108]. Upon detection of any pathological triggers, mediated by membrane receptors, microglia become activated and migrate to the area of the lesion. They change their shape to an amoeboid one and start releasing proinflammatory cytokines, such as tumour necrosis factor-α and interleukin-1β, and free oxygen radicals, such as nitric oxide and superoxide [109]. Both post mortem and preclinical data indicate that in AD the accumulation of Aβ plaques is the main trigger for neuroinflammation. Activated microglia surround Aβ plaques in an attempt to phagocyte them or degrade them through the secretion of proteolytic enzymes [110,111]. Although the initial microglial activation aims at clearance of Aβ plaques and might exert a neuroprotective effect, its continuous triggering and the inefficacy in the clearing process might lead to a vicious cycle of sustained chronic inflammation, with an ultimately neurotoxic effect [112]. This dual function of microglia has been exemplified in the M1/M2 theory, which postulates that microglia switch from a M1 proinflammatory phenotype to a M2 anti-inflammatory one [113]. However, this theory seems to be over-simplistic, and it is likely that microglial phenotype switching and its dual function are a dynamic process.

Once activated, microglia express the Translocator Protein 18 kDa (TSPO), formerly known as peripheral benzodiazepine receptor (PBR). In physiologic conditions, TSPO expression is low within the CNS, primarily confined to endothelial cells, ependyma, choroid plexus, olfactory bulb, and glial cells. Following any brain injuries, TSPO expression on microglial outer mitochondrial membrane markedly increases, making it a suitable marker of glial activation [114]. Over the last decades, several TSPO radioligands have been developed, the most widely used being [11C]-PK11195. This tracer was initially used as a racemate, but the R-enantiomer has a greater affinity for TSPO than the S-enantiomer, and subsequent studies only used [11C]-(R)-PK11195 to investigate neuroinflammation in vivo [109,115]. Although [11C]-(R)-PK11195 has been widely used in several neurological diseases associated with neuroinflammation [116,117], this tracer suffers major limitations, such as a poor signal-to-noise ratio due to high nonspecific binding, high plasma protein binding, and the use of ^{11}C, which limits its use to PET research centers and hospitals with an on-site cyclotron. These difficulties led to the development of second-generation TSPO ligands, with higher TSPO affinity and better kinetics, such as [11C]-PBR28, [11C]-DAA1106, [18F]-DPA714, [18F]-FEPPA, and [18F]-GE180. However, the binding affinity of second generation TSPO tracers is affected by a single-nucleotide polymorphism (SNP) rs6971 in the TSPO gene, which causes an Alanine-to-Threonine substitution in the protein. Based on this, individuals are classified into high-affinity binders (HABs), mixed-affinity binders (MABs), and low-affinity binders (LABs), so that genotyping is essential for appropriate tracer quantification [118].

In AD, Cagnin et al. were the first to report an increase in [11C]-PK11195 binding in the temporal lobe [119], while other groups found no differences between AD patients and controls [120]. Using second-generation TSPO radioligands, other researchers have demonstrated a significant increase in AD subjects with [11C]-DAA1106 [121], [11C]-PBR28 [122], and [18F]-FEPPA [123]. The relationship between microglial activation and amyloid deposition in AD has also been evaluated, finding clusters of significant correlation in most cases [124,125]. Combined PET studies provided evidence for a significant inverse correlation between microglia activation and glucose metabolism in AD patients [126] as well as with hippocampal volume [127]. When looking at cognitive function, the results are varied: some authors have found a significant inverse correlation between TSPO binding and Mini-Mental State Examination (MMSE) scores [124,128], others found no correlation [125], and another group found a positive correlation between the global cortical index and MMSE score [122]. Using different cognitive measures, a negative correlation has been observed between [11C]-PBR28 binding in the inferior parietal lobule and performance on Block Design [123], as well as between [18F]-FEPPA binding in the parietal and prefrontal cortices and visuospatial tasks [129]. A PET multitracer study has recently demonstrated significant widespread correlation between levels of microglial activation and tau aggregation in both MCI and AD subjects, suggesting that these pathologies increase together as the disease progresses. Moreover, microglial activation and amyloid load were also correlated, with a different spatial distribution. The three processes seem to be often found in similar areas of the association cortex [130]. Results are more controversial in the MCI population: some studies have reported increased [11C]-PK11195 uptake in 38% of MCI subjects, while others have shown no differences compared to healthy controls. Similarly, using second-generation radioligands, Yasuno et al. showed significant increases in [11C]-DAA1106 binding in the cerebellum, medial prefrontal cortex, parietal cortex, lateral temporal cortex, anterior cingulate cortex, and striatum in MCI [129], while Kreisl et al. found no differences between MCI patients and controls using [11C]-PBR28 [122].

There are only few studies that have evaluated the longitudinal changes in microglial activation in the AD continuum. Fan et al. demonstrated that microglial activation detected by [11C]-PK11195 increases in AD as the disease progresses, while it is reduced in MCI [131]. A recent study on prodromal AD or MCI subjects using [11C]-PBR28 reported increased longitudinal binding in patients but not in controls, on average equal to 2.5%–7.5% per year [132]. In a study of 64 AD patients, significantly higher global cortical [18F]-DPA-714 binding has been demonstrated in slower decliners compared to fast decliners, further substantiating the concept that early microglial activation could be protective [125].

5.2. *Imaging Astrocytes*

Astrocytes are star-shaped glial cells, conventionally divided in two categories: protoplasmic astrocytes, located in the grey matter, and fibrous astrocytes, located in the white matter. Their main function is to provide nutritional support to neurons and insulate synaptic connections, regulating extracellular concentrations of ions and neurotransmitters. When activated, astrocytes increase the expression of the glial fibrillary acidic protein (GFAP), and the process of reactive astrogliosis aims at neuroprotection. In AD, it seems that astrocytes play an important role in the clearance of Aβ, and after exposure to Aβ they can release cytokines, interleukins, and reactive oxygen species, contributing to the neuroinflammatory process [106].

During neuroinflammation, monoamine oxidase B (MAO B) is up-regulated in reactive astrocytes, and can be targeted in vivo using different PET tracers, such as [11C]-deuterium-L-deprenyl-[11C]-DED- and [11C]-deprenyl-D2 [105]. In a study on AD subjects and amyloid-positive MCI, increased [11C]-DED binding was observed in the frontal, parietal, and temporal cortices, and regional correlation between [11C]-DED uptake and amyloid burden was reported [133]. Results from a multitracer PET study using [11C]-DED, [11C]-PIB, and [18F]-FDG in genetic and sporadic AD patients showed divergent patterns of amyloid deposition and astrocytosis, with the latter being elevated in the early presymptomatic stages of the disease, and the former increasing with disease progression [134]. Astrocytosis has also been imaged using ligands for the I2-imidazoline receptor, such as [11C]-BU99008. Studies with this PET tracer are underway in AD and MCI subjects.

Figure 2 shows the chemical structures of some of the most commonly used PET tracers mentioned so far [135].

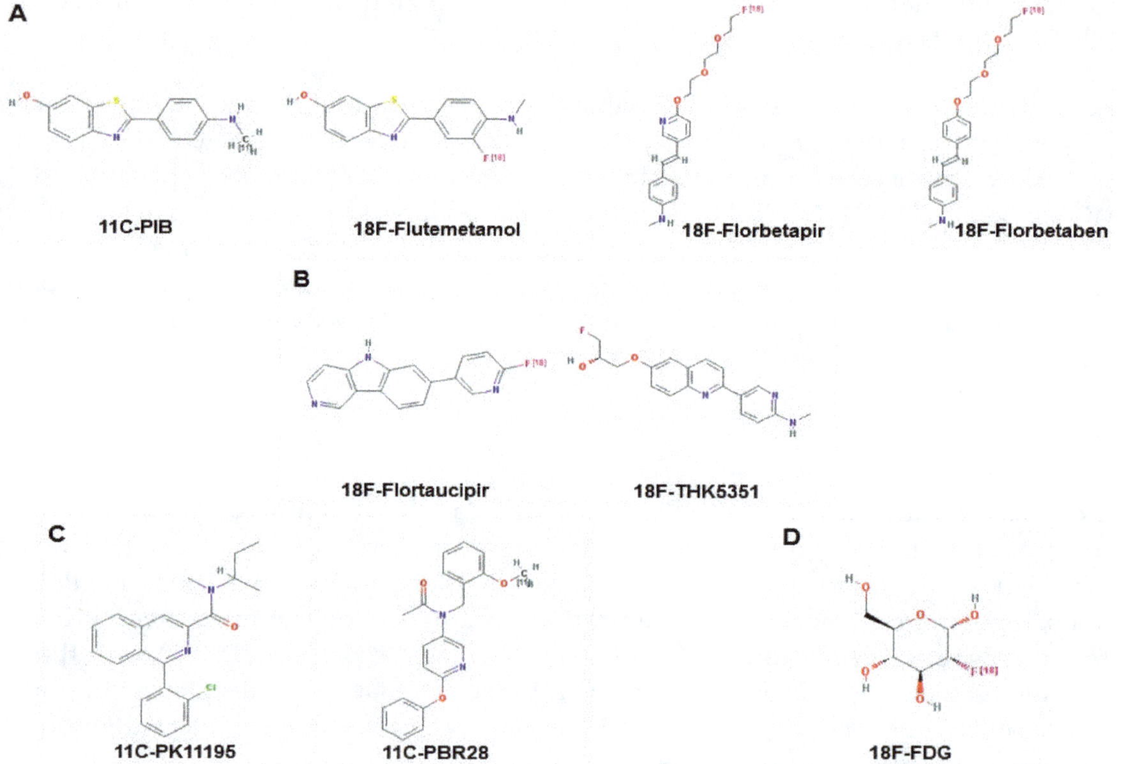

Figure 2. Chemical structure of some PET tracers. Panel **A** shows amyloid PET tracers, Panel **B** shows Tau tracers. Microglial tracers are shown in Panel **C**, and 18F-FDG is shown in Panel **D** (structures downloaded from [135]).

6. Imaging of Blood–Brain Barrier Dysfunction

The blood–brain barrier (BBB) is a highly functional, specialised barrier separating the intravascular system from the neurons, representing a fundamental interface between circulating cells in the bloodstream and the neuronal system. The BBB operates as part of the neurovascular unit (NVU), a multilayer barrier formed by endothelial cells expressing tight junction proteins, a basal lamina of extracellular proteins, astrocyte end-feet, and pericytes [136]. While low permeability is the usual state of the BBB, where protein and cell transport is led by the tight junction proteins (TJPs) and transporters [136], a breach in integrity and impaired function is a common finding in several diseases [137]. In AD, the deposition of Aβ fibrils in the vessel elicits the release of pro-inflammatory cytokines, contributing to BBB damage and an increase in its permeability [137]; moreover, cerebral amyloid angiopathy affects smooth muscle cells, pericytes, and endothelial cells, increasing the damage [137]. The timing of the BBB disruption and AD progression has been widely studied: an indirect measure of BBB breach is the CSF albumin index, demonstrating structural disruption in Alzheimer's and vascular dementia [138]. Post mortem studies reported BBB damage in subjects with AD, demonstrating the accumulation of several proteins in the hippocampus and the cortex and the degeneration of pericytes [139]. AD is also characterised by vascular changes in the endothelial and smooth muscle cells, partially secondary to amyloid toxicity; around amyloid deposits in the vessels, endothelial cells are less viable, and microvascular cerebral tissues showed reduced mitochondrial content and a higher concentration of pinocytotic vesicles [140].

While in case of tumour, strokes, or inflammatory diseases like multiple sclerosis the breach in the BBB permeability is to a major extent, in dementia it is more subtle and requires specific MRI imaging sequences [136] since other imaging techniques (PET and CT) failed to demonstrate any difference between patients with dementia and healthy controls [141,142]. A study conducted with a PET tracer [68Ga]ethylene-diamine-tetraacetic acid ([68Ga]EDTA) did not demonstrate a difference in

CNS permeability between a small group of AD subjects and healthy controls [142]. Similarly, a CT study with meglumine iothalamate failed to show any difference in BBB abnormality between AD and HC [141]. The measurement of BBB permeability with MRI is based on the use of paramagnetic contrast agent Gadolinium-based compounds and the measurement of its leakage from the intravascular space. The techniques used are either dynamic susceptibility contrast-enhanced MRI (DSC-MRI) or dynamic contrast-enhanced MRI (DCE-MRI) [136]. Very few studies have been conducted on small cohorts of AD or MCI patients. Degeneration of the BBB has been demonstrated in the hippocampus with the ageing process; however, that has been seen to appear earlier in subjects with Mild Cognitive Impairment when compared with cognitively intact subjects [139]. This evaluation was conducted using a DCE-MRI; with this technique, grey and white matter regions were simultaneously analysed. In a different MCI population compared to HC, DCE-MRI showed a lower contrast enhancement and slower contrast decay, respectively indicating lower vascular volume and higher BBB permeability in the hippocampi, suggesting impairment in the vasculature and possible BBB disruption [140]. Interestingly, the same difference was not seen in the cerebellum, but, considering that the cerebellum is spared by AD pathology, this is not surprising [140].

To investigate if the leakage could contribute to AD, a pilot study with a dynamic contrast-enhanced MRI was conducted on a population of MCI due to AD and early AD by Maastricht ad Leiden Universities [143]. The imaging protocol was designed with a resolution able to separate the vessel filling from the leakage. The authors also evaluated the relationship between BBB permeability and cognitive performance. The results of the study demonstrated a significantly higher BBB leakage rate in the patient group compared to the controls in the grey matter; the leakage volume was significantly higher in the grey matter, in the normal-appearing white matter, and in the cortex [143]. Considering all the subjects together, the leakage volume in the deep gray matter was higher when the MMSE was lower; a significantly higher leakage volume in the deep gray matter was found in the MCI group when compared to the controls. The overall results of the study supported the theory of BBB impairment as a contributing factor to the AD pathology, especially considering the association with the cognitive performance and the early phases of the subjects enrolled [143]. A case control MRI study was conducted on a cohort of 15 AD subjects and 15 healthy volunteers; for this dynamic contrast-enhanced MRI, regions of interest in the deep grey matter, cortical grey matter, white matter, CSF, and carotid and basilary arteries were selected [144]. In this study, the BBB permeability across the two groups did not differ significantly; however, a difference was seen in the temporal pattern after the injection, suggesting an early occurrence of the BBB permeability difference between healthy control and AD subjects [144]. Others have demonstrated that BBB permeability is increased in major dementia disorders but does not relate to amyloid pathology [145].

The evaluation of BBB damage and permeability is an interesting challenge, especially considering the complexity of the analysis required; certainly, more studies are needed to develop a reliable MRI protocol acquisition, and robust data results are necessary to be able to apply the technique on the larger scale of the clinical setting.

7. Limitations and Future Perspectives

Early diagnosis of sporadic neurodegenerative conditions can be very difficult, especially when patients present with nonspecific symptoms that can be attributable to any form of dementia or neurodegenerative disease. Recently, the NIA-AA research framework criteria for AD have developed the concept that diagnosis should be made based on the measurement of integrated biomarkers, moving towards a more biological definition of the disease. These biomarkers not only concern the presence of Aβ but also must include the tau status of the individual [146]. As the diagnostic criteria for AD continue to develop, the use of amyloid and tau PET imaging is likely to be at the forefront of use in clinical practice.

It is important to note, however, that PET imaging bears several methodological limitations, from the poor resolution of the PET itself to the presence of brain atrophy, which is certainly a crucial feature to be considered in AD imaging. Particularly regarding the latter, unfortunately, there is a lack of homogeneity in the approach to the atrophy [147]. Some studies' approach considered the partial volume effect, proportionate to the atrophy, applying partial volume correction; this has been done with different toolboxes or codes [148,149] and for different tracers [148–152]. Some other studies included the grey matter volume as a covariate in the analysis or excluded relative atrophy. The poor spatial resolution of the PET is also a limitation, especially when analysing small areas or areas where the cortical thickness and the voxel area have similar dimensions [147]. A possible solution is the use of combined PET and MR, which allows a better anatomical accuracy and a partial volume correction to the PET findings [153]. Another factor limiting broader and more routine use of PET imaging is the methodological quantification of the signal. Different techniques have been used in research, with various advantages and caveats to be considered. The standardised uptake value (SUV) technique, applicable to static images, is simple and practical to use; however, it is subjective to different variables, such as the tracer uptake time, dose measurement, and receiving body characteristics. More accurate estimates certainly come from kinetic parameters analysis; this is, however, less practical to use, requiring dynamic images and arterial input [154]. Despite the advances in imaging techniques, no single biomarker is likely to be able to provide the diagnostic certainty needed for early detection of neurodegenerative diseases. Identification or diagnosis requires a multimodal approach that combines biochemical and neuroimaging markers of pathology and neurodegeneration [155]. These biomarkers have now been incorporated into the new diagnostic criteria for the prodromal, preclinical, and overt stages of AD [156,157]. Furthermore, AD-specific interventional trials have been able to implement short-duration trials with smaller samples sizes due to the use of Aβ and/or tau biomarkers to confirm target and treatment efficacy [158]. Interpretation of amyloid positivity through PET is done either visually or quantitatively. Amyloid positivity is defined based on the presence of absence of tracer uptake in brain cortical regions compared to the cerebellum due to a lack of amyloid accumulation in this region. Visual analysis is usually performed using a binary scale while quantitative analysis involves receiver operating characteristic analysis without prespecified cut-off values. This causes data to over-fit which could result in sensitivity and specificity values that are overly optimistic [159]. Conversely, visual interpretation is dependent on the reader's experience, and while most scans are read by multiple readers to confirm positivity or negativity, this is against everyday clinical practice and will have an effect on diagnosis.

Multimodality imaging is the way forward in both research and clinical contexts in AD, suggesting that a combined use of MRI and PET may increase the accuracy of diagnosis due to the ability to detect pathological brain changes associated with AD in the earliest of stages (Tables 1 and 2). Moreover, in a research setting, and in particular in clinical trials with drugs targeting biomarkers, multimodal imaging also has the added value of allowing the monitoring of potential side effects of experimental drugs, which could be hindered by the cognitive impairment [160]. Even though in the diagnostic process of a neurodegenerative disease the results of imaging techniques have to be related to the clinical picture, there are some images with a very strong diagnostic power on their own, such as hippocampal atrophy for AD or DaTScan for Lewy Body Dementia [161]. However, studies have shown that high amyloid load or grey matter atrophy is not enough to give a clear predictive sign of AD, with many healthy individuals showing no signs of AD even with the hallmarks of the neuropathological changes [162,163]. The lack of actual multitracer studies, conducted longitudinally and exploring all the biomarkers at the same time-point, needs to be addressed, together with a strictly homogenous methodological protocol, to better facilitate a more detailed insight into disease pathology. Interest is now increasing in the use of plasma biomarkers for global organ diseases, which may be relevant in neurodegenerative disease, especially considering the link between nutrition, diet, and ageing. In particular, genomic, lipidomic, and proteomic biomarkers are increasingly interesting [164]. In particular, the study of genomics, i.e., the calorie-sensitive gene Sirt1, related to lipidomic and proteomic biomarkers, could be a sensitive tool in the assessment of a few chronic diseases which have showed association with AD (such as obesity and diabetes) [165]. Also, plasma biomarkers, due to their easy access, hold potential in terms of early diagnosis. Plasma Aβ levels seem to correlate with cognitive function and with CSF biomarkers [166], and the combination of clinical, imaging, and plasma markers can predict progression in MCI subjects [167]. This once again highlights the need for a clearer diagnostic route that does not rely solely on neuroimaging biomarkers.

Table 1. PET tracers in AD.

Target	Tracer	Clinical Correlates in AD	Ref.
Amyloid-β	18F-Florebetapir	Has demonstrated high sensitivity and specificity (92% and 100%, respectively) in detecting Aβ pathology	[13,14]
	18F-Florbetaben	High affinity for fibrillary Aβ, selectively labelled Aβ plaques, and cerebral amyloid angiopathy in tissue sections from patients with AD	[15]
	18F-Flutemetamol	In phase I and II studies, was able to differentiate between patients with AD and healthy controls	[17,18]
Tau protein	18F-flortaucipir, 18F-THK5351, 18F-THK5317, 11C-PBB3	Bind to neurofibrillary tangles with high selectivity and high signal-to-background ratio. Used for early detection of nerve fiber lesions in patients with AD	[39]
Microglial activation	11C-PK11195	Used to investigate neuroinflammation in vivo. There is an increase of binding in the temporal lobe of AD patients.	[73,74]
	11C-DAA1106, 11C-PBR28, 18F-FEPPA	Inverse correlation between microglia activation and glucose metabolism in AD patients as well as with hippocampal volume	[80,81]
	18F-DPA-714	Showed significantly higher global cortical binding in slower AD decliners compared to fast decliners	[79]
Astrocytes	[11C]-deuterium-L-deprenyl-[11C]-DED, [11C]-deprenyl-D2	In AD and amyloid-positive MCI, increased binding was observed in the frontal, parietal, and temporal cortices and regional correlation between 11C-DED uptake and amyloid burden	[59,86]
Glucose Metabolism	18F-FDG	Reduced uptake in posterior cingulate, hippocampi, and medial temporal structures is typical in AD and MCI, with a subsequent spreading to the whole cortex as the disease progresses. The reduction in glucose metabolism in regions like precuneus and posterior cingulate has been demonstrated to be associated with the severity of the cognitive impairment	[121, 126]

Table 2. MRI correlates in AD.

Target	Sequences	Clinical Correlates in AD	Ref.
Blood–brain barrier (BBB)	Dynamic susceptibility contrast-enhanced MRI (DSC-MRI)	Degeneration of the BBB has been demonstrated in the hippocampus with the ageing process; however, that has been seen to appear earlier in subjects with MCI when compared with cognitively intact subjects	[91]
	Dynamic contrast-enhanced MRI (DCE-MRI)	Significantly higher BBB leakage rate in AD compared to controls in the grey matter; the leakage volume was significantly higher in the grey matter, in the normal-appearing white matter, and in the cortex	[95]
Brain atrophy	Three-dimensional (3D) T1-weighted magnetisation-prepared rapid acquisition gradient-echo (T1-MPRAGE) sequence	Structural brain changes are accurately consistent with Braak stages of neurofibrillary tangle deposition and neuropsychological deficits. Rates of change in several structural measures, including whole-brain, entorhinal cortex, hippocampus, and temporal lobe volumes, correlate closely with changes in cognitive performance, validating atrophy in these regions as markers of AD.	[98–104]

References

1. Prince, M.; Wimo, A.; Guerchet, M.; Ali, G.; Wu, Y.; Prina, M. *World Alzheimer Report 2015—The Global Impact of Dementia: An Analysis of Prevalence, Incidence, Cost and Trends*; Alzheimer's Disease International (ADI): London, UK, 2015.
2. Alzheimer's Association. 2018 Alzheimer's disease facts and figures. *Alzheimer's Dement.* **2018**, *14*, 367–429. [CrossRef]
3. Scheltens, P.; Blennow, K.; Breteler, M.M.; de Strooper, B.; Frisoni, G.B.; Salloway, S.; Van der Flier, W.M. Alzheimer's disease. *Lancet* **2016**, *388*, 505–517. [CrossRef]
4. McKhann, G.M.; Knopman, D.S.; Chertkow, H.; Hyman, B.T.; Jack, C.R., Jr.; Kawas, C.H.; Klunk, W.E.; Koroshetz, W.J.; Manly, J.J.; Mayeux, R.; et al. The diagnosis of dementia due to Alzheimer's disease: Recommendations from the National Institute on Aging-Alzheimer's Association workgroups on diagnostic guidelines for Alzheimer's disease. *Alzheimer's Dement.* **2011**, *7*, 263–269. [CrossRef] [PubMed]
5. Selkoe, D.J.; Hardy, J. The amyloid hypothesis of Alzheimer's disease at 25 years. *EMBO Mol. Med.* **2016**, *8*, 595–608. [CrossRef] [PubMed]
6. Small, S.A.; Duff, K. Linking Abeta and tau in late-onset Alzheimer's disease: A dual pathway hypothesis. *Neuron* **2008**, *60*, 534–542. [CrossRef] [PubMed]
7. Frisoni, G.B.; Boccardi, M.; Barkhof, F.; Blennow, K.; Cappa, S.; Chiotis, K.; Demonet, J.F.; Garibotto, V.; Giannakopoulos, P.; Gietl, A.; et al. Strategic roadmap for an early diagnosis of Alzheimer's disease based on biomarkers. *Lancet Neurol.* **2017**, *16*, 661–676. [CrossRef]
8. Kollack-Walker, S.; Liu, C.Y.; Fleisher, A.S. The Role of Neuroimaging in the Assessment of the Cognitively Impaired Elderly. *Neurol. Clin.* **2017**, *35*, 231–262. [CrossRef] [PubMed]
9. Frisoni, G.B.; Fox, N.C.; Jack, C.R., Jr.; Scheltens, P.; Thompson, P.M. The clinical use of structural MRI in Alzheimer disease. *Nat. Rev. Neurol.* **2010**, *6*, 67–77. [CrossRef] [PubMed]
10. Whitwell, J.L.; Josephs, K.A.; Murray, M.E.; Kantarci, K.; Przybelski, S.A.; Weigand, S.D.; Vemuri, P.; Senjem, M.L.; Parisi, J.E.; Knopman, D.S.; et al. MRI correlates of neurofibrillary tangle pathology at autopsy: A voxel-based morphometry study. *Neurology* **2008**, *71*, 743–749. [CrossRef] [PubMed]
11. Vemuri, P.; Wiste, H.J.; Weigand, S.D.; Shaw, L.M.; Trojanowski, J.Q.; Weiner, M.W.; Knopman, D.S.; Petersen, R.C.; Jack, C.R., Jr.; Alzheimer's Disease Neuroimaging Initiative. MRI and CSF biomarkers in normal, MCI, and AD subjects: Predicting future clinical change. *Neurology* **2009**, *73*, 294–301. [CrossRef] [PubMed]

12. Vemuri, P.; Whitwell, J.L.; Kantarci, K.; Josephs, K.A.; Parisi, J.E.; Shiung, M.S.; Knopman, D.S.; Boeve, B.F.; Petersen, R.C.; Dickson, D.W.; et al. Antemortem MRI based STructural Abnormality iNDex (STAND)-scores correlate with postmortem Braak neurofibrillary tangle stage. *Neuroimage* **2008**, *42*, 559–567. [CrossRef] [PubMed]
13. Sluimer, J.D.; van der Flier, W.M.; Karas, G.B.; Fox, N.C.; Scheltens, P.; Barkhof, F.; Vrenken, H. Whole-brain atrophy rate and cognitive decline: Longitudinal MR study of memory clinic patients. *Radiology* **2008**, *248*, 590–598. [CrossRef] [PubMed]
14. Cardenas, V.A.; Chao, L.L.; Studholme, C.; Yaffe, K.; Miller, B.L.; Madison, C.; Buckley, S.T.; Mungas, D.; Schuff, N.; Weiner, M.W. Brain atrophy associated with baseline and longitudinal measures of cognition. *Neurobiol. Aging* **2011**, *32*, 572–580. [CrossRef] [PubMed]
15. Jack, C.R., Jr.; Shiung, M.M.; Gunter, J.L.; O'Brien, P.C.; Weigand, S.D.; Knopman, D.S.; Boeve, B.F.; Ivnik, R.J.; Smith, G.E.; Cha, R.H.; et al. Comparison of different MRI brain atrophy rate measures with clinical disease progression in AD. *Neurology* **2004**, *62*, 591–600. [CrossRef] [PubMed]
16. Hua, X.; Lee, S.; Yanovsky, I.; Leow, A.D.; Chou, Y.Y.; Ho, A.J.; Gutman, B.; Toga, A.W.; Jack, C.R., Jr.; Bernstein, M.A.; et al. Optimizing power to track brain degeneration in Alzheimer's disease and mild cognitive impairment with tensor-based morphometry: An ADNI study of 515 subjects. *Neuroimage* **2009**, *48*, 668–681. [CrossRef] [PubMed]
17. Jack, C.R., Jr.; Lowe, V.J.; Weigand, S.D.; Wiste, H.J.; Senjem, M.L.; Knopman, D.S.; Shiung, M.M.; Gunter, J.L.; Boeve, B.F.; Kemp, B.J.; et al. Serial PIB and MRI in normal, mild cognitive impairment and Alzheimer's disease: Implications for sequence of pathological events in Alzheimer's disease. *Brain* **2009**, *132*, 1355–1365. [CrossRef] [PubMed]
18. Josephs, K.A.; Whitwell, J.L.; Ahmed, Z.; Shiung, M.M.; Weigand, S.D.; Knopman, D.S.; Boeve, B.F.; Parisi, J.E.; Petersen, R.C.; Dickson, D.W.; et al. Beta-amyloid burden is not associated with rates of brain atrophy. *Ann. Neurol.* **2008**, *63*, 204–212. [CrossRef] [PubMed]
19. Engler, H.; Forsberg, A.; Almkvist, O.; Blomquist, G.; Larsson, E.; Savitcheva, I.; Wall, A.; Ringheim, A.; Langstrom, B.; Nordberg, A. Two-year follow-up of amyloid deposition in patients with Alzheimer's disease. *Brain* **2006**, *129*, 2856–2866. [CrossRef] [PubMed]
20. Giorgio, A.; De Stefano, N. Clinical use of brain volumetry. *J. Magn. Reson. Imaging* **2013**, *37*, 1–14. [CrossRef] [PubMed]
21. Bozzali, M.; Filippi, M.; Magnani, G.; Cercignani, M.; Franceschi, M.; Schiatti, E.; Castiglioni, S.; Mossini, R.; Falautano, M.; Scotti, G.; et al. The contribution of voxel-based morphometry in staging patients with mild cognitive impairment. *Neurology* **2006**, *67*, 453–460. [CrossRef] [PubMed]
22. Dickerson, B.C.; Feczko, E.; Augustinack, J.C.; Pacheco, J.; Morris, J.C.; Fischl, B.; Buckner, R.L. Differential effects of aging and Alzheimer's disease on medial temporal lobe cortical thickness and surface area. *Neurobiol. Aging* **2009**, *30*, 432–440. [CrossRef] [PubMed]
23. Barnes, J.; Lewis, E.B.; Scahill, R.I.; Bartlett, J.W.; Frost, C.; Schott, J.M.; Rossor, M.N.; Fox, N.C. Automated measurement of hippocampal atrophy using fluid-registered serial MRI in AD and controls. *J. Comput. Assist. Tomogr.* **2007**, *31*, 581–587. [CrossRef] [PubMed]
24. Bishop, C.A.; Jenkinson, M.; Andersson, J.; Declerck, J.; Merhof, D. Novel Fast Marching for Automated Segmentation of the Hippocampus (FMASH): Method and validation on clinical data. *Neuroimage* **2011**, *55*, 1009–1019. [CrossRef] [PubMed]
25. Jack, C.R., Jr.; Barkhof, F.; Bernstein, M.A.; Cantillon, M.; Cole, P.E.; Decarli, C.; Dubois, B.; Duchesne, S.; Fox, N.C.; Frisoni, G.B.; et al. Steps to standardization and validation of hippocampal volumetry as a biomarker in clinical trials and diagnostic criterion for Alzheimer's disease. *Alzheimer's Dement.* **2011**, *7*, 474–485.e4. [CrossRef] [PubMed]
26. Jack, C.R., Jr.; Bernstein, M.A.; Borowski, B.J.; Gunter, J.L.; Fox, N.C.; Thompson, P.M.; Schuff, N.; Krueger, G.; Killiany, R.J.; Decarli, C.S.; et al. Update on the magnetic resonance imaging core of the Alzheimer's disease neuroimaging initiative. *Alzheimer's Dement.* **2010**, *6*, 212–220. [CrossRef] [PubMed]
27. Kehoe, E.G.; McNulty, J.P.; Mullins, P.G.; Bokde, A.L. Advances in MRI biomarkers for the diagnosis of Alzheimer's disease. *Biomark. Med.* **2014**, *8*, 1151–1169. [CrossRef] [PubMed]
28. Steen, R.G.; Mull, C.; McClure, R.; Hamer, R.M.; Lieberman, J.A. Brain volume in first-episode schizophrenia: Systematic review and meta-analysis of magnetic resonance imaging studies. *Br. J. Psychiatry* **2006**, *188* 510–518. [CrossRef] [PubMed]

29. Arnone, D.; McIntosh, A.M.; Ebmeier, K.P.; Munafo, M.R.; Anderson, I.M. Magnetic resonance imaging studies in unipolar depression: Systematic review and meta-regression analyses. *Eur. Neuropsychopharmacol.* **2012**, *22*, 1–16. [CrossRef] [PubMed]
30. Frisoni, G.B.; Jack, C.R. Harmonization of magnetic resonance-based manual hippocampal segmentation: A mandatory step for wide clinical use. *Alzheimer's Dement.* **2011**, *7*, 171–174. [CrossRef] [PubMed]
31. Calsolaro, V.; Edison, P. Alterations in Glucose Metabolism in Alzheimer's Disease. *Recent Pat. Endocr. Metab. Immune Drug Discov.* **2016**, *10*, 31–39. [CrossRef] [PubMed]
32. Shah, K.; Desilva, S.; Abbruscato, T. The role of glucose transporters in brain disease: Diabetes and Alzheimer's Disease. *Int. J. Mol. Sci.* **2012**, *13*, 12629–12655. [CrossRef] [PubMed]
33. Femminella, G.D.; Edison, P. Evaluation of neuroprotective effect of glucagon-like peptide 1 analogs using neuroimaging. *Alzheimer's Dement.* **2014**, *10*, S55–S61. [CrossRef] [PubMed]
34. Herholz, K. Use of FDG PET as an imaging biomarker in clinical trials of Alzheimer's disease. *Biomark. Med.* **2012**, *6*, 431–439. [CrossRef] [PubMed]
35. Jack, C.R., Jr.; Knopman, D.S.; Jagust, W.J.; Shaw, L.M.; Aisen, P.S.; Weiner, M.W.; Petersen, R.C.; Trojanowski, J.Q. Hypothetical model of dynamic biomarkers of the Alzheimer's pathological cascade. *Lancet Neurol.* **2010**, *9*, 119–128. [CrossRef]
36. Chen, Z.C.; Zhong, C.J. Decoding Alzheimer's disease from perturbed cerebral glucose metabolism: Implications for diagnostic and therapeutic strategies. *Prog. Neurobiol.* **2013**, *108*, 21–43. [CrossRef] [PubMed]
37. Laforce, R., Jr.; Soucy, J.P.; Sellami, L.; Dallaire-Theroux, C.; Brunet, F.; Bergeron, D.; Miller, B.L.; Ossenkoppele, R. Molecular imaging in dementia: Past, present, and future. *Alzheimer's Dement.* **2018**, *14*, 1522–1552. [CrossRef] [PubMed]
38. Furst, A.J.; Rabinovici, G.D.; Rostomian, A.H.; Steed, T.; Alkalay, A.; Racine, C.; Miller, B.L.; Jagust, W.J. Cognition, glucose metabolism and amyloid burden in Alzheimer's disease. *Neurobiol. Aging* **2012**, *33*, 215–225. [CrossRef] [PubMed]
39. Edison, P.; Archer, H.A.; Hinz, R.; Hammers, A.; Pavese, N.; Tai, Y.F.; Hotton, G.; Cutler, D.; Fox, N.; Kennedy, A.; et al. Amyloid, hypometabolism, and cognition in Alzheimer disease: An [^{11}C]PIB and [^{18}F]FDG PET study. *Neurology* **2007**, *68*, 501–508. [CrossRef] [PubMed]
40. Langbaum, J.B.S.; Chen, K.; Lee, W.; Reschke, C.; Bandy, D.; Fleisher, A.S.; Alexander, G.E.; Foster, N.L.; Weiner, M.W.; Koeppe, R.A.; et al. Categorical and correlational analyses of baseline fluorodeoxyglucose positron emission tomography images from the Alzheimer's Disease Neuroimaging Initiative (ADNI). *Neuroimage* **2009**, *45*, 1107–1116. [CrossRef] [PubMed]
41. Ewers, M.; Insel, P.S.; Stern, Y.; Weiner, M.W.; Alzheimer's Disease Neuroimaging Initiative (ADNI). Cognitive reserve associated with FDG-PET in preclinical Alzheimer disease. *Neurology* **2013**, *80*, 1194–1201. [CrossRef] [PubMed]
42. Jagust, W.; Reed, B.; Mungas, D.; Ellis, W.; DeCarli, C. What does fluorodeoxyglucose PET imaging add to a clinical diagnosis of dementia? *Neurology* **2007**, *69*, 871–877. [CrossRef] [PubMed]
43. Drzezga, A.; Lautenschlager, N.; Siebner, H.; Riemenschneider, M.; Willoch, F.; Minoshima, S.; Schwaiger, M.; Kurz, A. Cerebral metabolic changes accompanying conversion of mild cognitive impairment into Alzheimer's disease: A PET follow-up study. *Eur. J. Nucl. Med. Mol. Imaging* **2003**, *30*, 1104–1113. [PubMed]
44. Anchisi, D.; Borroni, B.; Franceschi, M.; Kerrouche, N.; Kalbe, E.; Beuthien-Beumann, B.; Cappa, S.; Lenz, O.; Ludecke, S.; Marcone, A.; et al. Heterogeneity of brain glucose metabolism in mild cognitive impairment and clinical progression to Alzheimer disease. *Arch. Neurol.* **2005**, *62*, 1728–1733. [CrossRef] [PubMed]
45. Silverman, D.H.; Small, G.W.; Chang, C.Y.; Lu, C.S.; Kung De Aburto, M.A.; Chen, W.; Czernin, J.; Rapoport, S.I.; Pietrini, P.; Alexander, G.E.; et al. Positron emission tomography in evaluation of dementia: Regional brain metabolism and long-term outcome. *JAMA* **2001**, *286*, 2120–2127. [CrossRef] [PubMed]
46. Smailagic, N.; Vacante, M.; Hyde, C.; Martin, S.; Ukoumunne, O.; Sachpekidis, C. ^{18F}-FDG PET for the early diagnosis of Alzheimer's disease dementia and other dementias in people with mild cognitive impairment (MCI). *Cochrane Database Syst. Rev.* **2015**, *1*, CD010632. [CrossRef] [PubMed]
47. Pike, K.E.; Savage, G.; Villemagne, V.L.; Ng, S.; Moss, S.A.; Maruff, P.; Mathis, C.A.; Klunk, W.E.; Masters, C.L.; Rowe, C.C. Beta-amyloid imaging and memory in non-demented individuals: Evidence for preclinical Alzheimer's disease. *Brain* **2007**, *130*, 2837–2844. [CrossRef] [PubMed]

48. Johnson, K.A.; Minoshima, S.; Bohnen, N.I.; Donohoe, K.J.; Foster, N.L.; Herscovitch, P.; Karlawish, J.H.; Rowe, C.C.; Hedrick, S.; Pappas, V.; et al. Update on appropriate use criteria for amyloid PET imaging: Dementia experts, mild cognitive impairment, and education. Amyloid Imaging Task Force of the Alzheimer's Association and Society for Nuclear Medicine and Molecular Imaging. *Alzheimer's Dement.* **2013**, *9*, e106–e109. [CrossRef] [PubMed]
49. Villemagne, V.L.; Dore, V.; Burnham, S.C.; Masters, C.L.; Rowe, C.C. Imaging tau and amyloid-beta proteinopathies in Alzheimer disease and other conditions. *Nat. Rev. Neurol.* **2018**, *14*, 225–236. [CrossRef] [PubMed]
50. Johnson, K.A.; Minoshima, S.; Bohnen, N.I.; Donohoe, K.J.; Foster, N.L.; Herscovitch, P.; Karlawish, J.H.; Rowe, C.C.; Carrillo, M.C.; Hartley, D.M.; et al. Appropriate use criteria for amyloid PET: A report of the Amyloid Imaging Task Force, the Society of Nuclear Medicine and Molecular Imaging, and the Alzheimer's Association. *Alzheimer's Dement.* **2013**, *9*, E1–E16. [CrossRef] [PubMed]
51. Apostolova, L.G.; Haider, J.M.; Goukasian, N.; Rabinovici, G.D.; Chetelat, G.; Ringman, J.M.; Kremen, S.; Grill, J.D.; Restrepo, L.; Mendez, M.F.; et al. Critical review of the Appropriate Use Criteria for amyloid imaging: Effect on diagnosis and patient care. *Alzheimer's Dement.* **2016**, *5*, 15–22. [CrossRef] [PubMed]
52. Mathis, C.A.; Bacskai, B.J.; Kajdasz, S.T.; McLellan, M.E.; Frosch, M.P.; Hyman, B.T.; Holt, D.P.; Wang, Y.; Huang, G.F.; Debnath, M.L.; et al. A lipophilic thioflavin-T derivative for positron emission tomography (PET) imaging of amyloid in brain. *Bioorg. Med. Chem. Lett.* **2002**, *12*, 295–298. [CrossRef]
53. Lister-James, J.; Pontecorvo, M.J.; Clark, C.; Joshi, A.D.; Mintun, M.A.; Zhang, W.; Lim, N.; Zhuang, Z.; Golding, G.; Choi, S.R.; et al. Florbetapir f-18: A histopathologically validated Beta-amyloid positron emission tomography imaging agent. *Semin. Nucl. Med.* **2011**, *41*, 300–304. [CrossRef] [PubMed]
54. Sperling, R.A.; Johnson, K.A.; Doraiswamy, P.M.; Reiman, E.M.; Fleisher, A.S.; Sabbagh, M.N.; Sadowsky, C.H.; Carpenter, A.; Davis, M.D.; Lu, M.; et al. Amyloid deposition detected with florbetapir F 18 ((18)F-AV-45) is related to lower episodic memory performance in clinically normal older individuals. *Neurobiol. Aging* **2013**, *34*, 822–831. [CrossRef] [PubMed]
55. Fleisher, A.S.; Chen, K.; Liu, X.; Roontiva, A.; Thiyyagura, P.; Ayutyanont, N.; Joshi, A.D.; Clark, C.M.; Mintun, M.A.; Pontecorvo, M.J.; et al. Using positron emission tomography and florbetapir F18 to image cortical amyloid in patients with mild cognitive impairment or dementia due to Alzheimer disease. *Arch. Neurol.* **2011**, *68*, 1404–1411. [CrossRef] [PubMed]
56. Clark, C.M.; Schneider, J.A.; Bedell, B.J.; Beach, T.G.; Bilker, W.B.; Mintun, M.A.; Pontecorvo, M.J.; Hefti, F.; Carpenter, A.P.; Flitter, M.L.; et al. Use of florbetapir-PET for imaging beta-amyloid pathology. *JAMA* **2011**, *305*, 275–283. [CrossRef] [PubMed]
57. Clark, C.M.; Pontecorvo, M.J.; Beach, T.G.; Bedell, B.J.; Coleman, R.E.; Doraiswamy, P.M.; Fleisher, A.S.; Reiman, E.M.; Sabbagh, M.N.; Sadowsky, C.H.; et al. Cerebral PET with florbetapir compared with neuropathology at autopsy for detection of neuritic amyloid-beta plaques: A prospective cohort study. *Lancet Neurol.* **2012**, *11*, 669–678. [CrossRef]
58. Zhang, W.; Oya, S.; Kung, M.P.; Hou, C.; Maier, D.L.; Kung, H.F. F-18 stilbenes as PET imaging agents for detecting beta-amyloid plaques in the brain. *J. Med. Chem.* **2005**, *48*, 5980–5988. [CrossRef] [PubMed]
59. Rowe, C.C.; Ackerman, U.; Browne, W.; Mulligan, R.; Pike, K.L.; O'Keefe, G.; Tochon-Danguy, H.; Chan, G.; Berlangieri, S.U.; Jones, G.; et al. Imaging of amyloid beta in Alzheimer's disease with 18F-BAY94-9172, a novel PET tracer: Proof of mechanism. *Lancet Neurol.* **2008**, *7*, 129–135. [CrossRef]
60. Vandenberghe, R.; Van Laere, K.; Ivanoiu, A.; Salmon, E.; Bastin, C.; Triau, E.; Hasselbalch, S.; Law, I.; Andersen, A.; Korner, A.; et al. 18F-flutemetamol amyloid imaging in Alzheimer disease and mild cognitive impairment: A phase 2 trial. *Ann. Neurol.* **2010**, *68*, 319–329. [CrossRef] [PubMed]
61. Nelissen, N.; Van Laere, K.; Thurfjell, L.; Owenius, R.; Vandenbulcke, M.; Koole, M.; Bormans, G.; Brooks, D.J.; Vandenberghe, R. Phase 1 study of the Pittsburgh compound B derivative 18F-flutemetamol in healthy volunteers and patients with probable Alzheimer disease. *J. Nucl. Med.* **2009**, *50*, 1251–1259. [CrossRef] [PubMed]
62. Thurfjell, L.; Lotjonen, J.; Lundqvist, R.; Koikkalainen, J.; Soininen, H.; Waldemar, G.; Brooks, D.J.; Vandenberghe, R. Combination of biomarkers: PET [^{18}F]flutemetamol imaging and structural MRI in dementia and mild cognitive impairment. *Neurodegener. Dis.* **2012**, *10*, 246–249. [CrossRef] [PubMed]

63. Ye, L.; Morgenstern, J.L.; Gee, A.D.; Hong, G.; Brown, J.; Lockhart, A. Delineation of positron emission tomography imaging agent binding sites on beta-amyloid peptide fibrils. *J. Biol. Chem.* **2005**, *280*, 23599–23604. [CrossRef] [PubMed]
64. Cohen, A.D.; Rabinovici, G.D.; Mathis, C.A.; Jagust, W.J.; Klunk, W.E.; Ikonomovic, M.D. Using Pittsburgh Compound B for in vivo PET imaging of fibrillar amyloid-beta. *Adv. Pharmacol.* **2012**, *64*, 27–81. [PubMed]
65. Braak, H.; Braak, E. Frequency of stages of Alzheimer-related lesions in different age categories. *Neurobiol. Aging* **1997**, *18*, 351–357. [CrossRef]
66. Villain, N.; Chetelat, G.; Grassiot, B.; Bourgeat, P.; Jones, G.; Ellis, K.A.; Ames, D.; Martins, R.N.; Eustache, F.; Salvado, O.; et al. Regional dynamics of amyloid-beta deposition in healthy elderly, mild cognitive impairment and Alzheimer's disease: A voxelwise PiB-PET longitudinal study. *Brain* **2012**, *135*, 2126–2139. [CrossRef] [PubMed]
67. Vlassenko, A.G.; Mintun, M.A.; Xiong, C.; Sheline, Y.I.; Goate, A.M.; Benzinger, T.L.; Morris, J.C. Amyloid-beta plaque growth in cognitively normal adults: Longitudinal [^{11}C]Pittsburgh compound B data. *Ann. Neurol.* **2011**, *70*, 857–861. [CrossRef] [PubMed]
68. Ng, S.Y.; Villemagne, V.L.; Masters, C.L.; Rowe, C.C. Evaluating atypical dementia syndromes using positron emission tomography with carbon 11 labeled Pittsburgh Compound B. *Arch. Neurol.* **2007**, *64*, 1140–1144. [CrossRef] [PubMed]
69. Rabinovici, G.D.; Jagust, W.J.; Furst, A.J.; Ogar, J.M.; Racine, C.A.; Mormino, E.C.; O'Neil, J.P.; Lal, R.A.; Dronkers, N.F.; Miller, B.L.; et al. Abeta amyloid and glucose metabolism in three variants of primary progressive aphasia. *Ann. Neurol.* **2008**, *64*, 388–401. [CrossRef] [PubMed]
70. Drzezga, A.; Grimmer, T.; Henriksen, G.; Stangier, I.; Perneczky, R.; Diehl-Schmid, J.; Mathis, C.A.; Klunk, W.E.; Price, J.; DeKosky, S.; et al. Imaging of amyloid plaques and cerebral glucose metabolism in semantic dementia and Alzheimer's disease. *Neuroimage* **2008**, *39*, 619–633. [CrossRef] [PubMed]
71. Engler, H.; Santillo, A.F.; Wang, S.X.; Lindau, M.; Savitcheva, I.; Nordberg, A.; Lannfelt, L.; Langstrom, B.; Kilander, L. In vivo amyloid imaging with PET in frontotemporal dementia. *Eur. J. Nucl. Med. Mol. Imaging* **2008**, *35*, 100–106. [CrossRef] [PubMed]
72. Edison, P.; Rowe, C.C.; Rinne, J.O.; Ng, S.; Ahmed, I.; Kemppainen, N.; Villemagne, V.L.; O'Keefe, G.; Nagren, K.; Chaudhury, K.R.; et al. Amyloid load in Parkinson's disease dementia and Lewy body dementia measured with [^{11}C]PIB positron emission tomography. *J. Neurol. Neurosurg. Psychiatry* **2008**, *79*, 1331–1338. [CrossRef] [PubMed]
73. Kalaitzakis, M.E.; Walls, A.J.; Pearce, R.K.; Gentleman, S.M. Striatal Abeta peptide deposition mirrors dementia and differentiates DLB and PDD from other parkinsonian syndromes. *Neurobiol. Dis.* **2011**, *41*, 377–384. [CrossRef] [PubMed]
74. Delacourte, A.; Sergeant, N.; Wattez, A.; Maurage, C.A.; Lebert, F.; Pasquier, F.; David, J.P. Tau aggregation in the hippocampal formation: An ageing or a pathological process? *Exp. Gerontol.* **2002**, *37*, 1291–1296. [CrossRef]
75. Chiotis, K.; Saint-Aubert, L.; Rodriguez-Vieitez, E.; Leuzy, A.; Almkvist, O.; Savitcheva, I.; Jonasson, M.; Lubberink, M.; Wall, A.; Antoni, G.; et al. Longitudinal changes of tau PET imaging in relation to hypometabolism in prodromal and Alzheimer's disease dementia. *Mol. Psychiatry* **2018**, *23*, 1666–1673. [CrossRef] [PubMed]
76. Chiotis, K.; Saint-Aubert, L.; Savitcheva, I.; Jelic, V.; Andersen, P.; Jonasson, M.; Eriksson, J.; Lubberink, M.; Almkvist, O.; Wall, A.; et al. Imaging in-vivo tau pathology in Alzheimer's disease with THK5317 PET in a multimodal paradigm. *Eur. J. Nucl. Med. Mol. Imaging* **2016**, *43*, 1686–1699. [CrossRef] [PubMed]
77. Saint-Aubert, L.; Almkvist, O.; Chiotis, K.; Almeida, R.; Wall, A.; Nordberg, A. Regional tau deposition measured by [^{18}F]THK5317 positron emission tomography is associated to cognition via glucose metabolism in Alzheimer's disease. *Alzheimer's Res. Ther.* **2016**, *8*, 38. [CrossRef] [PubMed]
78. Royall, D.R. Location, location, location! *Neurobiol. Aging* **2007**, *28*, 1481–1482, discussion 1483. [CrossRef] [PubMed]
79. Delacourte, A.; David, J.P.; Sergeant, N.; Buee, L.; Wattez, A.; Vermersch, P.; Ghozali, F.; Fallet-Bianco, C.; Pasquier, F.; Lebert, F.; et al. The biochemical pathway of neurofibrillary degeneration in aging and Alzheimer's disease. *Neurology* **1999**, *52*, 1158–1165. [CrossRef] [PubMed]
80. Scholl, M.; Lockhart, S.N.; Schonhaut, D.R.; O'Neil, J.P.; Janabi, M.; Ossenkoppele, R.; Baker, S.L.; Vogel, J.W.; Faria, J.; Schwimmer, H.D.; et al. PET Imaging of Tau Deposition in the Aging Human Brain. *Neuron* **2016**, *89*, 971–982. [CrossRef] [PubMed]

81. Pontecorvo, M.J.; Devous, M.D., Sr.; Navitsky, M.; Lu, M.; Salloway, S.; Schaerf, F.W.; Jennings, D.; Arora, A.K.; McGeehan, A.; Lim, N.C.; et al. Relationships between flortaucipir PET tau binding and amyloid burden, clinical diagnosis, age and cognition. *Brain* **2017**, *140*, 748–763. [CrossRef] [PubMed]
82. Johnson, K.A.; Schultz, A.; Betensky, R.A.; Becker, J.A.; Sepulcre, J.; Rentz, D.; Mormino, E.; Chhatwal, J.; Amariglio, R.; Papp, K.; et al. Tau positron emission tomographic imaging in aging and early Alzheimer disease. *Ann. Neurol.* **2016**, *79*, 110–119. [CrossRef] [PubMed]
83. Lockhart, S.N.; Baker, S.L.; Okamura, N.; Furukawa, K.; Ishiki, A.; Furumoto, S.; Tashiro, M.; Yanai, K.; Arai, H.; Kudo, Y.; et al. Dynamic PET Measures of Tau Accumulation in Cognitively Normal Older Adults and Alzheimer's Disease Patients Measured Using [^{18}F] THK-5351. *PLoS ONE* **2016**, *11*, e0158460. [CrossRef] [PubMed]
84. Harada, R.; Okamura, N.; Furumoto, S.; Furukawa, K.; Ishiki, A.; Tomita, N.; Tago, T.; Hiraoka, K.; Watanuki, S.; Shidahara, M.; et al. 18F-THK5351: A Novel PET Radiotracer for Imaging Neurofibrillary Pathology in Alzheimer Disease. *J. Nucl. Med.* **2016**, *57*, 208–214. [CrossRef] [PubMed]
85. Cho, H.; Choi, J.Y.; Hwang, M.S.; Lee, J.H.; Kim, Y.J.; Lee, H.M.; Lyoo, C.H.; Ryu, Y.H.; Lee, M.S. Tau PET in Alzheimer disease and mild cognitive impairment. *Neurology* **2016**, *87*, 375–383. [CrossRef] [PubMed]
86. Ossenkoppele, R.; Cohn-Sheehy, B.I.; La Joie, R.; Vogel, J.W.; Moller, C.; Lehmann, M.; van Berckel, B.N.; Seeley, W.W.; Pijnenburg, Y.A.; Gorno-Tempini, M.L.; et al. Atrophy patterns in early clinical stages across distinct phenotypes of Alzheimer's disease. *Hum. Brain Mapp.* **2015**, *36*, 4421–4437. [CrossRef] [PubMed]
87. Tomlinson, B.E.; Blessed, G.; Roth, M. Observations on the brains of demented old people. *J. Neurol. Sci.* **1970**, *11*, 205–242. [CrossRef]
88. Jellinger, K.A.; Alafuzoff, I.; Attems, J.; Beach, T.G.; Cairns, N.J.; Crary, J.F.; Dickson, D.W.; Hof, P.R.; Hyman, B.T.; Jack, C.R., Jr.; et al. PART, a distinct tauopathy, different from classical sporadic Alzheimer disease. *Acta Neuropathol.* **2015**, *129*, 757–762. [CrossRef] [PubMed]
89. Wang, L.; Benzinger, T.L.; Su, Y.; Christensen, J.; Friedrichsen, K.; Aldea, P.; McConathy, J.; Cairns, N.J.; Fagan, A.M.; Morris, J.C.; et al. Evaluation of Tau Imaging in Staging Alzheimer Disease and Revealing Interactions Between beta-Amyloid and Tauopathy. *JAMA Neurol.* **2016**, *73*, 1070–1077. [CrossRef] [PubMed]
90. Price, J.L.; Morris, J.C. Tangles and plaques in nondemented aging and "preclinical" Alzheimer's disease. *Ann. Neurol.* **1999**, *45*, 358–368. [CrossRef]
91. Ishiki, A.; Harada, R.; Okamura, N.; Tomita, N.; Rowe, C.C.; Villemagne, V.L.; Yanai, K.; Kudo, Y.; Arai, H.; Furumoto, S.; et al. Tau imaging with [^{18}F]THK-5351 in progressive supranuclear palsy. *Eur. J. Neurol.* **2017**, *24*, 130–136. [CrossRef] [PubMed]
92. Josephs, K.A.; Holton, J.L.; Rossor, M.N.; Godbolt, A.K.; Ozawa, T.; Strand, K.; Khan, N.; Al-Sarraj, S.; Revesz, T. Frontotemporal lobar degeneration and ubiquitin immunohistochemistry. *Neuropathol. Appl. Neurobiol.* **2004**, *30*, 369–373. [CrossRef] [PubMed]
93. Ikonomovic, M.D.; Abrahamson, E.E.; Price, J.C.; Mathis, C.A.; Klunk, W.E. [F-18]AV-1451 positron emission tomography retention in choroid plexus: More than "off-target" binding. *Ann. Neurol.* **2016**, *80*, 307–308. [CrossRef] [PubMed]
94. Marquie, M.; Normandin, M.D.; Meltzer, A.C.; Siao Tick Chong, M.; Andrea, N.V.; Anton-Fernandez, A.; Klunk, W.E.; Mathis, C.A.; Ikonomovic, M.D.; Debnath, M.; et al. Pathological correlations of [F-18]-AV-1451 imaging in non-alzheimer tauopathies. *Ann. Neurol.* **2017**, *81*, 117–128. [CrossRef] [PubMed]
95. Chen, R.; Chen, C.P.; Preston, J.E. Effects of transthyretin on thyroxine and beta-amyloid removal from cerebrospinal fluid in mice. *Clin. Exp. Pharmacol. Physiol.* **2016**, *43*, 844–850. [CrossRef] [PubMed]
96. Lowe, V.J.; Curran, G.; Fang, P.; Liesinger, A.M.; Josephs, K.A.; Parisi, J.E.; Kantarci, K.; Boeve, B.F.; Pandey, M.K.; Bruinsma, T.; et al. An autoradiographic evaluation of AV-1451 Tau PET in dementia. *Acta Neuropathol. Commun.* **2016**, *4*, 58. [CrossRef] [PubMed]
97. Beach, T.G.; Monsell, S.E.; Phillips, L.E.; Kukull, W. Accuracy of the clinical diagnosis of Alzheimer disease at National Institute on Aging Alzheimer Disease Centers, 2005–2010. *J. Neuropathol. Exp. Neurol.* **2012**, *71* 266–273. [CrossRef] [PubMed]
98. Marquie, M.; Normandin, M.D.; Vanderburg, C.R.; Costantino, I.M.; Bien, E.A.; Rycyna, L.G.; Klunk, W.E.; Mathis, C.A.; Ikonomovic, M.D.; Debnath, M.L.; et al. Validating novel tau positron emission tomography tracer [F-18]-AV-1451 (T807) on postmortem brain tissue. *Ann. Neurol.* **2015**, *78*, 787–800. [CrossRef] [PubMed]

99. Ng, K.P.; Pascoal, T.A.; Mathotaarachchi, S.; Therriault, J.; Kang, M.S.; Shin, M.; Guiot, M.C.; Guo, Q.; Harada, R.; Comley, R.A.; et al. Monoamine oxidase B inhibitor, selegiline, reduces ^{18}F-THK5351 uptake in the human brain. *Alzheimer's Res. Ther.* **2017**, *9*, 25. [CrossRef] [PubMed]
100. Gobbi, L.C.; Knust, H.; Korner, M.; Honer, M.; Czech, C.; Belli, S.; Muri, D.; Edelmann, M.R.; Hartung, T.; Erbsmehl, I.; et al. Identification of Three Novel Radiotracers for Imaging Aggregated Tau in Alzheimer's Disease with Positron Emission Tomography. *J. Med. Chem.* **2017**, *60*, 7350–7370. [CrossRef] [PubMed]
101. Walji, A.M.; Hostetler, E.D.; Selnick, H.; Zeng, Z.; Miller, P.; Bennacef, I.; Salinas, C.; Connolly, B.; Gantert, L.; Holahan, M.; et al. Discovery of 6-(Fluoro-(18)F)-3-(1H-pyrrolo[2,3-c]pyridin-1-yl)isoquinolin-5-amine ([(18)F]-MK-6240): A Positron Emission Tomography (PET) Imaging Agent for Quantification of Neurofibrillary Tangles (NFTs). *J. Med. Chem.* **2016**, *59*, 4778–4789. [CrossRef] [PubMed]
102. Stephens, A.; Kroth, H.; Berndt, M.; Capotosti, F.; Mueller, A. Characterization of novel PET tracers for the assessment of tau pathology in Alzheimer's disease and other tauopathies. *Neurodegener. Dis.* **2017**, *17*.
103. Calsolaro, V.; Edison, P. Neuroinflammation in Alzheimer's disease: Current evidence and future directions. *Alzheimer's Dement.* **2016**, *12*, 719–732. [CrossRef] [PubMed]
104. Cuyvers, E.; Sleegers, K. Genetic variations underlying Alzheimer's disease: Evidence from genome-wide association studies and beyond. *Lancet Neurol.* **2016**, *15*, 857–868. [CrossRef]
105. Cerami, C.; Iaccarino, L.; Perani, D. Molecular Imaging of Neuroinflammation in Neurodegenerative Dementias: The Role of In Vivo PET Imaging. *Int. J. Mol. Sci.* **2017**, *18*, 993. [CrossRef] [PubMed]
106. Edison, P.; Brooks, D.J. Role of Neuroinflammation in the Trajectory of Alzheimer's Disease and in vivo Quantification Using PET. *J. Alzheimer's Dis.* **2018**, *64*, S339–S351. [CrossRef] [PubMed]
107. Heppner, F.L.; Ransohoff, R.M.; Becher, B. Immune attack: The role of inflammation in Alzheimer disease. *Nat. Rev. Neurosci.* **2015**, *16*, 358–372. [CrossRef] [PubMed]
108. Heneka, M.T.; Carson, M.J.; El Khoury, J.; Landreth, G.E.; Brosseron, F.; Feinstein, D.L.; Jacobs, A.H.; Wyss-Coray, T.; Vitorica, J.; Ransohoff, R.M.; et al. Neuroinflammation in Alzheimer's disease. *Lancet Neurol.* **2015**, *14*, 388–405. [CrossRef]
109. Knezevic, D.; Mizrahi, R. Molecular imaging of neuroinflammation in Alzheimer's disease and mild cognitive impairment. *Prog. Neuropsychopharmacol. Biol. Psychiatry* **2018**, *80*, 123–131. [CrossRef] [PubMed]
110. Schwab, C.; McGeer, P.L. Inflammatory aspects of Alzheimer disease and other neurodegenerative disorders. *J. Alzheimer's Dis.* **2008**, *13*, 359–369. [CrossRef]
111. Rogers, J.; Luber-Narod, J.; Styren, S.D.; Civin, W.H. Expression of immune system-associated antigens by cells of the human central nervous system: Relationship to the pathology of Alzheimer's disease. *Neurobiol. Aging* **1988**, *9*, 339–349. [CrossRef]
112. Heneka, M.T.; Kummer, M.P.; Latz, E. Innate immune activation in neurodegenerative disease. *Nat. Rev. Immunol.* **2014**, *14*, 463–477. [CrossRef] [PubMed]
113. Ransohoff, R.M. A polarizing question: Do M1 and M2 microglia exist? *Nat. Neurosci.* **2016**, *19*, 987–991. [CrossRef] [PubMed]
114. Lagarde, J.; Sarazin, M.; Bottlaender, M. In vivo PET imaging of neuroinflammation in Alzheimer's disease. *J. Neural Transm.* **2018**, *125*, 847–867. [CrossRef] [PubMed]
115. Vivash, L.; O'Brien, T.J. Imaging Microglial Activation with TSPO PET: Lighting Up Neurologic Diseases? *J. Nucl. Med.* **2016**, *57*, 165–168. [CrossRef] [PubMed]
116. Politis, M.; Giannetti, P.; Su, P.; Turkheimer, F.; Keihaninejad, S.; Wu, K.; Waldman, A.; Malik, O.; Matthews, P.M.; Reynolds, R.; et al. Increased PK11195 PET binding in the cortex of patients with MS correlates with disability. *Neurology* **2012**, *79*, 523–530. [CrossRef] [PubMed]
117. Gerhard, A.; Pavese, N.; Hotton, G.; Turkheimer, F.; Es, M.; Hammers, A.; Eggert, K.; Oertel, W.; Banati, R.B.; Brooks, D.J. In vivo imaging of microglial activation with [^{11}C](R)-PK11195 PET in idiopathic Parkinson's disease. *Neurobiol. Dis.* **2006**, *21*, 404–412. [CrossRef] [PubMed]
118. Owen, D.R.; Yeo, A.J.; Gunn, R.N.; Song, K.; Wadsworth, G.; Lewis, A.; Rhodes, C.; Pulford, D.J.; Bennacef, I.; Parker, C.A.; et al. An 18-kDa translocator protein (TSPO) polymorphism explains differences in binding affinity of the PET radioligand PBR28. *J. Cereb. Blood Flow Metab.* **2012**, *32*, 1–5. [CrossRef] [PubMed]
119. Cagnin, A.; Brooks, D.J.; Kennedy, A.M.; Gunn, R.N.; Myers, R.; Turkheimer, F.E.; Jones, T.; Banati, R.B. In-vivo measurement of activated microglia in dementia. *Lancet* **2001**, *358*, 461–467. [CrossRef]

120. Wiley, C.A.; Lopresti, B.J.; Venneti, S.; Price, J.; Klunk, W.E.; DeKosky, S.T.; Mathis, C.A. Carbon 11-labeled Pittsburgh Compound B and carbon 11-labeled (R)-PK11195 positron emission tomographic imaging in Alzheimer disease. *Arch. Neurol.* **2009**, *66*, 60–67. [CrossRef] [PubMed]
121. Yasuno, F.; Ota, M.; Kosaka, J.; Ito, H.; Higuchi, M.; Doronbekov, T.K.; Nozaki, S.; Fujimura, Y.; Koeda, M.; Asada, T.; et al. Increased binding of peripheral benzodiazepine receptor in Alzheimer's disease measured by positron emission tomography with [11C]DAA1106. *Biol. Psychiatry* **2008**, *64*, 835–841. [CrossRef] [PubMed]
122. Kreisl, W.C.; Lyoo, C.H.; McGwier, M.; Snow, J.; Jenko, K.J.; Kimura, N.; Corona, W.; Morse, C.L.; Zoghbi, S.S.; Pike, V.W.; et al. In vivo radioligand binding to translocator protein correlates with severity of Alzheimer's disease. *Brain* **2013**, *136*, 2228–2238. [CrossRef] [PubMed]
123. Suridjan, I.; Pollock, B.G.; Verhoeff, N.P.; Voineskos, A.N.; Chow, T.; Rusjan, P.M.; Lobaugh, N.J.; Houle, S.; Mulsant, B.H.; Mizrahi, R. In-vivo imaging of grey and white matter neuroinflammation in Alzheimer's disease: A positron emission tomography study with a novel radioligand, [18F]-FEPPA. *Mol. Psychiatry* **2015**, *20*, 1579–1587. [CrossRef] [PubMed]
124. Edison, P.; Archer, H.A.; Gerhard, A.; Hinz, R.; Pavese, N.; Turkheimer, F.E.; Hammers, A.; Tai, Y.F.; Fox, N.; Kennedy, A.; et al. Microglia, amyloid, and cognition in Alzheimer's disease: An [11C](R)PK11195-PET and [11C]PIB-PET study. *Neurobiol. Dis.* **2008**, *32*, 412–419. [CrossRef] [PubMed]
125. Hamelin, L.; Lagarde, J.; Dorothee, G.; Leroy, C.; Labit, M.; Comley, R.A.; de Souza, L.C.; Corne, H.; Dauphinot, L.; Bertoux, M.; et al. Early and protective microglial activation in Alzheimer's disease: A prospective study using 18F-DPA-714 PET imaging. *Brain* **2016**, *139*, 1252–1264. [CrossRef] [PubMed]
126. Fan, Z.; Aman, Y.; Ahmed, I.; Chetelat, G.; Landeau, B.; Ray Chaudhuri, K.; Brooks, D.J.; Edison, P. Influence of microglial activation on neuronal function in Alzheimer's and Parkinson's disease dementia. *Alzheimer's Dement.* **2015**, *11*, 608–621.e7. [CrossRef] [PubMed]
127. Femminella, G.D.; Ninan, S.; Atkinson, R.; Fan, Z.; Brooks, D.J.; Edison, P. Does Microglial Activation Influence Hippocampal Volume and Neuronal Function in Alzheimer's Disease and Parkinson's Disease Dementia? *J. Alzheimer's Dis.* **2016**, *51*, 1275–1289. [CrossRef] [PubMed]
128. Yokokura, M.; Mori, N.; Yagi, S.; Yoshikawa, E.; Kikuchi, M.; Yoshihara, Y.; Wakuda, T.; Sugihara, G.; Takebayashi, K.; Suda, S.; et al. In vivo changes in microglial activation and amyloid deposits in brain regions with hypometabolism in Alzheimer's disease. *Eur. J. Nucl. Med. Mol. Imaging* **2011**, *38*, 343–351. [CrossRef] [PubMed]
129. Yasuno, F.; Kosaka, J.; Ota, M.; Higuchi, M.; Ito, H.; Fujimura, Y.; Nozaki, S.; Takahashi, S.; Mizukami, K.; Asada, T.; et al. Increased binding of peripheral benzodiazepine receptor in mild cognitive impairment-dementia converters measured by positron emission tomography with [^{11}C]DAA1106. *Psychiatry Res.* **2012**, *203*, 67–74. [CrossRef] [PubMed]
130. Dani, M.; Wood, M.; Mizoguchi, R.; Fan, Z.; Walker, Z.; Morgan, R.; Hinz, R.; Biju, M.; Kuruvilla, T.; Brooks, D.J.; et al. Microglial activation correlates in vivo with both tau and amyloid in Alzheimer's disease. *Brain* **2018**, *141*, 2740–2754. [CrossRef] [PubMed]
131. Fan, Z.; Brooks, D.J.; Okello, A.; Edison, P. An early and late peak in microglial activation in Alzheimer's disease trajectory. *Brain* **2017**, *140*, 792–803. [CrossRef] [PubMed]
132. Kreisl, W.C.; Lyoo, C.H.; Liow, J.S.; Wei, M.; Snow, J.; Page, E.; Jenko, K.J.; Morse, C.L.; Zoghbi, S.S.; Pike, V.W.; et al. ^{11}C-PBR28 binding to translocator protein increases with progression of Alzheimer's disease. *Neurobiol. Aging* **2016**, *44*, 53–61. [CrossRef] [PubMed]
133. Santillo, A.F.; Gambini, J.P.; Lannfelt, L.; Langstrom, B.; Ulla-Marja, L.; Kilander, L.; Engler, H. In vivo imaging of astrocytosis in Alzheimer's disease: An ^{11}C-L-deuteriodeprenyl and PIB PET study. *Eur. J. Nucl. Med. Mol. Imaging* **2011**, *38*, 2202–2208. [CrossRef] [PubMed]
134. Rodriguez-Vieitez, E.; Saint-Aubert, L.; Carter, S.F.; Almkvist, O.; Farid, K.; Scholl, M.; Chiotis, K.; Thordardottir, S.; Graff, C.; Wall, A.; et al. Diverging longitudinal changes in astrocytosis and amyloid PET in autosomal dominant Alzheimer's disease. *Brain* **2016**, *139*, 922–936. [CrossRef] [PubMed]
135. Kim, S.; Thiessen, P.A.; Bolton, E.E.; Chen, J.; Fu, G.; Gindulyte, A.; Han, L.; He, J.; He, S.; Shoemaker, B.A.; et al. PubChem Substance and Compound databases. *Nucleic Acids Res.* **2016**, *44*, D1202–D1213. [CrossRef] [PubMed]
136. Raja, R.; Rosenberg, G.A.; Caprihan, A. MRI measurements of Blood-Brain Barrier function in dementia: A review of recent studies. *Neuropharmacology* **2018**, *134*, 259–271. [CrossRef] [PubMed]
137. Zenaro, E.; Piacentino, G.; Constantin, G. The blood-brain barrier in Alzheimer's disease. *Neurobiol. Dis.* **2017**, *107*, 41–56. [CrossRef] [PubMed]

138. Bowman, G.L.; Kaye, J.A.; Quinn, J.F. Dyslipidemia and blood-brain barrier integrity in Alzheimer's disease. *Curr. Gerontol. Geriatr. Res.* **2012**, *2012*, 184042. [CrossRef] [PubMed]
139. Montagne, A.; Barnes, S.R.; Sweeney, M.D.; Halliday, M.R.; Sagare, A.P.; Zhao, Z.; Toga, A.W.; Jacobs, R.E.; Liu, C.Y.; Amezcua, L.; et al. Blood-brain barrier breakdown in the aging human hippocampus. *Neuron* **2015**, *85*, 296–302. [CrossRef] [PubMed]
140. Wang, H.; Golob, E.J.; Su, M.Y. Vascular volume and blood-brain barrier permeability measured by dynamic contrast enhanced MRI in hippocampus and cerebellum of patients with MCI and normal controls. *J. Magn. Reson. Imaging* **2006**, *24*, 695–700. [CrossRef] [PubMed]
141. Caserta, M.T.; Caccioppo, D.; Lapin, G.D.; Ragin, A.; Groothuis, D.R. Blood-brain barrier integrity in Alzheimer's disease patients and elderly control subjects. *J. Neuropsychiatry Clin. Neurosci.* **1998**, *10*, 78–84. [CrossRef] [PubMed]
142. Schlageter, N.L.; Carson, R.E.; Rapoport, S.I. Examination of blood-brain barrier permeability in dementia of the Alzheimer type with [68Ga]EDTA and positron emission tomography. *J. Cereb. Blood Flow Metab.* **1987**, *7*, 1–8. [CrossRef] [PubMed]
143. Van de Haar, H.J.; Burgmans, S.; Jansen, J.F.; van Osch, M.J.; van Buchem, M.A.; Muller, M.; Hofman, P.A.; Verhey, F.R.; Backes, W.H. Blood-Brain Barrier Leakage in Patients with Early Alzheimer Disease. *Radiology* **2016**, *281*, 527–535. [CrossRef] [PubMed]
144. Starr, J.M.; Farrall, A.J.; Armitage, P.; McGurn, B.; Wardlaw, J. Blood-brain barrier permeability in Alzheimer's disease: A case-control MRI study. *Psychiatry Res.* **2009**, *171*, 232–241. [CrossRef] [PubMed]
145. Janelidze, S.; Hertze, J.; Nagga, K.; Nilsson, K.; Nilsson, C.; Swedish Bio, F.S.G.; Wennstrom, M.; van Westen, D.; Blennow, K.; Zetterberg, H.; et al. Increased blood-brain barrier permeability is associated with dementia and diabetes but not amyloid pathology or APOE genotype. *Neurobiol. Aging* **2017**, *51*, 104–112. [CrossRef] [PubMed]
146. Jack, C.R., Jr.; Bennett, D.A.; Blennow, K.; Carrillo, M.C.; Dunn, B.; Haeberlein, S.B.; Holtzman, D.M.; Jagust, W.; Jessen, F.; Karlawish, J.; et al. NIA-AA Research Framework: Toward a biological definition of Alzheimer's disease. *Alzheimer's Dement.* **2018**, *14*, 535–562. [CrossRef] [PubMed]
147. Habib, M.; Mak, E.; Gabel, S.; Su, L.; Williams, G.; Waldman, A.; Wells, K.; Ritchie, K.; Ritchie, C.; O'Brien, J.T. Functional neuroimaging findings in healthy middle-aged adults at risk of Alzheimer's disease. *Ageing Res. Rev.* **2017**, *36*, 88–104. [CrossRef] [PubMed]
148. Baker, S.L.; Maass, A.; Jagust, W.J. Considerations and code for partial volume correcting [^{18}F]-AV-1451 tau PET data. *Data Brief* **2017**, *15*, 648–657. [CrossRef] [PubMed]
149. Gonzalez-Escamilla, G.; Lange, C.; Teipel, S.; Buchert, R.; Grothe, M.J.; Alzheimer's Disease Neuroimaging Initiative. PETPVE12: An SPM toolbox for Partial Volume Effects correction in brain PET—Application to amyloid imaging with AV45-PET. *Neuroimage* **2017**, *147*, 669–677. [CrossRef] [PubMed]
150. Minhas, D.S.; Price, J.C.; Laymon, C.M.; Becker, C.R.; Klunk, W.E.; Tudorascu, D.L.; Abrahamson, E.E.; Hamilton, R.L.; Kofler, J.K.; Mathis, C.A.; et al. Impact of partial volume correction on the regional correspondence between in vivo [C-11]PiB PET and postmortem measures of A beta load. *Neuroimage-Clin.* **2018**, *19*, 182–189. [CrossRef] [PubMed]
151. Rullmann, M.; Dukart, J.; Hoffmann, K.T.; Luthardt, J.; Tiepolt, S.; Patt, M.; Gertz, H.J.; Schroeter, M.L.; Seiby, J.; Schulz-Schaeffer, W.J.; et al. Partial-Volume Effect Correction Improves Quantitative Analysis of F-18-Florbetaben beta-Amyloid PET Scans. *J. Nucl. Med.* **2016**, *57*, 198–203. [CrossRef] [PubMed]
152. Shidahara, M.; Thomas, B.A.; Okamura, N.; Ibaraki, M.; Matsubara, K.; Oyama, S.; Ishikawa, Y.; Watanuki, S.; Iwata, R.; Furumoto, S.; et al. A comparison of five partial volume correction methods for Tau and Amyloid PET imaging with [F-18]THK5351 and [C-11]PIB. *Ann. Nucl. Med.* **2017**, *31*, 563–569. [CrossRef] [PubMed]
153. Jena, A.; Renjen, P.N.; Taneja, S.; Gambhir, A.; Negi, P. Integrated (18)F-fluorodeoxyglucose positron emission tomography magnetic resonance imaging ((18)F-FDG PET/MRI), a multimodality approach for comprehensive evaluation of dementia patients: A pictorial essay. *Indian J. Radiol. Imaging* **2015**, *25*, 342–352. [PubMed]
154. Wangerin, K.A.; Muzi, M.; Peterson, L.M.; Linden, H.M.; Novakova, A.; Mankoff, D.A.; Kinahan, P.E. A virtual clinical trial comparing static versus dynamic PET imaging in measuring response to breast cancer therapy. *Phys. Med. Biol.* **2017**, *62*, 3639–3655. [CrossRef] [PubMed]

155. Shaw, L.M.; Korecka, M.; Clark, C.M.; Lee, V.M.; Trojanowski, J.Q. Biomarkers of neurodegeneration for diagnosis and monitoring therapeutics. *Nat. Rev. Drug Discov.* **2007**, *6*, 295–303. [CrossRef] [PubMed]
156. Dubois, B.; Hampel, H.; Feldman, H.H.; Scheltens, P.; Aisen, P.; Andrieu, S.; Bakardjian, H.; Benali, H.; Bertram, L.; Blennow, K.; et al. Preclinical Alzheimer's disease: Definition, natural history, and diagnostic criteria. *Alzheimer's Dement.* **2016**, *12*, 292–323. [CrossRef] [PubMed]
157. Jack, C.R., Jr.; Bennett, D.A.; Blennow, K.; Carrillo, M.C.; Feldman, H.H.; Frisoni, G.B.; Hampel, H.; Jagust, W.J.; Johnson, K.A.; Knopman, D.S.; et al. A/T/N: An unbiased descriptive classification scheme for Alzheimer disease biomarkers. *Neurology* **2016**, *87*, 539–547. [CrossRef] [PubMed]
158. Ostrowitzki, S.; Deptula, D.; Thurfjell, L.; Barkhof, F.; Bohrmann, B.; Brooks, D.J.; Klunk, W.E.; Ashford, E.; Yoo, K.; Xu, Z.X.; et al. Mechanism of amyloid removal in patients with Alzheimer disease treated with gantenerumab. *Arch. Neurol.* **2012**, *69*, 198–207. [CrossRef] [PubMed]
159. Altman, D.G.; Lausen, B.; Sauerbrei, W.; Schumacher, M. Dangers of using "optimal" cutpoints in the evaluation of prognostic factors. *J. Natl. Cancer Inst.* **1994**, *86*, 829–835. [CrossRef] [PubMed]
160. Johnson, K.A.; Fox, N.C.; Sperling, R.A.; Klunk, W.E. Brain Imaging in Alzheimer Disease. *CSH Perspect. Med.* **2012**, *2*, a006213. [CrossRef] [PubMed]
161. Scheltens, P. Imaging in Alzheimer's disease. *Dialogues Clin. Neurosci.* **2009**, *11*, 191–199. [PubMed]
162. Wolk, D.A.; Price, J.C.; Saxton, J.A.; Snitz, B.E.; James, J.A.; Lopez, O.L.; Aizenstein, H.J.; Cohen, A.D.; Weissfeld, L.A.; Mathis, C.A.; et al. Amyloid imaging in mild cognitive impairment subtypes. *Ann. Neurol.* **2009**, *65*, 557–568. [CrossRef] [PubMed]
163. Bourgeat, P.; Chetelat, G.; Villemagne, V.L.; Fripp, J.; Raniga, P.; Pike, K.; Acosta, O.; Szoeke, C.; Ourselin, S.; Ames, D.; et al. Beta-amyloid burden in the temporal neocortex is related to hippocampal atrophy in elderly subjects without dementia. *Neurology* **2010**, *74*, 121–127. [CrossRef] [PubMed]
164. Martins, I.J. The future of biomarkers tests and genomic medicine in global organ disease. *Int. J. Microbiol. Infect. Dis.* **2017**, *1*, 1–6.
165. Martins, I.J. The Role of Clinical Proteomics, Lipidomics, and Genomics in the Diagnosis of Alzheimer's Disease. *Proteomes* **2016**, *4*, 14. [CrossRef] [PubMed]
166. Hanon, O.; Vidal, J.S.; Lehmann, S.; Bombois, S.; Allinquant, B.; Treluyer, J.M.; Gele, P.; Delmaire, C.; Blanc, F.; Mangin, J.F.; et al. Plasma amyloid levels within the Alzheimer's process and correlations with central biomarkers. *Alzheimer's Dement.* **2018**, *14*, 858–868. [CrossRef] [PubMed]
167. Korolev, I.O.; Symonds, L.L.; Bozoki, A.C.; Alzheimer's Disease Neuroimaging Initiative. Predicting Progression from Mild Cognitive Impairment to Alzheimer's Dementia Using Clinical, MRI, and Plasma Biomarkers via Probabilistic Pattern Classification. *PLoS ONE* **2016**, *11*, e0138866. [CrossRef] [PubMed]

Permissions

All chapters in this book were first published by MDPI; hereby published with permission under the Creative Commons Attribution License or equivalent. Every chapter published in this book has been scrutinized by our experts. Their significance has been extensively debated. The topics covered herein carry significant findings which will fuel the growth of the discipline. They may even be implemented as practical applications or may be referred to as a beginning point for another development.

The contributors of this book come from diverse backgrounds, making this book a truly international effort. This book will bring forth new frontiers with its revolutionizing research information and detailed analysis of the nascent developments around the world.

We would like to thank all the contributing authors for lending their expertise to make the book truly unique. They have played a crucial role in the development of this book. Without their invaluable contributions this book wouldn't have been possible. They have made vital efforts to compile up to date information on the varied aspects of this subject to make this book a valuable addition to the collection of many professionals and students.

This book was conceptualized with the vision of imparting up-to-date information and advanced data in this field. To ensure the same, a matchless editorial board was set up. Every individual on the board went through rigorous rounds of assessment to prove their worth. After which they invested a large part of their time researching and compiling the most relevant data for our readers.

The editorial board has been involved in producing this book since its inception. They have spent rigorous hours researching and exploring the diverse topics which have resulted in the successful publishing of this book. They have passed on their knowledge of decades through this book. To expedite this challenging task, the publisher supported the team at every step. A small team of assistant editors was also appointed to further simplify the editing procedure and attain best results for the readers.

Apart from the editorial board, the designing team has also invested a significant amount of their time in understanding the subject and creating the most relevant covers. They scrutinized every image to scout for the most suitable representation of the subject and create an appropriate cover for the book.

The publishing team has been an ardent support to the editorial, designing and production team. Their endless efforts to recruit the best for this project, has resulted in the accomplishment of this book. They are a veteran in the field of academics and their pool of knowledge is as vast as their experience in printing. Their expertise and guidance has proved useful at every step. Their uncompromising quality standards have made this book an exceptional effort. Their encouragement from time to time has been an inspiration for everyone.

The publisher and the editorial board hope that this book will prove to be a valuable piece of knowledge for researchers, students, practitioners and scholars across the globe.

List of Contributors

Marzia Bianchi and Melania Manco
Research Unit for Multi-factorial Diseases, Obesity and Diabetes, Bambino Gesù Children's Hospital IRCCS (Istituto di Ricovero e Cura a Carattere Scientifico), viale di San Paolo 15, 00146 Rome, Italy

Rebecca Power, John M. Nolan, Alfonso Prado-Cabrero, Warren Roche and Tommy Power
Nutrition Research Centre Ireland, School of Health Sciences, Carriganore House, Waterford Institute of Technology West Campus, X91 K0EK Waterford, Ireland

Robert Coen
Mercer's Institute for Research on Ageing, St. James's Hospital, D08 NHY1 Dublin, Ireland

Alan N. Howard
Howard Foundation, 7 Marfleet Close, Great Shelford, Cambridge CB22 5LA, UK

Ríona Mulcahy
Age-Related Care Unit, Health Service Executive, University Hospital Waterford, Dunmore Road, X91 ER8E Waterford, Ireland
Royal College of Surgeons Ireland, 123 Stephen's Green, Saint Peter's, D02 YN77 Dublin, Ireland

Syed Haris Omar and John Preddy
Rural Clinical School, Faculty of Medicine, University of New South Wales, Wagga Wagga, NSW 2650, Australia
Murrumbidgee Local Health District, NSW Health, Wagga Wagga, NSW 2650, Australia

Catia Scassellati
Genetics Unit, IRCCS Istituto Centro San Giovanni di Dio Fatebenefratelli, 25123 Brescia, Italy
Biological Psychiatry Unit, IRCCS Istituto Centro San Giovanni di Dio Fatebenefratelli, 25123 Brescia, Italy

Miriam Ciani and Cristian Bonvicini
Molecular Markers Laboratory, IRCCS Istituto Centro San Giovanni di Dio Fatebenefratelli, 25123 Brescia, Italy

Carlo Maj
Genetics Unit, IRCCS Istituto Centro San Giovanni di Dio Fatebenefratelli, 25123 Brescia, Italy
Institute of Genomic Statistics and Bioinformatics, University of Bonn, 53127 Bonn, Germany

Cristina Geroldi and Orazio Zanetti
Alzheimer's Research Unit-Memory Clinic, IRCCS Istituto Centro San Giovanni di Dio Fatebenefratelli, 25123 Brescia, Italy

Massimo Gennarelli
Genetics Unit, IRCCS Istituto Centro San Giovanni di Dio Fatebenefratelli, 25123 Brescia, Italy
Section of Biology and Genetic, Department of Molecular and Translational Medicine, University of Brescia, 25123 Brescia, Italy

Walter J. Lukiw
LSU Neuroscience Center, Louisiana State University Health Science Center, New Orleans, LA 70112, USA
Department of Cell Biology and Anatomy, LSU-HSC, New Orleans, LA 70112, USA
Department of Ophthalmology, LSU Neuroscience Center, LSU-HSC, New Orleans, LA 70112, USA
Department Neurology, LSU Neuroscience Center, LSU-HSC, New Orleans, LA 70112, USA

Andrea Vergallo and Harald Hampel
Sorbonne University, GRC no 21, Alzheimer Precision Medicine (APM), AP-HP, Pitié-Salpêtrière hospital, F-75013 Paris, France

Simone Lista
Sorbonne University, GRC no 21, Alzheimer Precision Medicine (APM), AP-HP, Pitié-Salpêtrière hospital, F-75013 Paris, France
Brain & Spine Institute (ICM), INSERM U 1127, CNRS UMR 7225, Boulevard de l'Hôpital, F-75013 Paris, France
Department of Neurology, Institute of Memory and Alzheimer's Disease (IM2A), Pitié-Salpêtrière Hospital, AP-HP, F-75013 Paris, France

Yuhai Zhao
LSU Neuroscience Center, Louisiana State University Health Science Center, New Orleans, LA 70112, USA
Department of Cell Biology and Anatomy, LSU-HSC, New Orleans, LA 70112, USA

Marco Canevelli
Department of Human Neuroscience, Sapienza University, 00185 Rome, Italy
National Center for Disease Prevention and Health Promotion, Italian National Institute of Health, 00161 Rome, Italy

Giulia Remoli, Martina Valletta, Marco Toccaceli Blasi, Francesco Sciancalepore and Giuseppe Bruno
Department of Human Neuroscience, Sapienza University, 00185 Rome, Italy

Ilaria Bacigalupo and Nicola Vanacore
National Center for Disease Prevention and Health Promotion, Italian National Institute of Health, 00161 Rome, Italy

Matteo Cesari
Department of Clinical Sciences and Community Health, University of Milan, 20122 Milan, Italy
Geriatric Unit, Fondazione IRCCS Ca' Granda Ospedale Maggiore Policlinico, 20122 Milan, Italy

Yasuhisa Ano
Research Laboratories for Health Science & Food Technologies, Kirin Company Ltd., 1-13-5 Fukuura Kanazawa-ku, Yokohama-shi, Kanagawa 236-0004, Japan

Hiroyuki Nakayama
Laboratory of Veterinary Pathology, Graduate School of Agricultural and Life Sciences, the University of Tokyo, 1-1-1 Yayoi, Bunkyo-ku, Tokyo 113-8657, Japan

Sean X Naughton and Urdhva Raval
Department of Neurology, Icahn School of Medicine at Mount Sinai, New York, NY 10029, USA

Eva Ausó, Violeta Gómez-Vicente and Gema Esquiva
Department of Optics, Pharmacology and Anatomy, University of Alicante, 03690 Alicante, Spain

Paola Pizzo, Emy Basso, Riccardo Filadi, Elisa Greotti, Diana Pendin and Nicola Vajente
Department of Biomedical Sciences, University of Padua, Via U. Bassi 58/B, 35131 Padua, Italy
Neuroscience Institute, Italian National Research Council (CNR), Via U. Bassi 58/B, 35131 Padua, Italy

Alessandro Leparulo, Nelly Redolfi, Michela Rossini and Cristina Fasolato
Department of Biomedical Sciences, University of Padua, Via U. Bassi 58/B, 35131 Padua, Italy

Tullio Pozzan
Department of Biomedical Sciences, University of Padua, Via U. Bassi 58/B, 35131 Padua, Italy
Neuroscience Institute, Italian National Research Council (CNR), Via U. Bassi 58/B, 35131 Padua, Italy
Venetian Institute of Molecular Medicine (VIMM), Via G. Orus 2B, 35131 Padua, Italy

Simon M. Bell, Matteo De Marco, Katy Barnes, Pamela J. Shaw, Laura Ferraiuolo, Daniel J. Blackburn, Heather Mortiboys and Annalena Venneri
Sheffield Institute for Translational Neuroscience (SITraN), University of Sheffield, 385a Glossop Road, Sheffield S10 2HQ, UK

Mounia Chami and Frédéric Checler
Team Labelled "Laboratory of Excellence (LABEX) DistAlz", INSERM, CNRS, IPMC, Université Côte d'Azur, 660 route des Lucioles, Sophia-Antipolis, 06560 Valbonne, France

Giulio M. Pasinetti
Department of Neurology, Icahn School of Medicine at Mount Sinai, New York, NY 10029, USA
James J. Peters Veterans Affairs Medical Center, Bronx, NY 10468, USA

Grazia Daniela Femminella and Valeria Calsolaro
Neurology Imaging Unit, Imperial College London, London W12 0NN, UK

Tony Thayanandan
Imperial Memory Unit, Charing Cross Hospital, Imperial College London, London W6 8RF, UK

Klara Komici and Graziamaria Corbi
Department of Medicine and Health Sciences, University of Molise, 86100 Campobasso, Italy

Giuseppe Rengo and Nicola Ferrara
Department of Translational Medical Sciences, Federico II University of Naples, 80131 Naples, Italy
Istituti Clinici Scientifici Maugeri SPA – Società Benefit, IRCCS, 82037 Telese Terme, Italy

Index

Printed in the USA
CPSIA information can be obtained
at www.ICGtesting.com
LVHW080048211023
761596LV00010BA/1971